CLI
DR
20

EDITORS

Leonard G. Gomella, MD, FACS
Steven A. Haist, MD, MS, FACP
Aimee G. Adams, PharmD

www.eDrugbook.com
www.thescutmonkey.com

Medical

New York Chicago San Francisco Lisbon
London Madrid Mexico City Milan New Delhi
San Juan Seoul Singapore Sydney Toronto

ISBN 978-0-07-160280-8
MHID 0-07-160280-1
ISSN 1540-6725

The book was set in Times by International Typesetting and Composition.
The editors were Jim Shanahan and Harriet Lebowitz.
The senior production supervisor was Sherri Souffrance.
Project management was provided by Vipra Fauzdar.
Transcontinental was printer and binder.

This book is printed on acid-free paper.

CONTENTS

Contents

TIPS FOR SAFE PRESCRIPTION WRITING
Inside Front Cover

EMERGENCY CARDIAC CARE MEDICATIONS
Back Page and Inside Back Cover

EDITORS

Leonard G. Gomella, MD, FACS
The Bernard W. Godwin, Jr, Professor
Chairman, Department of Urology
Jefferson Medical College
Associate Director of Clinical Affairs
Kimmel Cancer Center
Thomas Jefferson University
Philadelphia, Pennsylvania

Steven A. Haist, MD, MS, FACP
Clinical Professor
Department of Medicine
Drexel University College of Medicine,
Philadelphia, Pennsylvania

Aimee G. Adams, PharmD
Clinical Pharmacist Specialist, Ambulatory Care
Adjunct Assistant Professor
College of Pharmacy and Department of Internal Medicine
University of Kentucky HealthCare
Lexington, Kentucky

CONSULTING EDITORS

Carol Beck, PhD
Assistant Dean, Jefferson College of
Graduate Studies
Assistant Professor, Department of
Pharmacology and Experimental
Therapeutics
Thomas Jefferson University
Philadelphia, Pennsylvania

Vincenzo Berghella, MD
Professor, Department of Obstetrics
and Gynecology
Director, Division of Maternal-Fetal
Medicine
Thomas Jefferson University
Philadelphia, Pennsylvania

Tricia L. Gomella, MD
Part-Time Clinical Assistant
Professor of Pediatrics
Johns Hopkins University School of
Medicine
Baltimore, Maryland

Nick A. Pavona, MD
Professor, Department of Surgery
Division of Urology
Benjamin Franklin University
Medical Center
Chadds Ford, Pennsylvania

Kelly M. Smith, PharmD, FASHP
Associate Professor
Department of Pharmacy Practice
and Science
University of Kentucky College of
Pharmacy
Clinical Specialist, Medication Use
Policy
University of Kentucky Medical
Center
Lexington, Kentucky

CONTRIBUTORS

Emily B. Borders, PharmD
Clinical Assistant Professor
University of Oklahoma Health
Sciences Center
Oklahoma City, Oklahoma

**William R. Judd, PharmD,
BCPS**
Postgraduate Year Two Infectious
Diseases Resident
College of Pharmacy
University of Kentucky HealthCare
Lexington, Kentucky

**Mandy Jones, PharmD, PA-C,
BCPS**
Clinical Assistant Professor
University of Kentucky College of
Pharmacy
Department of Family and
Community Medicine
Lexington, Kentucky

Mikael Jones, PharmD, BCPS
Clinical Assistant Professor
University of Kentucky College of
Pharmacy and
College of Nursing
Lexington, Kentucky

Neil Seligman, MD
Fellow, Maternal-Fetal Medicine
Department of Obstetrics and
Gynecology
Thomas Jefferson University
Philadelphia, Pennsylvania

Bojana Stevich, PharmD, MS
Clinical Pharmacist Specialist
University of Texas MD Anderson
Cancer Center
Houston, Texas

**William Vincent, PharmD,
BCPS**
Assistant Professor, Pharmacy
Practice
Arnold & Marie Schwartz College of
Pharmacy and Health Sciences
Long Island University
Brooklyn, New York

Ann M. Wiesner, PharmD
Postgraduate Year Two Ambulatory
Care Resident
College of Pharmacy
University of Kentucky HealthCare
Lexington, Kentucky

PREFACE

We are pleased to present the 8th edition of the *Clinician's Pocket Drug Reference*. This book is based on the drug presentation style used since 1983 in the *Clinician's Pocket Reference*, popularly known as the Scut Monkey Book. Our goal is to identify the most frequently used and clinically important medications, including branded, generic, and OTC products. The book includes well over 1000 medications and is designed to represent a cross-section of commonly used products in medical practices across the country.

Our style of drug presentation includes key "must-know" facts of commonly used medications, essential for both the student and practicing physician. The inclusion of common uses of medications rather than just the official FDA-labeled indications are based on the uses of the medication supported by publications and community standards of care. All uses have been reviewed by our editorial board.

It is essential that students and residents in training learn more than the name and dose of the medications they prescribe. Certain common side effects and significant warnings and contraindications are associated with prescription medications. Although health-care providers should ideally be completely familiar with the entire package insert of any medication prescribed, such a requirement is unreasonable. References such as the *Physician's Desk Reference* and the drug manufacturer's Web site make package inserts readily available for many medications, but may not highlight clinically significant facts or key data for generic drugs and those available over the counter.

The limitations of difficult-to-read package inserts were acknowledged by the Food and Drug Administration in 2001, when it noted that physicians do not have time to read the many pages of small print in the typical package insert. Newer drugs are now producing more user-friendly package insert summaries that highlight important drug information for easier practitioner reference. Although useful, these summaries do not commingle with similarly approved generic or "competing" similar products.

The editorial board and contributors have analyzed the information on both brand and generic medications and has made this key prescribing information available in this pocket-sized book. Information in this book is meant for use by health-care professionals who are familiar with these commonly prescribed medications.

This 2009 edition has been completely reviewed and updated by our editorial board and technical contributors. More than 45 new drugs have been added, and dozens of changes in other medications based on FDA actions have been incorporated, including deletions of discontinued brand names and compounds. Where appropriate, emergency cardiac care (ECC) guidelines are provided based on the latest recommendations from the American Heart Association (*Circulation*, Volume 112, Issue 24 Supplement; December 13, 2005). New for this edition is a convenient emergency medication summary in the back of the book for more rapid reference.

Editions of this book are also available in a variety of electronic or eBook formats. Visit www.eDrugbook.com for a link to the electronic versions currently available. Additionally, this web site has enhanced content features such as a comprehensive listing of "look alike–sound alike" medications that can contribute to prescribing errors.

We express special thanks to our spouses and families for their long-term support of this book and the entire Scut Monkey project (www.thescutmonkey.com). The Scut Monkey Project is designed to provide new medical students and those in the allied health professions with the basic tools needed when entering the world of hands-on patient care.

The contributions of the members of the editorial board, contributors and the team at McGraw-Hill are deeply appreciated. Your comments and suggestions are always welcome and encouraged because improvements to this and all our books would be impossible without the interest and feedback of our readers. We hope this book will help you learn some of the key elements in prescribing medications and allow you to care for your patients in the best way possible.

Leonard G. Gomella, MD, FACS
Philadelphia, Pennsylvania
Leonard.Gomella@jefferson.edu

Steven A. Haist, MD, MS, FACP
Philadelphia, Pennsylvania

Aimee G. Adams, PharmD
Lexington, Kentucky
argelh1@email.uky.edu

MEDICATION KEY

Medications are listed by prescribing class and the individual medications are then listed in alphabetical order by generic name. Some of the more commonly recognized trade names are listed for each medication (in parentheses after the generic name) or if available without prescription, noted as OTC (over-the-counter).

> **Generic Drug Name (Selected Common Brand Names) [Controlled Substance]** **WARNING:** Summarized versions of the "Black Box" precautions deemed necessary by the FDA. These are significant precautions and contraindications concerning the individual medication. **Uses:** This includes both FDA-labeled indications bracketed by * and other "off-label" uses of the medication. Because many medications are used to treat various conditions based on the medical literature and not listed in their package insert, we list common uses of the medication in addition the official "labeled indications" (FDA approved) based on input from our editorial board **Action:** How the drug works. This information is helpful in comparing classes of drugs and understanding side effects and contraindications. *Spectrum:* Specifies activity against selected microbes for antimicrobials **Dose:** *Adults.* Where no specific pediatric dose is given, the implication is that this drug is not commonly used or indicated in that age group. At the end of the dosing line, important dosing modifications may be noted (ie, take with food, avoid antacids, etc) **Caution:** [pregnancy/fetal risk categories, breast-feeding (as noted below)] cautions concerning the use of the drug in specific settings **CI:** Contraindications **Disp:** Common dosing forms **SE:** Common or significant side effects **Notes:** Other key useful information about the drug.

CONTROLLED SUBSTANCE CLASSIFICATION

Medications under the control of the US Drug Enforcement Agency (Schedules I–V controlled substances) are indicated by the symbol [C]. Most medications are "uncontrolled" and do not require a DEA prescriber number on the prescription. The following is a general description for the schedules of DEA-controlled substances:

Schedule (C-I) I: All nonresearch use forbidden (eg, heroin, LSD, mescaline).

Schedule (C-II) II: High addictive potential; medical use accepted. No telephone call-in prescriptions; no refills. Some states require special prescription form (eg, cocaine, morphine, methadone).

Schedule (C-III) III: Low to moderate risk of physical dependence, high risk of psychologic dependence; prescription must be rewritten after 6 months or 5 refills (eg, acetaminophen plus codeine).

Schedule (C-IV) IV: Limited potential for dependence; prescription rules same as for schedule III (eg, benzodiazepines, propoxyphene).

Schedule (C-V) V: Very limited abuse potential; prescribing regulations often same as for uncontrolled medications; some states have additional restrictions.

FDA FETAL RISK CATEGORIES

Category A: Adequate studies in pregnant women have not demonstrated a risk to the fetus in the first trimester of pregnancy; there is no evidence of risk in the last two trimesters.

Category B: Animal studies have not demonstrated a risk to the fetus, but no adequate studies have been done in pregnant women.

or

Animal studies have shown an adverse effect, but adequate studies in pregnant women have not demonstrated a risk to the fetus during the first trimester of pregnancy, and there is no evidence of risk in the last two trimesters.

Category C: Animal studies have shown an adverse effect on the fetus, but no adequate studies have been done in humans. The benefits from the use of the drug in pregnant women may be acceptable despite its potential risks.

or

No animal reproduction studies and no adequate studies in humans have been done.

Category D: There is evidence of human fetal risk, but the potential benefits from the use of the drug in pregnant women may be acceptable despite its potential risks.

Category X: Studies in animals or humans or adverse reaction reports, or both, have demonstrated fetal abnormalities. The risk of use in pregnant women clearly outweighs any possible benefit.

Category ?: No data available (not a formal FDA classification; included to provide complete dataset).

BREAST-FEEDING CLASSIFICATION

No formally recognized classification exists for drugs and breast-feeding. This shorthand was developed for the *Clinician's Pocket Drug Reference*.

+	Compatible with breast-feeding
M	Monitor patient or use with caution
±	Excreted, or likely excreted, with unknown effects or at unknown concentrations
?/–	Unknown excretion, but effects likely to be of concern
–	Contraindicated in breast-feeding
?	No data available

ABBREVIATIONS

√ check, follow, or monitor
Ab: antibody, abortion
Abd: abdominal
ABMT: autologous bone marrow transplantation
ac: before meals (*ante cibum*)
ACE: angiotensin-converting enzyme
ACH: acetylcholine
ACLS: advanced cardiac life support
ACS: acute coronary syndrome, American Cancer Society, American College of Surgeons
ACT: activated coagulation time
ADH: antidiuretic hormone
ADHD: attention-deficit hyperactivity disorder
ADR: adverse drug reaction
AF: atrial fibrillation
AHA: American Heart Association
ALL: acute lymphocytic leukemia
ALT: alanine aminotransferase
AMI: acute myocardial infarction
AML: acute myelogenous leukemia
amp: ampule
ANA: antinuclear antibody
ANC: absolute neutrophil count
APAP: acetaminophen [*N*-acetyl-*p*-aminophenol]
aPTT: activated partial thromboplastin time
ARB: angiotensin II receptor blocker
ARDS: adult respiratory distress syndrome
ARF: acute renal failure
AS: aortic stenosis

ASA: aspirin (acetylsalicylic acid)
AST: aspartate aminotransferase
ATP: adenosine triphosphate
AUC: area under the curve
AUB: abnormal uterine/vaginal bleeding
AV: atrioventricular
AVM: arteriovenous malformation
BCL: B-cell lymphoma
BPM: beats per minute
BID: twice daily
BM: bone marrow, bowel movement
↓BM: bone marrow suppression, myelosuppression
BMD: bone mineral density
BMT: bone marrow transplantation
BOO: bladder outlet obstruction
BP: blood pressure
↓BP: hypotension
BPH: benign prostatic hyperplasia
BSA: body surface area
BUN: blood urea nitrogen
Ca: calcium
CA: cancer
CABG: coronary artery bypass graft
CAD: coronary artery disease
CAP: community-acquired pneumonia
caps: capsule
cardiotox: cardiotoxicity
CBC: complete blood count
CCB: calcium channel blocker
CDC: Centers for Disease Control and Prevention
CF: cystic fibrosis

CHF: congestive heart failure
CI: contraindicated
CLL: chronic lymphocytic leukemia
CML: chronic myelogenous leukemia
CMV: cytomegalovirus
CNS: central nervous system
combo: combination
comp: complicated
conc: concentration
cont: continuous
COPD: chronic obstructive
  pulmonary disease
COX: cyclooxygenase
CP: chest pain
CPP: central precocious puberty
CR: controlled release
CrCl: creatinine clearance
CRF: chronic renal failure
CSF: cerebrospinal fluid
CV: cardiovascular
CVA: cerebrovascular accident,
  costovertebral angle
CVH: common variable
  hypergammaglobulinemia
CYP: cytochrome P450 enzyme
÷ : divided
D: diarrhea
d: day
DA: dopamine
DBP: diastolic blood pressure
D/C: discontinue
derm: dermatologic
D$_5$LR: 5% dextrose in lactated
  Ringer solution
D$_5$NS: 5% dextrose in normal saline
D$_5$W: 5% dextrose in water
DI: diabetes insipidus
Disp: dispensed as; how the drug is
  supplied
DKA: diabetic ketoacidosis
dL: deciliter
DM: diabetes mellitus

DMARD: disease-modifying
  antirheumatic drug; drugs in
  randomized trials to decrease
  erosions and joint space narrowing
  in rheumatoid arthritis (eg,
  D-penicillamine, methotrexate,
  azathioprine)
DN: diabetic nephropathy
DOT: directly observed therapy
DR: delayed release
DVT: deep venous thrombosis
Dz: disease
EC: enteric coated
ECC: emergency cardiac care
ECG: electrocardiogram
ED: erectile dysfunction
EGFR: epidermal growth factor
  receptor
EIB: exercise induced
  bronchoconstriction
ELISA: enzyme-linked
  immunosorbent assay
EMG: electromyelogram
EMIT: enzyme-multiplied
  immunoassay test
epi: epinephrine
EPS: extrapyramidal symptoms
  (tardive dyskinesia, tremors and
  rigidity, restlessness [akathisia],
  muscle contractions [dystonia],
  changes in breathing and heart rate)
ER: extended release
ESRD: end-stage renal disease
ET: endotracheal
EtOH: ethanol
extrav: extravasation
FAP: familial adenomatous polyposis
FSH: follicle-stimulating hormone
5-FU: fluorouracil
Fxn: function
g: gram
GABA: gamma-aminobutyric acid

G-CSF: granulocyte colony-stimulating factor
GC: gonorrhea
gen: generation
GERD: gastroesophageal reflux disease
GF: growth factor
GFR: glomerular filtration rate
GI: gastrointestinal
GIST: Gastrointestinal stromal tumor
GM-CSF: granulocyte-macrophage colony-stimulating factor
GnRH: gonadotropin-releasing hormone
G6PD: glucose-6-phosphate dehydrogenase
gtt: drop, drops (*gutta*)
GU: genitourinary
GVHD: graft-versus-host disease
h: hour(s)
HA: headache
HBsAg: hepatitis B surface antigen
HBV: hepatitis B virus
HCL: hairy cell leukemia
Hct: hematocrit
HCTZ: hydrochlorothiazide
HD: hemodialysis
hep: hepatitis
hepatotox: hepatotoxicity
Hgb: hemoglobin
HIT: heparin-induced thrombocytopenia
HITTS: heparin-induced thrombosis-thrombocytopenia syndrome
HIV: human immunodeficiency virus
HMG-CoA: hydroxymethylglutaryl coenzyme A
HPV: human papillomavirus
HR: heart rate
↑HR: increased heart rate (tachycardia)
hs: at bedtime (*hora somni*)

HSV: herpes simplex virus
5-HT: 5-hydroxytryptamine
HTN: hypertension
Hx: history of
IBD: irritable bowel disease
IBS: irritable bowel syndrome
IBW: ideal body weight
ICP: intracranial pressure
IFIS: intraoperative floppy iris syndrome
Ig: immunoglobulin
IGF: insulin-like growth factor
IHSS: idiopathic hypertropic subaortic stenosis
IL: interleukin
IM: intramuscular
impair: impairment
Inf: infusion
Infxn: infection
Inh: inhalation
INH: isoniazid
Inj: injection
INR: international normalized ratio
Insuff: insufficiency
Intravag: intravaginal
IO: intraosseous
IOP: intraocular pressure
IR: immediate release
ISA: intrinsic sympathomimetic activity
IT: intrathecal
ITP: idiopathic thrombocytopenic purpura
Int units: international units
IUD: intrauterine device
IV: intravenous
JRA: juvenile rheumatoid arthritis
K/K⁺: potassium
LA: long-acting
LDL: low-density lipoprotein
LFT: liver function test
LH: luteinizing hormone

LHRH: luteinizing hormone-releasing hormone
liq: liquid(s)
LMW: low molecular weight
LP: lumbar puncture
LVD: left ventricular dysfunction
LVEF: left ventricular ejection fraction
LVSD: left ventricular systolic dysfunction
lytes: electrolytes
MAC: *Mycobacterium avium* complex
maint: maintenance dose/drug
MAO/MAOI: monoamine oxidase/inhibitor
max: maximum
mcg: microgram(s)
mcL: microliter(s)
MDD: major depressive disorder
MDI: multidose inhaler
MDS: myeoldysplasia syndrome
meds: medicines
mEq: milliequivalent
met: metastatic
mg: milligram(s)
Mg/Mg^{+2}: magnesium
MI: myocardial infarction, mitral insufficiency
min: minute(s)
mL: milliliter(s)
mo: month(s)
MoAb: monoclonal antibody
mod: moderate
MRSA: methicillin-resistant *Staphylococcus aureus*
msec: millisecond(s)
MS: multiple sclerosis, musculoskeletal
MSSA: methicillin-sensitive *Staphylococcus aureus*
MTT: monotetrazolium

MTX: methotrexate
MyG: myasthenia gravis
N: nausea
NA: narrow angle
NAG: narrow angle glaucoma
nephrotox: nephrotoxicity
neurotox: neurotoxicity
ng: nanogram(s)
NG: nasogastric
NHL: non-Hodgkin lymphoma
NIAON: nonischemic arterial optic neuritis
nl: normal
NO: nitric oxide
NPO: nothing by mouth (*nil per os*)
NRTI: nucleoside reverse transcriptase inhibitor
NS: normal saline
NSAID: nonsteroidal anti-inflammatory drug
NSCLC: non-small cell lung cancer
N/V: nausea and vomiting
N/V/D: nausea, vomiting, diarrhea
NYHA: New York Heart Association
OA: osteoarthritis
OAB: overactive bladder
obst: obstruction
OCP: oral contraceptive pill
OD: overdose
ODT: orally disintegrating tablets
OK: recommended
oint: ointment
ophthal: ophthalmic
OTC: over the counter
ototox: ototoxicity
PAT: paroxysmal atrial tachycardia
pc: after eating (*post cibum*)
PCa: cancer of the prostate
PCI: percutaneous coronary intervention
PCN: penicillin

PCP: *Pneumocystis jiroveci* (formerly *carinii*) pneumonia

PCWP: pulmonary capillary wedge pressure

PDE5: phosphodiesterase type 5

PDGF: platelet-derived growth factor

PE: pulmonary embolus, physical examination, pleural effusion

PEA: pulseless electrical activity

PFT: pulmonary function test

pg: picogram(s)

Ph: Philadelphia chromosome

PID: pelvic inflammatory disease

plt: platelet

PMDD: premenstrual dysphoric disorder

PML: progressive multifocal leukoencephalopathy

PMS: premenstrual syndrome

PO: by mouth (*per os*)

PPD: purified protein derivative

PR: by rectum

PRG: pregnancy

PRN: as often as needed (*pro re nata*)

PSA: prostate-specific antigen

PSVT: paroxysmal supraventricular tachycardia

pt: patient

PT: prothrombin time

PTCA: percutaneous transluminal coronary angioplasty

PTH: parathyroid hormone

PTT: partial thromboplastin time

PUD: peptic ulcer disease

PVD: peripheral vascular disease

pulm: pulmonary

PVC: premature ventricular contraction

PWP: pulmonary wedge pressure

Px: prevention

q: every (*quaque*)

q_h: every _ hours

q day: every day

qh: every hour

qhs: every hour of sleep (before bedtime)

QID: four times a day (*quater in die*)

q other day: every other day

RA: rheumatoid arthritis

RAS: renin-angiotensin system

RBC: red blood cell(s) (count)

RCC: renal cell carcinoma

RDA: recommended dietary allowance

RDS: respiratory distress syndrome

resp: respiratory

RHuAb: recombinant human antibody

RIA: radioimmune assay

RR: respiratory rate

RSV: respiratory syncytial virus

RT: reverse transcriptase

RTA: renal tubular acidosis

Rx: prescription or therapy

Rxn: reaction

s: second(s)

SAE: serious adverse event

SBE: subacute bacterial endocarditis

SBP: systolic blood pressure

SCr: serum creatinine

SCLC: small cell lung cancer

SDV: single-dose vial

SE: side effect(s)

SIADH: syndrome of inappropriate antidiuretic hormone

sig: significant

SL: sublingual

SLE: systemic lupus erythematosus

SNRIs: serotonin-norepinephrine reuptake inhibitors

Sol/soln: solution

sp: species

SPAG: small particle aerosol generator

SQ: subcutaneous

SR: sustained release

SSRI: selective serotonin reuptake inhibitor
SSS: sick sinus syndrome
S/Sys: signs & symptoms
stat: immediately (*statim*)
STD: sexually transmitted disease
supl: supplement
supp: suppository
susp: suspension
SVT: supraventricular tachycardia
synth: synthesis
Sx: symptom
Sz: seizure
tab/tabs: tablet/tablets
TB: tuberculosis
TCA: tricyclic antidepressant
TFT: thyroid function test
TIA: transient ischemic attack
TID: three times a day (*ter in die*)
TKI: tyrosine kinase inhibitors
TMP: trimethoprim
TMP—SMX: trimethoprim—sulfamethoxazole
TNF: tumor necrosis factor
tox: toxicity
TPA: tissue plasminogen activator
tri: trimester
TTP: thrombotic thrombocytopenic purpura

TTS: transdermal therapeutic system
Tx: treatment
UGT: uridine 5′ diphosphoglucuronosyl transferase
UC: ulcerative colitis
ULN: upper limits of normal
uncomp: uncomplicated
URI: upper respiratory infection
UTI: urinary tract infection
V: vomiting
Vag: vaginal
VEGF: vascular endothelial growth factor
VF: ventricular fibrillation
vit: vitamin
vol: volume
VPA: valproic acid
VRE: vancomycin-resistant *Enterococcus*
VT: ventricular tachycardia
WBC: white blood cell(s) (count)
Wgt: weight
WHI: Women's Health Initiative
wk: week(s)
WNL: within normal limits
WPW: Wolff–Parkinson–White syndrome
XR: extended release
ZE: Zollinger–Ellison (syndrome)

CLASSIFICATION (Generic and common brand names)

ALLERGY

Antihistamines

Azelastine (Astelin, Optivar)
Cetirizine (Zyrtec, Zyrtec D)
Chlorpheniramine (Chlor-Trimeton)

Clemastine Fumarate (Tavist)
Cyproheptadine (Periactin)
Desloratadine (Clarinex)
Diphenhydramine (Benadryl)

Fexofenadine (Allegra)
Hydroxyzine (Atarax, Vistaril)
Levocetirizine (Xyzal)
Loratadine (Claritin, Alavert)

Miscellaneous Antiallergy Agents

Budesonide (Rhinocort, Pulmicort)

Cromolyn Sodium (Intal, NasalCrom, Opticrom)

Montelukast (Singulair)

ANTIDOTES

Acetylcysteine (Acetadote, Mucomyst)
Amifostine (Ethyol)
Atropine (AtroPen)
Charcoal (SuperChar, Actidose, Liqui-Char Activated)

Deferasirox (Exjade)
Dexrazoxane (Totect, Zinecard)
Digoxin Immune Fab (Digibind, DigiFab)
Flumazenil (Romazicon)
Hydroxocobalamin (Cyanokit)

Ipecac Syrup (OTC Syrup)
Mesna (Mesnex)
Naloxone
Physostigmine (Antilirium)
Succimer (Chemet)

ANTIMICROBIAL AGENTS

Antibiotics

AMINOGLYCOSIDES

Amikacin (Amikin)
Gentamicin (Garamycin, G-Mycitin)

Neomycin
Streptomycin

Tobramycin (Nebcin)

1

CARBAPENEMS

Doripenem (Doribax)
Ertapenem (Invanz)

Imipenem-Cilastatin
(Primaxin)

Meropenem (Merrem)

CEPHALOSPORINS, FIRST GENERATION

Cefadroxil (Duricef,
Ultracef)

Cefazolin (Ancef,
Kefzol)

Cephalexin (Keflex,
Panixine DisperDose)

CEPHALOSPORINS, SECOND GENERATION

Cefaclor (Ceclor)
Cefotetan (Cefotan)

Cefoxitin (Mefoxin)
Cefprozil (Cefzil)

Cefuroxime (Ceftin [oral],
Zinacef [parenteral])

CEPHALOSPORINS, THIRD GENERATION

Cefdinir (Omnicef)
Cefditoren (Spectracef)
Cefixime (Suprax)
Cefoperazone (Cefobid)
Cefotaxime (Claforan)

Cefpodoxime (Vantin)
Ceftazidime (Fortaz,
Ceptaz, Tazidime,
Tazicef)

Ceftibuten (Cedax)
Ceftizoxime (Cefizox)
Ceftriaxone (Rocephin)

CEPHALOSPORINS, FOURTH GENERATION

Cefepime (Maxipime)

FLUOROQUINOLONES

Ciprofloxacin (Cipro,
Proquin XR)
Gemifloxacin (Factive)

Levofloxacin (Levaquin)
Lomefloxacin (Maxaquin)
Moxifloxacin (Avelox)

Norfloxacin (Noroxin)
Ofloxacin (Floxin)

KETOLIDE

Telithromycin (Ketek)

MACROLIDES

Azithromycin
(Zithromax)
Clarithromycin (Biaxin)

Erythromycin
(E-Mycin, E.E.S.,
Ery-Tab)

Erythromycin &
Sulfisoxazole
(Eryzole, Pediazole)

PENICILLINS

Amoxicillin (Amoxil, Polymox)
Amoxicillin & Clavulanic Acid (Augmentin)
Ampicillin (Amcill, Omnipen)
Ampicillin-Sulbactam (Unasyn)
Dicloxacillin (Dynapen, Dycill)

Nafcillin (Nallpen, Unipen)
Oxacillin (Bactocill, Prostaphlin)
Penicillin G, Aqueous (Potassium or Sodium) (Pfizerpen, Pentids)
Penicillin G Benzathine (Bicillin)

Penicillin G Procaine (Wycillin)
Penicillin V (Pen-Vee K, Veetids)
Piperacillin (Pipracil)
Piperacillin-Tazobactam (Zosyn)
Ticarcillin/Potassium Clavulanate (Timentin)

TETRACYCLINES

Doxycycline (Adoxa, Periostat, Oracea, Vibramycin, Vibra-Tabs)

Minocycline (Dynacin, Minocin, Solodyn)

Tetracycline (Achromycin V, Sumycin)
Tigecycline (Tygacil)

Miscellaneous Antibiotic Agents

Aztreonam (Azactam)
Clindamycin (Cleocin, Cleocin-T)
Fosfomycin (Monurol)
Linezolid (Zyvox)
Metronidazole (Flagyl, MetroGel)
Mupirocin (Bactroban, Bactroban Nasal)

Nitrofurantoin (Furadantin, Macrodantin, Macrobid)
Quinupristin-Dalfopristin (Synercid)
Rifaximin (Xifaxan)
Retapamulin (Altabax)

Trimethoprim (Primsol, Proloprim)
Trimethoprim–Sulfamethoxazole [Co-Trimoxazole] (Bactrim, Septra)
Vancomycin (Vancocin, Vancoled)

Antifungals

Amphotericin B (Fungizone)
Amphotericin B Cholesteryl (Amphotec)
Amphotericin B Lipid Complex (Abelcet)

Amphotericin B Liposomal (AmBisome)
Anidulafungin (Eraxis)
Caspofungin (Cancidas)
Clotrimazole (Lotrimin, Mycelex)

Clotrimazole & Betamethasone (Lotrisone)
Econazole (Spectazole)
Fluconazole (Diflucan)
Itraconazole (Sporanox)

Ketoconazole, oral (Nizoral)
Ketoconazole, topical (Extina, Kuric, Xolegel, Nizoral A-D Shampoo) [Shampoo–OTC]

Miconazole (Monistat 1 combo, Monistat 3, Monistat 7) [OTC] (Monistat-Derm)
Nystatin (Mycostatin)
Oxiconazole (Oxistat)

Sertaconazole (Ertaczo)
Terbinafine (Lamisil, Lamisil AT)
Triamcinolone & Nystatin (Mycolog-II)
Voriconazole (VFEND)

Antimycobacterials

Dapsone, oral
Ethambutol (Myambutol)

Isoniazid (INH)
Pyrazinamide
Rifabutin (Mycobutin)

Rifampin (Rifadin)
Rifapentine (Priftin)
Streptomycin

Antiprotozoals

Nitazoxanide (Alinia)

Tinidazole (Tindamax)

Antiretrovirals

Abacavir (Ziagen)
Daptomycin (Cubicin)
Delavirdine (Rescriptor)
Didanosine [ddI] (Videx)
Efavirenz (Sustiva)
Efavirenz/emtricitabine/ tenofovir (Atripla)
Etravirine (Intelence)
Fosamprenavir (Lexiva)
Indinavir (Crixivan)

Lamivudine (Epivir, Epivir-HBV, 3 TC [many combo regimens])
Lopinavir/Ritonavir (Kaletra)
Maraviroc (Selzentry)
Nelfinavir (Viracept)
Nevirapine (Viramune)
Raltegravir (Isentress)

Ritonavir (Norvir)
Saquinavir (Fortovase)
Stavudine (Zerit)
Tenofovir (Viread)
Tenofovir/Emtricitabine (Truvada)
Zidovudine (Retrovir)
Zidovudine & Lamivudine (Combivir)

Antivirals

Acyclovir (Zovirax)
Adefovir (Hepsera)
Amantadine (Symmetrel)
Atazanavir (Reyataz)
Cidofovir (Vistide)

Emtricitabine (Emtriva)
Enfuvirtide (Fuzeon)
Famciclovir (Famvir)
Foscarnet (Foscavir)
Ganciclovir (Cytovene, Vitrasert)

Interferon Alfa-2b & Ribavirin Combo (Rebetron)
Oseltamivir (Tamiflu)
Palivizumab (Synagis)

Peg Interferon Alfa 2a
(Peg Intron)
Penciclovir (Denavir)
Ribavirin (Virazole)

Rimantadine
(Flumadine)
Telbivudine (Tyzeka)
Valacyclovir (Valtrex)

Valganciclovir (Valcyte)
Zanamivir (Relenza)

Miscellaneous Antiviral Agents

Atovaquone (Mepron)
Atovaquone/Proguanil
(Malarone)

Daptomycin (Cubicin)
Pentamidine (Pentam
300, NebuPent)

Trimetrexate
(NeuTrexin)

ANTINEOPLASTIC AGENTS

Alkylating Agents

Altretamine (Hexalen)
Bendamustine (Treanda)
Busulfan (Myleran,
Busulfex)

Carboplatin (Paraplatin)
Cisplatin (Platinol)
Oxaliplatin (Eloxatin)

Procarbazine (Matulane)
Triethylenethiophosphor-
amide (Thio-Tepa)

NITROGEN MUSTARDS

Chlorambucil
(Leukeran)
Cyclophosphamide
(Cytoxan, Neosar)

Ifosfamide (Ifex,
Holoxan)
Mechlorethamine
(Mustargen)

Melphalan [L-PAM]
(Alkeran)

NITROSOUREAS

Carmustine [BCNU]
(BiCNU, Gliadel)

Streptozocin (Zanosar)

Antibiotics

Bleomycin Sulfate
(Blenoxane)
Dactinomycin (Cosmegen)
Daunorubicin
(Daunomycin,
Cerubidine)

Doxorubicin
(Adriamycin,
Rubex)
Epirubicin (Ellence)

Idarubicin
(Idamycin)
Mitomycin
(Mutamycin)

Antimetabolites

Clofarabine (Clolar)
Cytarabine [ARA-C] (Cytosar-U)
Cytarabine Liposome (DepoCyt)
Floxuridine (FUDR)
Fludarabine Phosphate (Flamp, Fludara)

Fluorouracil [5-FU] (Adrucil)
Gemcitabine (Gemzar)
Mercaptopurine [6-MP] (Purinethol)

Methotrexate (Folex, Rheumatrex)
Nelarabine (Arranon)
Pemetrexed (Alimta)
6-Thioguanine [6-TG]

Hormones

Anastrozole (Arimidex)
Bicalutamide (Casodex)
Estramustine Phosphate (Emcyt)
Exemestane (Aromasin)
Flutamide (Eulexin)

Fulvestrant (Faslodex)
Goserelin (Zoladex)
Leuprolide (Lupron, Viadur, Eligard)
Levamisole (Ergamisol)

Megestrol Acetate (Megace)
Nilutamide (Nilandron)
Tamoxifen
Triptorelin (Trelstar Depot, Trelstar LA)

Mitotic Inhibitors

Etoposide [VP-16] (VePesid)
Vinblastine (Velban, Velbe)

Vincristine (Oncovin, Vincasar PFS)

Vinorelbine (Navelbine)

Monoclonal Antibodies

Bevacizumab (Avastin)
Cetuximab (Erbitux)
Erlotinib (Tarceva)
Gemtuzumab Ozogamicin (Mylotarg)

Panitumumab (Vectibix)

Trastuzumab (Herceptin)

Proteasome inhibitor

Bortezomib (Velcade)

Tyrosine Kinase Inhibitors (TKI)

Dasatinib (Sprycel)
Gefitinib (Iressa)
Imatinib (Gleevec)

Nilotinib (Tasigna)
Sorafenib (Nexavar)

Sunitinib (Sutent)
Temsirolimus (Torisel)

Miscellaneous Antineoplastic Agents

Aldesleukin [Interleukin-2, IL-2] (Proleukin)
Aminoglutethimide (Cytadren)
L-Asparaginase (Elspar, Oncaspar)
BCG [Bacillus Calmette-Guérin] (TheraCys, Tice BCG)
Cladribine (Leustatin)
Dacarbazine (DTIC)
Docetaxel (Taxotere)

Hydroxyurea (Hydrea, Droxia)
Irinotecan (Camptosar)
Ixabepilone (Ixempra)
Letrozole (Femara)
Leucovorin (Wellcovorin)
Mitoxantrone (Novantrone)
Paclitaxel (Taxol, Abraxane)

Panitumumab (Vectibix)
Pemetrexed (Alimta)
Rasburicase (Elitek)
Thalidomide (Thalomid)
Topotecan (Hycamtin)
Tretinoin, Topical [Retinoic Acid] (Retin-A, Avita, Renova, Retin-A Micro)

CARDIOVASCULAR (CV) AGENTS
Aldosterone Antagonist

Eplerenone (Inspra)

Spironolactone (Aldactone)

Alpha₁-Adrenergic Blockers

Doxazosin (Cardura)

Prazosin (Minipress)

Terazosin (Hytrin)

Angiotensin-Converting Enzyme (ACE) Inhibitors

Benazepril (Lotensin)
Captopril (Capoten)
Enalapril (Vasotec)
Fosinopril (Monopril)

Lisinopril (Prinivil, Zestril)
Moexipril (Univasc)
Perindopril Erbumine (Aceon)

Quinapril (Accupril)
Ramipril (Altace)
Trandolapril (Mavik)

Angiotensin II Receptor Antagonists/Blockers

Amlodipine/Olmesartan (Azor)
Amlodipine/Valsartan (Exforge)

Candesartan (Atacand)
Eprosartan (Teveten)
Irbesartan (Avapro)
Losartan (Cozaar)

Telmisartan (Micardis)
Valsartan (Diovan)

Antiarrhythmic Agents

Adenosine (Adenocard)
Amiodarone (Cordarone, Pacerone)
Atropine
Digoxin (Digitek, Lanoxin, Lanoxicaps)

Disopyramide (NAPAmide, Norpace, Norpace CR, Rythmodan)
Dofetilide (Tikosyn)
Esmolol (Brevibloc)
Flecainide (Tambocor)
Ibutilide (Corvert)
Lidocaine (Xylocaine)

Mexiletine (Mexitil)
Procainamide (Pronestyl, Pronestyl SR, Procanbid)
Propafenone (Rythmol)
Quinidine (Quinidex, Quinaglute)
Sotalol (Betapace, Betapace AF)

Beta-Adrenergic Blockers

Acebutolol (Sectral)
Atenolol (Tenormin)
Atenolol & Chlorthalidone (Tenoretic)
Betaxolol (Kerlone)
Bisoprolol (Zebeta)

Carteolol (Cartrol, Ocupress Ophthalmic)
Carvedilol (Coreg, Coreg CR)
Labetalol (Trandate, Normodyne)
Metoprolol (Lopressor, Toprol XL)

Nadolol (Corgard)
Nebivolol (Bystolic)
Penbutolol (Levatol)
Pindolol (Visken)
Propranolol (Inderal)
Timolol (Blocadren)

Calcium Channel Antagonists/Blockers (CCB)

Amlodipine (Norvasc)
Amlodipine/Olmesartan (Azor)
Amlodipine/Valsartan (Exforge)
Diltiazem (Cardizem, Cardizem CD, Cardizem LA,

Cardizem SR, Cartia XT, Dilacor XR, Diltia XT, Taztia XT, Tiamate, Tiazac)
Felodipine (Plendil)
Isradipine (DynaCirc)
Nicardipine (Cardene)

Nifedipine (Procardia, Procardia XL, Adalat CC)
Nimodipine (Nimotop)
Nisoldipine (Sular)
Verapamil (Calan, Isoptin, Verelan)

Centrally Acting Antihypertensive Agents

Clonidine (Catapres) Methyldopa (Aldomet)

Diuretics

Acetazolamide (Diamox)
Amiloride (Midamor)
Bumetanide (Bumex)
Chlorothiazide (Diuril)
Chlorthalidone
  (Hygroton)
Furosemide (Lasix)
Hydrochlorothiazide
  (HydroDIURIL,
  Esidrix)

Hydrochlorothiazide &
  Amiloride
  (Moduretic)
Hydrochlorothiazide &
  Spironolactone
  (Aldactazide)
Hydrochlorothiazide &
  Triamterene (Dyazide,
  Maxzide)
Indapamide (Lozol)

Mannitol
Metolazone (Zaroxolyn)
Spironolactone
  (Aldactone)
Torsemide (Demadex)
Triamterene (Dyrenium)

Inotropic/Pressor Agents

Digoxin (Digitek,
  Lanoxin, Lanoxicaps)
Dobutamine
  (Dobutrex)
Dopamine (Intropin)

Epinephrine (Adrenalin,
  Sus-Phrine, EpiPen)
Inamrinone (Inocor)
Isoproterenol (Isuprel)
Milrinone (Primacor)

Nesiritide (Natrecor)
Norepinephrine
  (Levophed)
Phenylephrine
  (Neo-Synephrine)

Lipid-Lowering Agents

Atorvastatin (Lipitor)
Colesevelam (WelChol)
Colestipol (Colestid)
Cholestyramine
  (Questran, Questran
  Light, Prevalite)
Ezetimibe (Zetia)
Fenofibrate (TriCor,
  Antara, Lipofen,
  Triglide)

Fluvastatin (Lescol)
Gemfibrozil (Lopid)
Lovastatin (Mevacor,
  Altoprev)
Niacin (Niaspan,
  Slo-Niacin)
Niacin and Lovastatin
  (Advicor)
Niacin and Simvastatin
  (Simcor)

Omega-3 fatty acid [fish
  oil] (Lovaza)
Pravastatin (Pravachol)
Rosuvastatin (Crestor)
Simvastatin (Zocor)

Lipid-Lowering/Antihypertensive Combos

Amlodipine/Atorvastatin
  (Caduet)

Vasodilators

Alprostadil
[Prostaglandin E₁]
(Prostin VR)
Epoprostenol (Flolan)
Fenoldopam
(Corlopam)
Hydralazine
(Apresoline)
Iloprost (Ventavis)

Isosorbide Dinitrate
(Isordil, Sorbitrate,
Dilatrate-SR)
Isosorbide Mononitrate
(Ismo, Imdur)
Minoxidil, oral
Nitroglycerin (Nitrostat,
Nitrolingual,
Nitro-Bid Ointment,

Nitro-Bid IV,
Nitrodisc,
Transderm-Nitro,
NitroMist, others)
Nitroprusside (Nipride,
Nitropress)
Tolazoline (Priscoline)
Treprostinil Sodium
(Remodulin)

Miscellaneous Cardiovascular Agents

Aliskiren (Tekturna)
Aliskiren/Hydrochloroth-
iazide (Tekturna HCT)

Ambrisentan (Letairis)
Conivaptan (Vaprisol)

Ranolazine (Ranexa)
Sildenafil (Revatio)

CENTRAL NERVOUS SYSTEM AGENTS

Antianxiety Agents

Alprazolam (Xanax)
Buspirone (BuSpar)
Chlordiazepoxide
(Librium, Mitran,
Libritabs)

Clorazepate (Tranxene)
Diazepam (Valium,
Diastat)
Doxepin (Sinequan,
Adapin)

Hydroxyzine (Atarax,
Vistaril)
Lorazepam (Ativan)
Meprobamate (various)
Oxazepam

Anticonvulsants

Carbamazepine (Tegretol
XR, Carbatrol, Epitol,
Equetro)
Clonazepam (Klonopin)
Diazepam (Valium)
Ethosuximide (Zarontin)
Fosphenytoin (Cerebyx)
Gabapentin (Neurontin)

Lamotrigine (Lamictal)
Levetiracetam (Keppra)
Lorazepam (Ativan)
Oxcarbazepine
(Trileptal)
Pentobarbital
(Nembutal)
Phenobarbital

Phenytoin (Dilantin)
Tiagabine (Gabitril)
Topiramate (Topamax)
Valproic Acid
(Depakene, Depakote)
Zonisamide (Zonegran)

Antidepressants

Amitriptyline (Elavil)
Bupropion
hydrobromide
(Aplenzin)
Bupropion hydrochloride
(Wellbutrin,
Wellbutrin SR,
Wellbutrin XL,
Zyban)
Citalopram (Celexa)
Desipramine
(Norpramin)

Desvenlafaxine
(Pristiq)
Doxepin (Adapin)
Duloxetine (Cymbalta)
Escitalopram (Lexapro)
Fluoxetine (Prozac,
Sarafem)
Fluvoxamine (Luvox)
Imipramine (Tofranil)
Mirtazapine (Remeron)
Nefazodone (Serzone)
Nortriptyline (Pamelor)

Paroxetine (Paxil, Paxil
CR, Pexeva)
Phenelzine (Nardil)
Selegiline transdermal
(Emsam)
Sertraline (Zoloft)
Trazodone (Desyrel)
Venlafaxine (Effexor,
Effexor XR)

Antiparkinson Agents

Amantadine
(Symmetrel)
Apomorphine (Apokyn)
Benztropine (Cogentin)
Bromocriptine (Parlodel)
Carbidopa/Levodopa
(Sinemet)

Entacapone (Comtan)
Pramipexole (Mirapex)
Rasagiline mesylate
(Azilect)
Rivastigmine
transdermal (Exelon
Patch)

Ropinirole (Requip)
Selegiline (Eldepryl,
Zelapar)
Tolcapone (Tasmar)
Trihexyphenidyl

Antipsychotics

Aripiprazole (Abilify,
Abilify DISCMELT)
Chlorpromazine
(Thorazine)
Clozapine (Clozaril,
FazaClo)
Haloperidol (Haldol)
Lithium Carbonate
(Eskalith, Lithobid)

Molindone (Moban)
Olanzapine (Zyprexa,
Zyprexa Zydis)
Paliperidone (Invega)
Perphenazine (Trilafon)
Prochlorperazine
(Compazine)
Quetiapine (Seroquel,
Seroquel XR)

Risperidone (Risperdal,
Risperdal Consta,
Risperdal M-Tab)
Thioridazine (Mellaril)
Thiothixene (Navane)
Trifluoperazine
(Stelazine)
Ziprasidone (Geodon)

Sedative Hypnotics

Chloral Hydrate
(Aquachloral,
Supprettes)
Diphenhydramine
(Benadryl)
Estazolam (ProSom)
Eszopiclone (Lunesta)

Flurazepam (Dalmane)
Hydroxyzine (Atarax,
Vistaril)
Midazolam (various)
[C-IV]
Pentobarbital
(Nembutal)

Phenobarbital
Propofol (Diprivan)
Secobarbital (Seconal)
Temazepam (Restoril)
Triazolam (Halcion)
Zaleplon (Sonata)
Zolpidem (Ambien)

Stimulants

Armodafinil (Nuvigil)
Atomoxetine (Strattera)
Lisdexamfetamine
(Vyvanse)

Methylphenidate, Oral
(Concerta, Metadate
CD, Ritalin, Ritalin LA,
Ritalin SR, others) [CII]

Methylphenidate,
Transdermal (Daytrana)
Sibutramine (Meridia)

Miscellaneous CNS Agents

Donepezil (Aricept)
Galantamine (Razadyne)
Interferon beta 1a
(Rebif)

Meclizine
(Antivert) (Bonine,
Dramamine OTC)
Memantine (Namenda)

Sodium Oxybate (Xyrem)
Tacrine (Cognex)
Natalizumab (Tysabri)
Nimodipine (Nimotop)

DERMATOLOGIC AGENTS

Acitretin (Soriatane)
Acyclovir (Zovirax)
Alefacept (Amevive)
Anthralin (Anthra-Derm)
Amphotericin B
(Fungizone)
Bacitracin, Topical
(Baciguent)
Bacitracin & Polymyxin
B, Topical
(Polysporin)

Bacitracin, Neomycin, &
Polymyxin B, Topical
(Neosporin Ointment)
Bacitracin, Neomycin,
Polymyxin B, &
Hydrocortisone,
Topical (Cortisporin)
Bacitracin, Neomycin,
Polymyxin B, &
Lidocaine, Topical
(Clomycin)

Botulinum toxin type A
(Botox Cosmetic)
Calcipotriene (Dovonex)
Capsaicin (Capsin,
Zostrix)
Ciclopirox (Loprox)
Ciprofloxacin (Cipro)
Clindamycin (Cleocin)
Clotrimazole &
Betamethasone
(Lotrisone)

Dapsone Topical
(Aczone)
Dibucaine
(Nupercainal)
Doxepin, Topical
(Zonalon, Prudoxin)
Econazole
(Spectazole)
Efalizumab (Raptiva)
Erythromycin, Topical
(A/T/S, Eryderm,
Erycette, T-Stat)
Finasteride (Propecia)
Gentamicin, Topical
(Garamycin,
G-Mycitin)
Imiquimod Cream, 5%
(Aldara)
Isotretinoin [13-*cis*
Retinoic acid]
(Accutane,
Amnesteem, Claravis,
Sotret)
Ketoconazole (Nizoral)
Kunecatechins
[sinecatechins]
(Veregen)

Lactic Acid &
Ammonium
Hydroxide
[Ammonium Lactate]
(Lac-Hydrin)
Lindane (Kwell, others)
Metronidazole (Flagyl,
MetroGel)
Miconazole
(Monistat)
Miconazole/zinc
oxide/petrolatum
(Vusion)
Minocycline (Solodyn)
Minoxidil, topical
(Theroxidil,
Rogaine) [OTC]
Mupirocin
(Bactroban)
Naftifine (Naftin)
Nystatin (Mycostatin)
Oxiconazole (Oxistat)
Penciclovir (Denavir)
Permethrin (Nix,
Elimite)
Pimecrolimus
(Elidel)

Podophyllin (Podocon-
25, Condylox Gel
0.5%, Condylox)
Pramoxine (Anusol
Ointment,
ProctoFoam-NS)
Pramoxine & Hydro-
cortisone (Enzone,
ProctoFoam-HC)
Selenium Sulfide (Exsel
Shampoo, Selsun Blue
Shampoo, Selsun
Shampoo)
Silver Sulfadiazine
(Silvadene)
Steroids, Topical (Table 4,
page 252)
Tacrolimus (Prograf,
Protopic)
Tazarotene (Tazorac,
Avage)
Terbinafine (Lamisil)
Tolnaftate (Tinactin)
Tretinoin, Topical
[Retinoic Acid] (Retin-
A, Avita, Renova)
Vorinostat (Zolinza)

DIETARY SUPPLEMENTS

Calcium Acetate
(Calphron, Phos-Ex,
PhosLo)
Calcium Glubionate
(Neo-Calglucon)
Calcium Salts [Chloride,
Gluconate,
Gluceptate]
Cholecalciferol [Vitamin
D_3] (Delta D)

Cyanocobalamin
[Vitamin B_{12}]
(Nascobal)
Ferric Gluconate
Complex (Ferrlecit)
Ferrous Gluconate
(Fergon [OTC],
others)
Ferrous Sulfate
Fish Oil (Lovaza, OTC)

Folic Acid
Iron Dextran
(Dexferrum, INFeD)
Iron Sucrose (Venofer)
Magnesium Oxide
(Mag-Ox 400)
Magnesium Sulfate
Multivitamins (Table 13,
page 268)

Phytonadione [Vitamin K] (Aqua-MEPHYTON)
Potassium Supplements (Kaon, Kaochlor, K-Lor, Slow-K, Micro-K, Klorvess)

Pyridoxine [Vitamin B$_6$]
Sodium Bicarbonate [NaHCO$_3$]

Thiamine [Vitamin B$_1$]

EAR (OTIC) AGENTS

Acetic Acid & Aluminum Acetate (Otic Domeboro)
Benzocaine & Antipyrine (Auralgan)
Ciprofloxacin, Otic (Cipro HC Otic)
Ciprofloxacin and dexamethasone, Otic (Ciprodex Otic)

Ciprofloxacin and hydrocortisone, Otic (Cipro HC Otic)
Neomycin, Colistin, & Hydrocortisone (Cortisporin-TC Otic Drops)
Neomycin, Colistin, Hydrocortisone, & Thonzonium (Cortisporin-TC Otic Suspension)

Ofloxacin otic (generic)
Polymyxin B & Hydrocortisone (Otobiotic Otic)
Sulfacetamide & Prednisolone (Blephamide)
Triethanolamine (Cerumenex)

ENDOCRINE SYSTEM AGENTS

Antidiabetic Agents

Acarbose (Precose)
Chlorpropamide (Diabinese)
Glimepiride (Amaryl)
Glimepiride/pioglitazone (Duetact)
Glipizide (Glucotrol)
Glyburide (DiaBeta, Micronase, Glynase)

Glyburide/Metformin (Glucovance)
Insulins, Systemic (Table 5, page 255)
Metformin (Glucophage)
Miglitol (Glyset)
Nateglinide (Starlix)
Pioglitazone (Actos)

Pioglitazone/Metformin (ACTOplus Met)
Repaglinide (Prandin)
Rosiglitazone (Avandia)
Sitagliptin (Januvia)
Sitagliptin/Metformin (Janumet)
Tolazamide (Tolinase)
Tolbutamide (Orinase)

Hormone & Synthetic Substitutes

Calcitonin (Cibacalcin, Miacalcin)

Calcitriol (Rocaltrol, Calcijex)

Fluoxymesterone (Halotestin, Androxy)

Glucagon

Hydrocortisone Topical & Systemic (Cortef, Solu-Cortef)

Cortisone Systemic, Topical

Desmopressin (DDAVP, Stimate)

Methylprednisolone (Solu-Medrol)

Prednisolone

Prednisone

Testosterone (AndroGel, Androderm, Striant, Testim)

Dexamethasone (Decadron)

Fludrocortisone Acetate (Florinef)

Vasopressin [Antidiuretic Hormone, ADH] (Pitressin)

Hypercalcemia/Osteoporosis Agents

Alendronate (Fosamax)

Etidronate Disodium (Didronel)

Gallium Nitrate (Ganite)

Ibandronate (Boniva)

Pamidronate (Aredia)

Raloxifene (Evista)

Risedronate (Actonel, Actonel w/calcium)

Teriparatide (Forteo)

Zoledronic acid (Zometa, Reclast)

Obesity

Orlistat (Xenical, Alli [OTC])

Sibutramine (Meridia)

Thyroid/Antithyroid

Levothyroxine (Synthroid, Levoxyl)

Liothyronine (Cytomel)

Methimazole (Tapazole)

Potassium Iodide [Lugol Soln] (SSKI, Thyro-Block, Thyro Safe, ThyroShield)

Propylthiouracil [PTU]

Miscellaneous Endocrine Agents

Cinacalcet (Sensipar)

Demeclocycline (Declomycin)

Diazoxide (Proglycem)

EYE (OPHTHALMIC) AGENTS

Glaucoma Agents

Acetazolamide (Diamox)
Apraclonidine (Iopidine)
Betaxolol, Ophthalmic (Betoptic)
Brimonidine (Alphagan P)
Brimonidine/Timolol (Combigan)
Brinzolamide (Azopt)
Carteolol (Ocupress, Carteolol Ophthalmic)
Dipivefrin (Propine)
Dorzolamide (Trusopt)
Dorzolamide & Timolol (Cosopt)
Echothiophate Iodine (Phospholine Ophthalmic)
Latanoprost (Xalatan)
Levobunolol (A-K Beta, Betagan)
Timolol, Ophthalmic (Timoptic)

Ophthalmic Antibiotics

Azithromycin Ophthalmic (AzaSite)
Bacitracin, Ophthalmic (AK-Tracin Ophthalmic)
Bacitracin & Polymyxin B, Ophthalmic (AK-Poly-Bac Ophthalmic, Polysporin Ophthalmic)
Bacitracin, Neomycin, & Polymyxin B (AK Spore Ophthalmic, Neosporin Ophthalmic)
Bacitracin, Neomycin, Polymyxin B, & Hydrocortisone, Ophthalmic (AK Spore HC Ophthalmic, Cortisporin Ophthalmic)
Ciprofloxacin, Ophthalmic (Ciloxan)
Erythromycin, Ophthalmic (Ilotycin Ophthalmic)
Gentamicin, Ophthalmic (Garamycin, Genoptic, Gentacidin, Gentak)
Levofloxacin ophthalmic (Quixin, Iquix)
Moxifloxacin ophthalmic (Vigamox Ophthalmic)
Neomycin, Polymyxin, & Hydrocortisone (Cortisporin Ophthalmic & Otic)
Neomycin & Dexamethasone (AK-Neo-Dex Ophthalmic, NeoDecadron Ophthalmic)
Neomycin, Polymyxin B, & Dexamethasone (Maxitrol)
Neomycin, Polymyxin B, & Prednisolone (Poly-Pred Ophthalmic)
Norfloxacin ophthalmic (Chibroxin)
Ofloxacin ophthalmic (Ocuflox Ophthalmic)
Silver Nitrate (Dey-Drop)
Sulfacetamide (Bleph-10, Cetamide, Sodium Sulamyd)
Sulfacetamide & Prednisolone (Blephamide)
Tobramycin ophthalmic (AKTob, Tobrex)
Tobramycin & Dexamethasone (TobraDex)
Trifluridine (Viroptic)

Miscellaneous Ophthalmic Agents

Artificial Tears (Tears Naturale)
Atropine
Cromolyn Sodium (Opticrom)
Cyclopentolate (Cyclogyl, Cyclate)
Cyclopentolate with phenylephrine (Cyclomydril)
Cyclosporine Ophthalmic (Restasis)

Dexamethasone, Ophthalmic (AK-Dex Ophthalmic, Decadron Ophthalmic)
Diclofenac ophthalmic (Voltaren ophthalmic)
Emedastine (Emadine)
Epinastine (Elestat)
Ketotifen Ophthalmic (Alaway, Zaditor) [OTC]
Ketorolac Ophthalmic (Acular, Acular LS, Acular PF)

Levocabastine (Livostin)
Lodoxamide (Alomide)
Naphazoline (Albalon, Naphcon, others)
Naphazoline & Pheniramine Acetate (Naphcon A, Visine A)
Nepafenac (Nevanac)
Olopatadine ophthalmic (Patanol, Pataday)
Pemirolast (Alamast)
Rimexolone (Vexol Ophthalmic)
Scopolamine ophthalmic

GASTROINTESTINAL AGENTS

Antacids

Alginic Acid (Gaviscon)
Aluminum Hydroxide (Amphojel, AlternaGEL)
Aluminum Hydroxide with Magnesium Carbonate (Gaviscon)

Aluminum Hydroxide with Magnesium Hydroxide (Maalox)
Aluminum Hydroxide with Magnesium Hydroxide & Simethicone (Mylanta, Mylanta II, Maalox Plus)

Aluminum Hydroxide with Magnesium Trisilicate (Gaviscon, Gaviscon-2)
Calcium Carbonate (Tums, Alka-Mints)
Magaldrate (Riopan-Plus) [OTC]
Simethicone (Mylicon)

Antidiarrheals

Bismuth Subsalicylate (Pepto-Bismol)
Diphenoxylate with Atropine (Lomotil, Lonox)

Lactobacillus (Lactinex Granules)
Loperamide (Diamode, Imodium) [OTC]

Octreotide (Sandostatin, Sandostatin LAR)
Paregoric [Camphorated Tincture of Opium]

Antiemetics

Aprepitant (Emend)
Chlorpromazine (Thorazine)

Dimenhydrinate (Dramamine)
Dolasetron (Anzemet)
Dronabinol (Marinol)

Droperidol (Inapsine)
Fosaprepitant (Emend, Injection)
Granisetron (Kytril)

Meclizine (Antivert)
Metoclopramide
  (Reglan, Clopra,
  Octamide)
Nabilone (Cesamet)
Ondansetron (Zofran)

Palonosetron (Aloxi)
Prochlorperazine
  (Compazine)
Promethazine
  (Phenergan)
Scopolamine (Scopace)

Thiethylperazine
  (Torecan)
Trimethobenzamide
  (Tigan)

Antiulcer Agents

Cimetidine (Tagamet)
Esomeprazole (Nexium)
Famotidine (Pepcid,
  Pepcid AC)
Lansoprazole (Prevacid)

Nizatidine (Axid)
Omeprazole (Prilosec,
  Prilosec OTC,
  Zegerid)
Pantoprazole (Protonix)

Rabeprazole (AcipHex)
Ranitidine
  Hydrochloride
  (Zantac)
Sucralfate (Carafate)

Cathartics/Laxatives

Bisacodyl (Dulcolax)
Docusate Calcium
  (Surfak)
Docusate Potassium
  (Dialose)
Docusate Sodium (Doss,
  Colace)
Glycerin Suppository
Lactulose (Constulose,
  Generlac, Chronulac,
  Cephulac, Enulose)

Magnesium Citrate
  (Citroma, others)
  [OTC]
Magnesium Hydroxide
  (Milk of Magnesia)
Mineral Oil Enema
  (Fleet Mineral Oil)
  [OTC]
Polyethylene Glycol-
  Electrolyte Solution
  (GoLYTELY, CoLyte)

Psyllium (Metamucil,
  Serutan, Effer-
  Syllium)
Sodium Phosphate
  (Visicol)
Sorbitol

Enzymes

Pancreatin (Pancrease,
  Cotazym, Creon,
  Ultrase)

Miscellaneous GI Agents

Alosetron (Lotronex)
Budesonide (Entocort EC)
Balsalazide (Colazal)
Certolizumab (Cimzia)

Dexpanthenol (Ilopan-
  Choline Oral, Ilopan)
Dibucaine (Nupercainal)
Dicyclomine (Bentyl)

Mineral Oil-Pramoxine
  HCl-Zinc Oxide
  (Tucks Ointment)
  [OTC]

Hydrocortisone, Rectal
  (Anusol-HC
  Suppository,
  Cortifoam Rectal,
  Proctocort)
Hyoscyamine
  (Anaspaz, Cystospaz,
  Levsin)
Hyoscyamine,
  Atropine,
  Scopolamine, &
  Phenobarbital
  (Donnatal)
Infliximab (Remicade)
Lubiprostone (Amitiza)

Mesalamine (Asacol,
  Canasa, Lialda,
  Pentasa, Rowasa)
Methylnaltrexone
  bromide (Relistor)
Metoclopramide
  (Reglan, Clopra,
  Octamide)
Misoprostol (Cytotec)
Neomycin Sulfate
  (Neo-Fradin, generic)
Olsalazine (Dipentum)
Pramoxine (Anusol
  Ointment,
  ProctoFoam-NS)

Pramoxine with
  Hydrocortisone
  (Enzone,
  ProctoFoam-HC)
Propantheline
  (Pro-Banthine)
Starch, topical, rectal
  (Tucks Suppositories)
  [OTC]
Vasopressin (Pitressin)
Witch Hazel (Tucks
  Pads, others [OTC])

HEMATOLOGIC AGENTS

Anticoagulants

Argatroban (Acova)
Bivalirudin (Angiomax)
Dalteparin (Fragmin)
Enoxaparin (Lovenox)

Fondaparinux (Arixtra)
Heparin
Lepirudin (Refludan)
Protamine

Tinzaparin (Innohep)
Warfarin (Coumadin)

Antiplatelet Agents

Abciximab (ReoPro)
Aspirin (Bayer, Ecotrin,
  St. Joseph's)
Clopidogrel (Plavix)

Dipyridamole
  (Persantine)
Dipyridamole & Aspirin
  (Aggrenox)

Eptifibatide (Integrilin)
Ticlopidine (Ticlid)
Tirofiban (Aggrastat)

Antithrombotic Agents

Alteplase, Recombinant
  [tPA] (Activase)
Aminocaproic Acid
  (Amicar)
Anistreplase (Eminase)

Danaparoid (Orgaran)
Dextran 40 (Gentran 40,
  Rheomacrodex)
Reteplase (Retavase)

Streptokinase (Streptase,
  Kabikinase)
Tenecteplase (TNKase)
Urokinase (Abbokinase)

Hematopoietic Stimulants

Darbepoetin Alfa
(Aranesp)
Epoetin Alfa
[Erythropoietin, EPO]
(Epogen, Procrit)

Filgrastim [G-CSF]
(Neupogen)
Oprelvekin
(Neumega)

Pegfilgrastim (Neulasta)
Sargramostim
[GM-CSF]
(Leukine)

Volume Expanders

Albumin
(Albuminar,
Buminate, Albutein)

Dextran 40
(Rheomacrodex)
Hetastarch (Hespan)

Plasma Protein Fraction
(Plasmanate)

Miscellaneous Hematologic Agents

Antihemophilic Factor
VIII (Monoclate)
Antihemophilic Factor
(Recombinant)
(Xyntha)

Decitabine
(Dacogen)
Desmopressin
(DDAVP, Stimate)

Lenalidomide
(Revlimid)
Pentoxifylline
(Trental)

IMMUNE SYSTEM AGENTS

Immunomodulators

Abatacept (Orencia)
Adalimumab (Humira)
Anakinra (Kineret)
Etanercept (Enbrel)
Interferon Alfa
(Roferon-A, Intron A)

Interferon Alfacon-1
(Infergen)
Interferon Beta-1b
(Betaseron)
Interferon Gamma-1b
(Actimmune)

Natalizumab (Tysabri)
Peg Interferon Alfa-2b
(PEG-Intron)

Immunosuppressive Agents

Azathioprine
(Imuran)
Basiliximab
(Simulect)
Cyclosporine
(Sandimmune,
Gengraf, Neoral)
Daclizumab (Zenapax)

Lymphocyte Immune
Globulin
[Antithymocyte
Globulin, ATG] (Atgam)
Muromonab-CD3
(Orthoclone OKT3)
Mycophenolic Acid
(Myfortic)

Mycophenolate Mofetil
(CellCept)
Sirolimus
(Rapamune)
Steroids, Systemic
(Table 3, page 251)
Tacrolimus (Prograf,
Protopic)

Vaccines/Serums/Toxoids

Cytomegalovirus
Immune Globulin
[CMV-IG IV]
(CytoGam)
Diphtheria, Tetanus
Toxoids, & Acellular
Pertussis Adsorbed,
Hepatitis B
(recombinant), &
Inactivated Poliovirus
Vaccine (IPV)
Combined (Pediarix)
Haemophilus B
Conjugate Vaccine
(ActHIB, HibTITER,
PedvaxHIB, Prohibit)
Hepatitis A (Inactivated)
& Hepatitis B
Recombinant Vaccine
(Twinrix)
Hepatitis A Vaccine
(Havrix, Vaqta)
Hepatitis B Immune
Globulin (HyperHep,
HepaGam B, H-BIG)

Hepatitis B Vaccine
(Engerix-B,
Recombivax HB)
Human Papillomavirus
(Types 6, 11, 16, 18)
Recombinant Vaccine
(Gardasil)
Immune Globulin, IV
(Gamimune N,
Sandoglobulin,
Gammar IV)
Immune Globulin, Sub
Cutaneous
(Vivaglobin)
Influenza Vaccine
(Fluarix, FluLaval,
Fluzone, Fluvirin)
Influenza Virus Vaccine
Live, Intranasal
(FluMist)
Measles, Mumps,
Rubella, and
Varicella Virus
Vaccine Live
[MMRV] (ProQuad)

Meningococcal
conjugate vaccine
(Menactra, MCV4)
Meningococcal
Polysaccharide Vaccine
[MPSV4] (Menomune
A/C/Y/ W-135)
Pneumococcal 7-Valent
Conjugate Vaccine
(Prevnar)
Pneumococcal Vaccine,
Polyvalent
(Pneumovax-23)
Rotavirus vaccine, live,
oral, monovalent
(RotaRix)
Rotavirus vaccine, live,
oral, pentavalent
(RotaTeq)
Tetanus Immune Globulin
Tetanus Toxoid
Varicella Virus Vaccine
(Varivax)
Zoster vaccine, live
(Zostavax)

MUSCULOSKELETAL AGENTS

Antigout Agents

Allopurinol (Zyloprim,
Lopurin, Aloprim)

Colchicine

Probenecid (Benemid)

Muscle Relaxants

Baclofen (Lioresal
Intrathecal)
Carisoprodol (Soma)
Chlorzoxazone (Paraflex,
Parafon Forte DSC)
Cyclobenzaprine (Flexeril)

Cyclobenzaprine,
extended release
(Amrix)
Dantrolene (Dantrium)

Diazepam (Valium)
Metaxalone (Skelaxin)
Methocarbamol
(Robaxin)
Orphenadrine (Norflex)

Neuromuscular Blockers

Atracurium (Tracrium)   Succinylcholine   Vecuronium (Norcuron)
Pancuronium (Pavulon)   (Anectine, Quelicin,
Rocuronium (Zemuron)   Sucostrin)

Miscellaneous Musculoskeletal Agents

Edrophonium (Tensilon,   Leflunomide   Methotrexate (Folex,
Reversol)   (Arava)   Rheumatrex)

OB/GYN AGENTS
Contraceptives

Copper IUD   Etonogestrel/Ethinyl   Oral Contraceptives,
Contraceptive   Estradiol vaginal   Multiphasic (Table 6,
(ParaGard T 380A)   insert (NuvaRing)   page 258)
Estradiol Cypionate &   Medroxyprogesterone   Oral Contraceptives,
Medroxyprogesterone   (Provera, Depo   Progestin Only
Acetate (Lunelle)   Provera, Depo-Sub Q   (Table 6, page 259)
Etonogestrel Implant   Provera)   Oral Contraceptives,
(Implanon)   Oral Contraceptives,   Extended Cycle
Levonorgestrel   Monophasic (Table 6,   Combination (Table 6,
intrauterine device   page 256)   page 260)
(IUD) (Mirena)

Emergency Contraceptives

Levonorgestrel (Plan B)

Estrogen Supplementation
ESTROGEN ONLY

Estradiol (Estrace,   Estradiol, spray   Estrogen, Conjugated
Femtrace,   (Evamist)   (Premarin)
Delestrogen, others)   Estradiol, transdermal   Estrogen, Conjugated-
Estradiol gel   (Estraderm, Climara,   Synthetic (Cenestin,
(Divigel)   Vivelle)   Enjuvia)
Estradiol gel   Estradiol, vaginal (Estring, Esterified Estrogens
(Elestrin)   Femring, Vagifem)   (Estratab, Menest)

COMBINATION ESTROGEN/PROGESTIN

Esterified
  Estrogens with
  Methyltestosterone
  (Estratest, Estratest
  HS, Syntest DS, HS)
Estrogen,
  Conjugated with
  Medroxyprogesterone
  (Prempro,
  Premphase)

Estrogen, Conjugated
  with Methyl
  progesterone
  (Premarin with
  Methyl progesterone)
Estrogen,
  Conjugated with
  Methyltestosterone
  (Premarin with
  Methyltestosterone)

Estradiol/levonorgestrel,
  transdermal
  (Climara Pro)
Estradiol/Norethindrone
  acetate (Femhrt,
  Activella)
Norethindrone
  acetate/ethinyl
  Estradiol (Femhrt,
  Activella)

Vaginal Preparations

Amino-Cerv pH 5.5
  Cream

Miconazole (Monistat)
Nystatin (Mycostatin)

Terconazole (Terazol 7)
Tioconazole (Vagistat)

Miscellaneous Ob/Gyn Agents

Dinoprostone (Cervidil
  Vaginal Insert,
  Prepidil Vaginal Gel,
  Prostin E2)
Gonadorelin (Factrel)
Leuprolide (Lupron)
Lutropin Alfa (Luveris)

Magnesium Sulfate
Medroxyprogesterone
  (Provera,
  Depo-Provera)
Methylergonovine
  (Methergine)

Mifepristone [RU 486]
  (Mifeprex)
Oxytocin (Pitocin)
Terbutaline (Brethine,
  Bricanyl)

PAIN MEDICATIONS
Local Anesthetics (Table 2, page 250)

Benzocaine &
  Antipyrine
  (Auralgan)
Bupivacaine
  (Marcaine)
Capsaicin (Capsin,
  Zostrix)
Cocaine

Dibucaine
  (Nupercainal)
Lidocaine, Lidocaine
  with epinephrine
  (Anestacon Topical,
  Xylocaine, Xylocaine
  Viscous, Xylocaine
  MPF, others)

Lidocaine, powder
  intradermal injection
  system (Zingo)
Lidocaine & Prilocaine
  (EMLA, LMX)
Pramoxine (Anusol
  Ointment,
  ProctoFoam-NS)

Migraine Headache Medications

Acetaminophen with
   Butalbital w/ & w/o
   Caffeine (Fioricet,
   Medigesic, Repan,
   Sedapap-10,
   Two-Dyne, Triapin,
   Axocet, Phrenilin
   Forte)

Almotriptan (Axert)
Aspirin & Butalbital
   Compound (Fiorinal)
Aspirin with Butalbital,
   Caffeine, & Codeine
   (Fiorinal with
   Codeine)
Eletriptan (Relpax)

Frovatriptan (Frova)
Naratriptan (Amerge)
Sumatriptan (Imitrex)
Sumatriptan and
   Naproxen Sodium
   (Treximet)
Zolmitriptan (Zomig)

Narcotic Analgesics

Acetaminophen with
   Codeine (Tylenol No.
   2 3, 4)
Alfentanil
   (Alfenta)
Aspirin with Codeine
   (Empirin No. 2, 3, 4)
Buprenorphine
   (Buprenex)
Butorphanol (Stadol)
Codeine
Fentanyl (Sublimaze)
Fentanyl iontophoretic
   transdermal system
   (Ionsys)
Nalbuphine (Nubain)
Oxycodone (OxyContin,
   OxyIR, Roxicodone)
Oxycodone &
   Acetaminophen
   (Percocet, Tylox)
Oxycodone & Aspirin
   (Percodan)

Fentanyl, Transdermal
   (Duragesic)
Fentanyl, Transmucosal
   (Actiq, Fentora)
Hydrocodone &
   Acetaminophen
   (Lorcet, Vicodin,
   Hycet)
Hydrocodone & Aspirin
   (Lortab ASA)
Hydrocodone &
   Ibuprofen
   (Vicoprofen)
Hydromorphone
   (Dilaudid)
Oxymorphone (Opana,
   Opana ER)
Pentazocine (Talwin)
Propoxyphene
   (Darvon)
Propoxyphene &
   Acetaminophen
   (Darvocet)

Levorphanol
   (Levo-Dromoran)
Meperidine (Demerol,
   Meperitab) [C-II]
Methadone (Dolophine,
   Methadose) [C-II]
Morphine (Avinza XR,
   Astramorph/PF,
   Duramorph,
   Infumorph, MS
   Contin, Kadian SR,
   Oramorph SR,
   Roxanol) [C-II]
Morphine, Liposomal
   (DepoDur)
Propoxyphene & Aspirin
   (Darvon
   Compound-65,
   Darvon-N with
   Aspirin)

Nonnarcotic Analgesics

Acetaminophen
   [APAP] (Tylenol)
Aspirin (Bayer,
   Ecotrin, St. Joseph's)

Tramadol (Ultram,
   Ultram ER)

Tramadol/Acetaminophen
   (Ultracet)

Nonsteroidal Antiinflammatory Agents

Celecoxib (Celebrex)
Diclofenac (Arthrotec,
    Cataflam, Flector,
    Flector patch,
    Voltaren, Voltaren XR,
    Voltaren gel)
Diflunisal (Dolobid)
Etodolac
Fenoprofen
    (Nalfon)

Flurbiprofen (Ansaid,
    Ocufen)
Ibuprofen (Motrin,
    Rufen, Advil)
Indomethacin
    (Indocin)
Ketoprofen (Orudis,
    Oruvail)
Ketorolac (Toradol)
Meloxicam (Mobic)

Nabumetone
    (Relafen)
Naproxen (Aleve,
    Naprosyn, Anaprox)
Oxaprozin (Daypro)
Piroxicam
    (Feldene)
Sulindac (Clinoril)
Tolmetin
    (Tolectin)

Miscellaneous Pain Medications

Amitriptyline
    (Elavil)
Imipramine
    (Tofranil)

Pregabalin
    (Lyrica)
Tramadol
    (Ultram)

Ziconotide
    (Prialt)

RESPIRATORY AGENTS

Antitussives, Decongestants, & Expectorants

Acetylcysteine
    (Acetadote,
    Mucomyst)
Benzonatate
    (Tessalon Perles)
Codeine
Dextromethorphan
    (Mediquell, Benylin
    DM, PediaCare 1)
Guaifenesin
    (Robitussin)
Guaifenesin &
    Codeine (Robitussin
    AC, Brontex)

Guaifenesin &
    Dextromethorphan
Hydrocodone &
    Guaifenesin
    (Hycotuss
    Expectorant)
Hydrocodone &
    Homatropine
    (Hycodan,
    Hydromet)
Hydrocodone &
    Pseudoephedrine
    (Detussin,
    Histussin-D)

Hydrocodone,
    Chlorpheniramine,
    Phenylephrine,
    Acetaminophen, &
    Caffeine
    (Hycomine)
Potassium Iodide
    (SSKI, Thyro-
    Block)
Pseudoephedrine
    (Sudafed, Novafed,
    Afrinol)

Bronchodilators

Albuterol (Proventil, Ventolin, Volmax)

Albuterol & Ipratropium (Combivent)

Aminophylline

Arformoterol (Brovana)

Ephedrine

Epinephrine (Adrenalin, Sus-Phrine, EpiPen)

Formoterol (Foradil Aerolizer)

Isoproterenol (Isuprel)

Levalbuterol (Xopenex, Xopenex HFA)

Metaproterenol (Alupent, Metaprel)

Pirbuterol (Maxair)

Salmeterol (Serevent, Serevent Diskus)

Terbutaline (Brethine, Bricanyl)

Theophylline (Theo24, Theochron)

Respiratory Inhalants

Acetylcysteine (Acetadote, Mucomyst)

Beclomethasone (Beconase, Vancenase Nasal Inhaler)

Beclomethasone (QVAR)

Beractant (Survanta)

Budesonide (Rhinocort, Pulmicort)

Budesonide/formoterol (Symbicort)

Calfactant (Infasurf)

Ciclesonide, Inhalation (Alvesco)

Ciclesonide, Nasal (Omnaris)

Cromolyn Sodium (Intal, NasalCrom, Opticrom)

Dexamethasone, Nasal (Dexacort Phosphate Turbinaire)

Flunisolide (AeroBid, Aerospan, Nasarel)

Fluticasone Furoate Nasal (Veramyst)

Fluticasone Propionate, Nasal (Flonase)

Fluticasone Propionate, Inhalation (Flovent HFA, Flovent Diskus)

Fluticasone Propionate & Salmeterol Xinafoate (Advair Diskus, Advair HFA)

Formoterol Fumarate (Foradil, Perforomist)

Ipratropium (Atrovent HFA, Atrovent Nasal)

Olopatadine Nasal (Patanase)

Tiotropium (Spiriva)

Triamcinolone (Azmacort)

Miscellaneous Respiratory Agents

Alpha$_1$-Protease Inhibitor (Prolastin)

Dornase Alfa (Pulmozyme, DNase)

Montelukast (Singulair)

Omalizumab (Xolair)

Zafirlukast (Accolate)

Zileuton (Zyflo, Zyflo CR)

URINARY/GENITOURINARY AGENTS

Benign Prostatic Hyperplasia

Alfuzosin (Uroxatral)
Doxazosin (Cardura, Cardura XL)

Dutasteride (Avodart)
Finasteride (Proscar)
Tamsulosin (Flomax)

Terazosin (Hytrin)
Silodosin (Rapaflo)

Bladder Agents (Overactive Bladder, Other Anticholinergics)

Belladonna & Opium Suppositories (B & O Supprettes)
Bethanechol (Urecholine, Duvoid)
Butabarbital-Hyoscyamine Hydrobromide-Phenazopyridine (Pyridium Plus)
Darifenacin (Enablex)
Flavoxate (Urispas)

Hyoscyamine (Anaspaz, Cystospaz, Levsin)
Methenamine Hippurate (Hiprex)
Methenamine Mandelate (UROQUID-Acid No. 2)
Oxybutynin (Ditropan, Ditropan XL)
Oxybutynin Transdermal System (Oxytrol)

Phenazopyridine (Pyridium, Azo-Standard, Urogesic, many others)
Solifenacin (Vesicare)
Tolterodine (Detrol, Detrol LA)
Trospium Chloride (Sanctura, Sanctura XR)

Erectile Dysfunction

Alprostadil, Intracavernosal (Caverject, Edex)

Alprostadil, Urethral Suppository (Muse)
Sildenafil (Viagra)
Tadalafil (Cialis)

Vardenafil (Levitra)
Yohimbine (Yocon, Yohimex)

Urolithiasis

Potassium Citrate (Urocit-K)
Potassium Citrate & Citric Acid (Polycitra-K)

Sodium Citrate/Citric Acid (Bicitra, Oracit)

Trimethoprim (Trimpex, Proloprim)

Miscellaneous Urology Agents

Ammonium
  Aluminum Sulfate
  [Alum]
Dimethyl Sulfoxide
  [DMSO] (Rimso-50)

Neomycin-
  Polymyxin Bladder
  Irrigant
  [Neosporin GU
  Irrigant]

Nitrofurantoin
  (Macrodantin,
  Furadantin, Macrobid)
Pentosan Polysulfate
  (Elmiron)

WOUND CARE

Becaplermin
  (Regranex Gel)

Silver Nitrate
  (Dey-Drop)

MISCELLANEOUS THERAPEUTIC AGENTS

Acamprosate (Campral)
Alglucosidase Alfa
  (Myozyme)
Cilostazol (Pletal)
Drotrecogin Alfa
  (Xigris)
Eculizumab (Soliris)
Megestrol Acetate
  (Megace, Megace-ES)
Mecasermin (Increlex,
  Iplex)
Lanthanum Carbonate
  (Fosrenol)

Naltrexone (Depade,
  ReVia, Vivitrol)
Nicotine Gum
  (Nicorette, others)
Nicotine Nasal Spray
  (Nicotrol NS)
Nicotine Transdermal
  (Habitrol, Nicoderm
  CQ [OTC], others)
Palifermin (Kepivance)
Potassium Iodide [Lugol
  Solution] (SSKI,
  Thyro-Block)

Sevelamer HCl
  (Renagel)
Sevelamer carbonate
  (Renvela)
Sodium Polystyrene
  Sulfonate
  (Kayexalate)
Talc (Sterile Talc
  Powder)
Varenicline (Chantix)

NATURAL AND HERBAL AGENTS

Black Cohosh
Chamomile
Cranberry (Vaccinium
  macrocarpon)
Dong Quai (Angelica
  polymorpha, sinensis)
Echinacea (Echinacea
  purpurea)
Ephedra/Ma Huang
Evening Primrose Oil
Fish Oil
Garlic (Allium sativum)

Ginger (Zingiber
  officinale)
Ginkgo Biloba
Ginseng
Glucosamine Sulfate
  (Chitosamine) &
  Chondroitin Sulfate
Kava Kava
  (Kava Kava Root
  Extract, Piper
  methysticum)
Melatonin

Milk Thistle (Silybum
  marianum)
Saw Palmetto (Serenoa
  repens)
St. John's Wort
  (Hypericum
  perforatum)
Valerian (Valeriana
  officinalis)
Yohimbine
  (Pausinystalia
  yohimbe)

GENERIC AND SELECTED BRAND DRUG DATA

Abacavir (Ziagen) **WARNING:** Allergy (fever, rash, fatigue, GI, resp) reported; stop drug immediately & do not rechallenge; lactic acidosis & hepatomegaly/steatosis reported **Uses:** *HIV Infxn* **Action:** NRTI **Dose:** *Adults.* 300 mg PO bid or 600 mg PO daily *Peds.* 8 mg/kg bid/300 mg bid max **Caution:** [C, –] CDC recommends HIV-infected mothers not breast-feed (transmission risk) **Disp:** Tabs 300 mg; soln 20 mg/mL **SE:** See Warning, ↑ LFTs, fat redistribution **Notes:** Many drug interactions; HLA-B*5701 at ↑ risk for fatal hypersensitivity Rxn, genetic screen before use

Abatacept (Orencia) **Uses:** *Mod/severe RA w/ inadequate response to one or more DMARDs, juvenile idiopathic arthritis* **Action:** Selective costimulation modulator, ↓ T-cell activation **Dose:** *Adults.* Initial 500 mg (<60 kg), 750 mg (60–100 kg); 1 g (>100 kg) IV over 30 min; repeat at 2 and 4 wk, then Q 4 wk *Peds 6–17 y:* 10 mg/kg (<75 kg), 750 mg (75–100 kg), IV × 1 wk 0, 2, 4, then q4wk (>100 kg, adult dose) **Caution:** [C; ?/–] w/ TNF blockers; COPD; Hx recurrent/localized/chronic/predisposition to Infxn; w/ immunosuppressants **CI:** w/ live vaccines w/in 3 mo of D/C abatacept **Disp:** IV powder: 250 mg/10 mL **SE:** HA, URI, N, nasopharyngitis, Infxn, malignancy, Inf Rxns/hypersensitivity (dizziness, HA, HTN), COPD exacerbations, cough, dyspnea **Notes:** Screen for TB prior to use

Abciximab (ReoPro) **Uses:** *Prevent acute ischemic comps in PTCA,* MI **Action:** ↓ plt aggregation (glycoprotein IIb/IIIa inhibitor) **Dose:** *Unstable angina w/ planned PCI w/in 24 h of dose (ECC 2005):* 0.25 mg/kg bolus, then 10 mcg/min cont Inf × 18–24 h, stop 1 h after PCI; *PCI:* 0.25 mg/kg bolus 10–60 min pre-PTCA, then 0.125 mcg/kg/min (max = 10 mcg/min) cont inf for 12 h; **Caution:** [C, ?/–] **CI:** Active/recent (w/in 6 wk) internal hemorrhage, CVA w/in 2 y or CVA w/ sig neuro deficit, bleeding diathesis or PO anticoagulants w/in 7 d (unless PT <1.2 × control), ↓ plt (<100,000 cells/mcL), recent trauma or major surgery (w/in 6 wk), CNS tumor, AVM, aneurysm, severe uncontrolled HTN, vasculitis, use of dextran prior to or during PTCA, allergy to murine proteins, w/ other glycoprotein IIb/IIIa inhibitors **Disp:** Inj 2 mg/mL **SE:** ↓ BP, CP, allergic Rxns, bleeding, ↓ plt **Notes:** Use w/ heparin/ASA

Acamprosate (Campral) **Uses:** *Maintain abstinence from EtOH* **Action:** ↓ Glutamatergic transmission; modulates neuronal hyperexcitability; related to GABA **Dose:** 666 mg PO tid; CrCl 30–50 mL/min: 333 mg PO tid **Caution:** [C; ?/–] **CI:** CrCl <30 mL/min **Disp:** Tabs 333 mg EC **SE:** N/D, depression, anxiety, insomnia **Notes:** Does not eliminate EtOH withdrawal Sx; continue even if relapse occurs

Acarbose (Precose) Uses: *Type 2 DM* Action: α-Glucosidase inhibitor; delays carbohydrates digestion to ↓ glucose Dose: 25–100 mg PO tid w/ 1st bite each meal; 50 mg tid (<60 kg); 100 mg tid (>60 kg); usual maint 50–100 mg PO tid Caution: [B, ?] w/ CrCl <25 mL/min; can affect digoxin levels CI: IBD, colonic ulceration, partial intestinal obst; cirrhosis Disp: Tabs 25, 50, 100 mg SE: Abd pain, D, flatulence, ↑ LFTs, hypersensitivity Rxn Notes: OK w/ sulfonylureas; ✓ LFTs q3mo for 1st y

Acebutolol (Sectral) Uses: *HTN, arrhythmias* chronic stable angina Action: Blocks β-adrenergic receptors, β₁, & ISA Dose: HTN: 400–800 mg/d 2 ÷ doses; arrhythmia: 400–1200 mg/d 2 ÷ doses; ↓ if CrCl <50 mL/min or elderly; elderly initial 200–400 mg/d; max 800 mg/d Caution: [B, D in 2nd & 3rd tri, +] Can exacerbate ischemic heart Dz, do not D/C abruptly CI: 2nd-, 3rd-degree heart block Disp: Caps 200, 400 mg SE: Fatigue, HA, dizziness, bradycardia

Acetaminophen [APAP, N-acetyl-p-aminophenol] (Tylenol, other generic) [OTC] Uses: *Mild-mod pain, HA, fever* Action: Nonnarcotic analgesic; ↓ CNS synth of prostaglandins & hypothalamic heat-regulating center Dose: *Adults.* 650 mg PO or PR q4–6h or 1000 mg PO q6h; max 4 g/24 h. *Peds* <12 y: 10–15 mg/kg/dose PO or PR q4–6h; max 2.6 g/24 h. Quick dosing Table 1 Page 248. Administer q6h if CrCl 10–50 mL/min & q8h if CrCl <10 mL/min Caution: [B, +] Hepatotoxic in elderly & w/ EtOH use w/ >4 g/d; EtOH liver Dz, G6PD deficiency CI: Hypersensitivity Disp: Tabs melt away/dissolving 160 mg; Tabs: 325, 500, 650 mg; chew tabs 80, 160 mg; liq 100 mg/2.5 mL, 120 mg/2.5 mL, 120 mg/5 mL, 160 mg/5 mL, 167 mg/5 mL, 325 mg/5 mL, 500 mg/15 mL, 80 mg/0.8 mL; supp 80, 120, 125, 325, 650 mg SE: OD hepatotoxic at 10 g; 15 g can be lethal; Rx w/ N-acetylcysteine Notes: No anti-inflammatory or plt-inhibiting action; avoid EtOH

Acetaminophen + Butalbital ± Caffeine (Fioricet, Medigesic, Repan, Sedapap-10, Two-Dyne, Triapin, Axocet, Phrenilin Forte) [C-III] Uses: *Tension HA,* mild pain Action: Nonnarcotic analgesic w/ barbiturate Dose: 1–2 tabs or caps PO q4–6h PRN; ↓ in renal/hepatic impair; 4 g/24 h APAP max Caution: [C, D, +] Alcoholic liver Dz, G6PD deficiency CI: Hypersensitivity Disp: Caps *Dolgic Plus:* butalbital 50 mg, caffeine 40 mg, APAP 750 mg; Caps *Medigesic, Repan, Two-Dyne:* butalbital 50 mg, caffeine 40 mg, + APAP 325 mg; Caps *Axocet, Phrenilin Forte:* butalbital 50 mg + APAP 650 mg; Caps: *Esgic-Plus, Zebutal:* butalbital 50 mg, caffeine 40 mg, APAP 500 mg; Liq. *Dolgic LQ:* butalbital 50 mg, caffeine 40 mg, APAP 325 mg/15 mL. Tabs *Medigesic, Fioricet, Repan:* butalbital 50 mg, caffeine 40 mg, APAP 325 mg; *Phrenilin:* butalbital 50 mg + APAP 325 mg; *Sedapap-10:* butalbital 50 mg + APAP 650 mg SE: Drowsiness, dizziness, "hangover" effect, N/V Notes: Butalbital habit forming; avoid EtOH

Acetaminophen + Codeine (Tylenol No. 2, 3, No. 4) [C-III, C-V] Uses: *Mild-mod pain (No.2–3); mod–severe pain (No. 4)* Action: Combined

APAP & narcotic analgesic **Dose: *Adults.*** 1–2 tabs q3–4h PRN or 30–60 mg/ codeine q4–6h based on codeine content (max dose APAP = 4 g/d). ***Peds.*** APAP 10–15 mg/dose; codeine 0.5–1 mg/kg dose q4–6h (guide: 3–6 y, 5 mL/dose; 7–12 y, 10 mL/dose) max 2.6 g/d if <12 y; ↓ in renal/hepatic impair **Caution:** [C, +] Alcoholic liver Dz; G6PD deficiency **CI:** Hypersensitivity **Disp:** Tabs 300 mg APAP + codeine(No. 2 = 15 mg, No. 3 = 30 mg, No. 4 = 60 mg); caps 325 mg APAP + codeine; susp (C-V) APAP 120 mg + codeine 12 mg/5 mL **SE:** Drowsiness, dizziness, N/V

Acetazolamide (Diamox)
Uses: *Diuresis, drug and CHF edema, glaucoma, prevent high-altitude sickness, refractory epilepsy* metabolic alkalosis **Action:** Carbonic anhydrase inhibitor; ↓ renal excretion of hydrogen & ↑ renal excretion of Na^+, K^+, HCO_3^-, & H_2O **Dose: *Adults.*** *Diuretic:* 250–375 mg IV or PO q24h in ÷ doses. *Epilepsy:* 8–30 mg/kg PO q24h in ÷ doses. *Altitude sickness:* 250 mg PO q8–12h or SR 500 mg PO q12–24h start 24–48 h before & 48 h after highest ascent. Metabolic alkalosis 250 mg IV q6h × 4 or 500 mg IV × 1 ***Peds.*** *Epilepsy:* 8–30 mg/kg/24 h PO in ÷ doses; max 1 g/d. Diuretic: 5 mg/kg/24 h PO or IV. *Alkalinization of urine:* 5 mg/kg/dose PO bid-tid. *Glaucoma:* 8–30 mg/kg/24 h PO in 3 ÷ doses; max 1 g/d; ↓ dose w/ CrCl 10–50 mL/min; avoid if CrCl <10 mL/min **Caution:** [C, +] **CI:** Renal/hepatic/ adrenal failure, sulfa allergy, hyperchloremic acidosis **Disp:** Tabs 125, 250 mg; ER caps 500 mg; Inj 500 mg/vial, powder for recons **SE:** Malaise, metallic taste, drowsiness, photosensitivity, hyperglycemia **Notes:** Follow Na^+ & K^+; watch for metabolic acidosis; ✓ CBC & plts; SR forms not for epilepsy

Acetic Acid & Aluminum Acetate (Otic Domeboro)
Uses: *Otitis externa* **Action:** Anti-infective **Dose:** 4–6 gtt in ear(s) q2–3h **Caution:** [C, ?] **CI:** Perforated tympanic membranes **Disp:** 2% otic soln **SE:** Local irritation

Acetylcysteine (Acetadote, Mucomyst)
Uses: *Mucolytic, antidote to APAP hepatotox/OD* adjuvant Rx chronic bronchopulmonary Dzs & CF* prevent contrast-induced renal dysfunction **Action:** Splits mucoprotein disulfide linkages; restores glutathione in APAP OD to protect liver **Dose: *Adults & Peds.*** *Nebulizer:* 3–5 mL of 20% soln diluted w/ equal vol of H_2O or NS tid-qid. *Antidote:* PO or NG: 140 mg/kg load, then 70 mg/kg q4h × 17 doses (dilute 1:3 in carbonated beverage or OJ), repeat if emesis w/in 1 h of dosing *Acetadote:* 150 mg/kg IV over 60 min, then 50 mg/kg over 4 h, then 100 mg/kg over 16 h; Prevent renal dysfunction: 600–1200 mg PO bid × 2 d **Disp:** Soln, inhaled and oral 10%, 20%; Acetadote IV soln 20% **SE:** Bronchospasm (inhaled), N/V, drowsiness, anaphylactoid Rxns w/ IV **Notes:** Activated charcoal adsorbs PO acetylcysteine for APAP ingestion; start Rx for APAP OD w/in 6–8 h

Acitretin (Soriatane)
WARNING: Must not be used by females who are pregnant or who intend to become pregnant during or for 3 y following D/C of therapy; EtOH must not be ingested during or for 2 mo following cessation; do not donate blood for 3 y following cessation; Hepatotoxic **Uses:** *Severe psoriasis*;

other keratinization disorders (lichen planus, etc) **Action:** Retinoid-like activity **Dose:** 25–50 mg/d PO, w/ main meal; ↑ if no response by 4 wk to 75 mg/d **Caution:** [X, –] Renal/hepatic impair; in women of reproductive potential **CI:** See Warning; ↑ serum lipids; w/ MTX or tetracyclines **Disp:** Caps 10, 25 mg **SE:** Hyperesthesia, cheilitis, skin peeling, alopecia, pruritus, rash, arthralgia, GI upset, photosensitivity, thrombocytopenia, hypertriglyceridemia, ↑ Na, K, PO_4^- **Notes:** Follow LFTs, lytes, lipids; response takes up to 2–3 mo; informed consent prior to use; FDA guide w/ each Rx

Acyclovir (Zovirax)
Uses: *Herpes simplex(HSV)(genital/mucocutaneous), encephalitis, keratitis), Varicella zoster, Herpes zoster (shingles) Infxns* **Action:** Interferes w/ viral DNA synth **Dose:** *Adults.* Dose on IBW if obese >125% IBW PO: *Initial genital HSV:* 200 mg PO q4h while awake (5 caps/d) × 10 d or 400 mg PO tid × 7–10 d. *Chronic HSV suppression:* 400 mg PO bid. *Intermittent HSV Rx:* As initial Rx, except Rx for 5 d, or 800 mg PO bid, at prodrome. *Topical: Initial herpes genitalis:* Apply q3h (6×/d) for 7 d. *HSV encephalitis:* 10 mg/kg IV q8h × 10 d. *Herpes zoster:* 800 mg PO 5×/d for 7–10 d. *IV:* 5–10 mg/kg/dose IV q8h. *Peds. Genital HSV:* **3 mo–2 y:** 15 mg/kg/d IV ÷ q8h × 5–7 d, 60 mg/kg/d max. **2–12 y:** 1200 mg/d PO ÷ q8h × 7–10 d. **>12 y:** 1000–1200 mg PO ÷ q8h × 7–10 d. *HSV encephalitis:* **3 mo–2 12 y:** 60 mg/kg IV q8h × 10 d. **>12 y:** 30 mg/kg/d IV ÷ q8h × 10 d. *Chickenpox:* **≥2 y:** 20 mg/kg/dose PO qid × 5 d. *Shingles:* **<12 y:** 30 mg/kg/d PO or 1500 mg/ m²/d IV ÷ q8h × 7–10 d; ↓ w/ CrCl <50 mL/min **Caution:** [B, +] **CI:** Hypersensitivity to compound **Disp:** Caps 200 mg; tabs 400, 800 mg; susp 200 mg/5 mL; Inj 500 & 1000 mg/vial; Inj soln 25 mg/mL, 50 mg/mL oint 5% and cream 5% **SE:** Dizziness, lethargy, malaise, confusion, rash, IV site inflammation; transient ↑ Cr/BUN **Notes:** PO better than topical for herpes genitalis

Adalimumab (Humira)
WARNING: Cases of TB have been observed; ✓ TB skin test prior to use; Hep B reactivation possible, invasive fungal and other opportunistic Infxns reported; malignancies in children and young adults reported **Uses:** *Mod–severe RA w/ an inadequate response to one or more DMARDs, psoriatic arthritis (PA), juvenile idiopathic arthritis (JIA), plaque psoriasis, ankylosing spondylitis (AS), Crohn Dz* **Action:** TNF-α inhibitor **Dose:** *RA, PA, AS:* 40 mg SQ qOwk; may ↑ 40 mg qwk if not on MTX. *JIA* 15–30 kg 20 mg QOW. *Chron Dz:* 160 mg d 1, 80 mg 2 wk later, then 2 wk later start maint 40 mg q other wk **Caution:** [B, ?/–] See Warnings do not use w/ live vaccines **CI:** none **Disp:** Prefilled 0.4 mL (20 mg) & 0.8 mL (40 mg) syringe **SE:** Inj site Rxns, anaphylaxis, cytopenias demyelinating Dz **Notes:** Refrigerate prefilled syringe, rotate Inj sites, OK w/ other DMARDs

Adefovir (Hepsera)
WARNING: Acute exacerbations of hep seen after d/c therapy (monitor LFTs); nephrotoxic w/ underlying renal impair w/ chronic use (monitor renal Fxn); HIV resistance/untreated may emerge; lactic acidosis & severe hepatomegaly w/ steatosis reported **Uses:** *Chronic active hep B* **Action:** Nucleotide analog **Dose:** CrCl >50 mL/min: 10 mg PO daily; CrCl 20–49 mL/min:

10 mg PO q48h; CrCl 10–19 mL/min: 10 mg PO q72h; HD: 10 mg PO q7d post-dialysis; adjust w/ CrCl <50 mL/min **Caution:** [C, –] **Disp:** Tabs 10 mg **SE:** Asthenia, HA, Abd pain; see Warning **Notes:** ✓ HIV status before using

Adenosine (Adenocard) **Uses:** *PSVT*; including w/ WPW **Action:** Class IV antiarrhythmic; slows AV node conduction **Dose:** *Adults.* 6 mg over 1–3 s, then 20 mL NS bolus, elevate extremity; repeat 12 mg in 1–2 min PRN, max single dose 12 mg (*ECC 2005*) *Peds <50 kg:* 0.05–0.1 mg/kg IV bolus; may repeat q1–2min to 0.3 mg/kg max **Caution:** [C, ?] Hx bronchospasm **CI:** 2nd-3rd-degree AV block or SSS (w/o pacemaker); A flutter, A fibrillation, V tachycardia, recent MI or CNS bleed **Disp:** Inj 3 mg/mL **SE:** Facial flushing, HA, dyspnea, chest pressure, ↓ BP **Notes:** Doses >12 mg not OK; can cause momentary asystole with use; caffeine, theophylline antagonize effects

Albumin (Albuminar, Buminate, Albutein) **Uses:** *Plasma vol expansion for shock* (eg, burns, hemorrhage) **Action:** Maintain plasma colloid oncotic pressure **Dose:** *Adults.* Initial 25 g IV; then based on response; 250 g/48 h max. *Peds.* 0.5–1 g/kg dose; Inf at 0.05–0.1 g/min; max 6 g/kg/d **Caution:** [C, ?] Severe anemia; cardiac, renal, or hepatic Insuff due to protein load & hypervolemia **CI:** CHF, severe anemia **Disp:** Soln 5%, 25% **SE:** Chills, fever, CHF, tachycardia, ↓ BP, hypervolemia **Notes:** Contains 130–160 mEq Na$^+$/L; may cause pulm edema

Albuterol (Proventil, Ventolin, Volmax) **Uses:** *Asthma, COPD, prevent exercise-induced bronchospasm* **Action:** β-Adrenergic sympathomimetic bronchodilator; relaxes bronchial smooth muscle **Dose:** *Adults. Inhaler:* 2 Inh q4–6h PRN; 1 Rotacaps inhaled q4–6h. *PO:* 2–4 mg PO tid-qid. *Nebulizer:* 1.25–5 mg (0.25–1 mL of a 0.5% soln in 2–3 mL of NS) tid-qid. *Prevent exercise-induced asthma:* 2 puffs 5–30 min prior to activity *Peds. Inhaler:* 2 Inh q4–6h. *PO:* 0.1–0.2 mg/kg/dose PO; max 2–4 mg PO tid; *Nebulizer:* 0.05 mg/kg (max 2.5 mg) in 2–3 mL of NS tid-qid. 2–6 y 12 mg/d max, 6–12 y 24 mg/d max **Caution:** [C, +] **Disp:** Tabs 2, 4 mg; XR tabs 4, 8 mg; syrup 2 mg/5 mL; 90 mcg/dose metered-dose inhaler; soln for nebulizer 0.083, 0.5% **SE:** Palpitations, tachycardia, nervousness, GI upset

Albuterol & Ipratropium (Combivent, DuoNeb) **Uses:** *COPD* **Action:** Combo of β-adrenergic bronchodilator & quaternary anticholinergic **Dose:** 2 Inh qid; nebulizer 3 mL q 6 h; max 12 Inh/24h or 3 mL q4h **Caution:** [C, +] **CI:** Peanut/soybean allergy **Disp:** Metered-dose inhaler, 18 mcg ipratropium & 103 mcg albuterol/puff; nebulization soln (DuoNeb) ipratropium 0.5 mg & albuterol 2.5 mg/3 mL 0.042%, 0.21% **SE:** Palpitations, tachycardia, nervousness, GI upset, dizziness, blurred vision

Aldesleukin [IL-2] (Proleukin) **WARNING:** High dose associated w/ capillary leak syndrome w/ hypotension and ↓ organ perfusion; ↑ Ifxn due to poor neutrophil activity; D/C w/ mod–severe lethargy, may progress to coma **Uses:** *Met RCC & melanoma* **Action:** Acts via IL-2 receptor; many immunomodulatory effects **Dose:** 600,000 Int Units/kg q8h × 14 doses days 1–5 and days 15–19 of 28-d cycle (FDA-approved dose/schedule for RCC); other schedules (eg, "high dose" 24 × 10^6 Int Units/m² IV q8h on days 1–5 & 12–16) **Caution:** [C, ?/–] **CI:** Organ allografts **Disp:** Powder for recons 22 × 10^6 Int Units, when reconstituted 18 million Int Units/mL = 1.1 mg/mL **SE:** Flu-like syndromes (malaise, fever, chills), N/V/D, ↑ bilirubin; capillary leak syndrome; ↓ BP, tachycardia, pulm & peripheral edema, fluid retention, & wgt gain; renal & mild hematologic tox (↓ HgB, plt, WBC), eosinophilia; cardiac tox (ischemia, atrial arrhythmias); neuro tox (CNS depression, somnolence, delirium, rare coma); pruritic rashes, urticaria, & erythroderma common.

Alefacept (Amevive) WARNING: Monitor CD4 before each dose; w/hold if <250; D/C if <250 × 1 mo **Uses:** *Mod/severe chronic plaque psoriasis* **Action:** Fusion protein inhibitor **Dose:** 7.5 mg IV or 15 mg IM once/wk × 12 wk **Caution:** [B, ?/–] PRG registry; associated w/ serious Infxn **CI:** Lymphopenia, HIV **Disp:** 15-mg powder for recons **SE:** Pharyngitis, myalgia, Inj site Rxn, malignancy, Infxn **Notes:** IV or IM different formulations; may repeat course 12 wk later if CD4 OK

Alendronate (Fosamax, Fosamax Plus D) **Uses:** *Rx & prevent osteoporosis male & postmenopausal female, Rx steroid-induced osteoporosis, Paget Dz* **Action:** ↓ nl & abnormal bone resorption, ↓ osteoclast action **Dose:** *Osteoporosis:* Rx: 10 mg/d PO or 70 mg qwk; Fosamax plus D tab qwk. *Steroid-induced osteoporosis:* Rx: 5 mg/d PO, 10 mg/d postmenopausal not on estrogen. *Prevention:* 5 mg/d PO or 35 mg qwk. *Paget Dz:* 40 mg/d PO **Caution:** [C, ?] Not OK if CrCl <35 mL/min, w/ NSAID use **CI:** Esophageal anomalies, inability to sit/stand upright for 30 min, ↓ Ca^{2+} **Disp:** Tabs 5, 10, 35, 40, 70 mg, soln 70 mg/ 75 mL, Fosamax plus D: Alendronate 70 mg w/ cholecalciferol (vit D_3) 2800 or 5600 Int Units **SE:** Abd pain, acid regurgitation, constipation, D/N, dyspepsia, musculoskeletal pain, jaw osteonecrosis (w/ dental procedures, chemo) **Notes:** Take 1st thing in A.M. w/ H_2O (8 oz) >30 min before 1st food/beverage of the day; do not lie down for 30 min after. Ca^{2+} & vit D supl necessary for regular tab

Alfentanil (Alfenta) [C-II] **Uses:** *Adjunct in maint of anesthesia; analgesia* **Action:** Short-acting narcotic analgesic **Dose:** *Adults & Peds >12 y:* 75 mcg/kg (IBW) IV Inf; total depends on duration of procedure **Caution:** [C, +/–] ↑ ICP, resp depression **Disp:** Inj 500 mcg/mL **SE:** Bradycardia, ↓ BP arrhythmias, peripheral vasodilation, ↑ ICP, drowsiness, resp depression, N/V/constipation

Alfuzosin (Uroxatral) WARNING: May prolong QTc interval **Uses:** *symptomatic BPH* **Action:** α-Blocker **Dose:** 10 mg PO daily immediately after the same meal **Caution:** [B, –] **CI:** w/ CYP3A4 inhibitors; mod–severe hepatic impair **Disp:** Tabs 10 mg ER **SE:** Postural ↓ BP, dizziness, HA, fatigue **Notes:** Do not cut or crush; ↓ ejaculatory disorders compared w/ similar drugs

Alginic Acid + Aluminum Hydroxide & Magnesium Trisilicate (Gaviscon) [OTC] **Uses:** *Heartburn*; hiatal hernia pain **Action:** Protective layer blocks gastric acid **Dose:** Chew 2–4 tabs or 15–30 mL PO qid followed by H_2O; **Caution:** [B, –] Avoid in renal impair or Na^+-restricted diet **Disp:** Chew tabs, susp **SE:** D, constipation

Alglucosidase alfa (Myozyme) **WARNING:** Life-threatening anaphylactic Rxns seen w/ Inf; medical support measures should be immediately available **Uses:** *Rx Pompe DZ* **Action:** Recombinant acid α-glucosidase; degrades glycogen in lysosomes **Dose:** *Peds 1 mo–3.5 y* 20 mg/kg IV q 2 wk over 4 h (see insert) **Caution:** [B, ?/–] Illness at time of Inf may ↑ Inf Rxns **CI:** None **Disp:** Powder 50 mg/vial **SE:** Hypersensitivity, fever, rash, D,V, gastroenteritis, pneumonia, URI, cough, resp distress/failure, Infxns, cardiac arrhythmia w/ general anesthesia, tachy/bradycardia, flushing, anemia

Aliskiren (Tekturna) **WARNING:** May cause injury and death to a developing fetus; D/C immediately when PRG detected **Uses:** *HTN* **Action:** 1st direct renin inhibitor **Dose:** 150–300 mg/d PO **Caution:** [C (1st tri), D (2nd & 3rd tri); ?]; Avoid w/ CrCl <30 mL/min; ketoconazole and other CYP3A4 inhibitors may ↑ aliskiren levels **CI:** Anuria, sulfur sensitivity **Disp:** Tabs 150, 300 mg **SE:** D, Abd pain, dyspepsia, GERD, cough, ↑ K^+, angioedema, ↓ BP, dizziness

Aliskiren/Hydrochlorothiazide (Tekturna HCT) **WARNING:** May cause injury and death to a developing fetus; D/C immediately when PRG detected **Uses:** *HTN, not primary Rx* **Action:** Renin inhibitor w/ diuretic **Dose:** Monotherapy failure: 150 mg/12.5 mg PO q d; may ↑ to 150 mg/25 mg, 300 mg/12.5 mg q d after 2–4 wk; max: 300 mg/25 mg **Caution:** [D, ?] Avoid w/ CrCl ≤30 mL/min; avoid w/ lithium, ketoconazole, and other CYP3A4 inhibitors may ↑ aliskiren levels **Disp:** Tab: aliskiren mg/HCTZ mg: 150/12.5, 150/25, 300/12.5, 300/25 **SE:** Dizziness, influenza, D, cough, vertigo, asthenia, arthralgia, angioedema

Allopurinol (Zyloprim, Lopurin, Aloprim) **Uses:** *Gout, hyperuricemia of malignancy, uric acid urolithiasis* **Action:** Xanthine oxidase inhibitor; ↓ uric acid production **Dose:** *Adults.* PO: Initial 100 mg/d; usual 300 mg/d; max 800 mg/d; ÷ dose if >300 mg/d IV: 200–400 mg/m^2/d (max 600 mg/24 h); (after meal w/ plenty of fluid). *Peds.* Only for hyperuricemia of malignancy if <10 y: 10 mg/kg/24 h PO or 200 mg/m^2/d IV ÷ q6–8h; max 600 mg/24 h; ↓ in renal impair **Caution:** [C, M] **Disp:** Tabs 100, 300, Inj 500 mg/30 mL (Aloprim) **SE:** Rash, N/V, renal impair, angioedema **Notes:** Aggravates acute gout; begin after acute attack resolves; IV dose of 6 mg/mL final conc as single daily Inf or ÷ 6-, 8-, or 12-h intervals

Almotriptan (Axert) **Uses:** *Rx acute migraine* **Action:** Vascular serotonin receptor agonist **Dose:** *Adults.* PO: 6.25–12 mg PO, repeat in 2 h PRN; 2 dose/24 h max PO dose; max 12 or 24 mg/d; w/ hepatic/renal impair 6.25 mg single dose (max 12.5 mg/d) **Caution:** [C, ?/–] **CI:** Angina, ischemic heart Dz, coronary artery vasospasm, hemiplegic or basilar migraine, uncontrolled HTN, ergot use, MAOI use w/in 14 d **Disp:** Tabs 6.25, 12.5 mg **SE:** N, somnolence, paresthesias, HA, dry mouth, weakness, numbness, coronary vasospasm, HTN

Alosetron (Lotronex)   **WARNING:** Serious GI side effects, some fatal, including ischemic colitis reported. Prescribed only through participation in the prescribing program **Uses:** *Severe D—predominant IBS in women who fail conventional therapy* **Action:** Selective 5-HT$_3$ receptor antagonist **Dose:** *Adults.* 0.5 mg PO bid; ↑ to 1 mg bid max after 4 wk; D/C after 8 wk not controlled **Caution:** [B, ?/–] **CI:** Hx chronic/severe constipation, GI obst, strictures, toxic megacolon, GI perforation, adhesions, ischemic/ulcerative colitis, Crohn Dz, diverticulitis, thrombophlebitis, hypercoagulability **Disp:** Tabs 0.5, 1 mg **SE:** Constipation, Abd pain, N **Notes:** D/C immediately if constipation or Sxs of ischemic colitis develop; pt must sign informed consent prior to use "patient-physician agreement"

Alpha$_1$-Protease Inhibitor (Prolastin)   **Uses:** *α_1-Antitrypsin deficiency*; panacinar emphysema **Action:** Replace human α_1-protease inhibitor **Dose:** 60 mg/kg IV once/wk **Caution:** [C, ?] **CI:** Selective IgA deficiencies w/ known IgA antibodies **Disp:** Inj 500 mg/20 mL, 1000 mg/40 mL powder for Inj **SE:** HA, MS discomfort, fever, dizziness, flu-like Sxs, allergic Rxns, ↑ AST/ALT

Alprazolam (Xanax, Niravam) [C-IV]   **Uses:** *Anxiety & panic disorders,* anxiety w/ depression **Action:** Benzodiazepine; antianxiety agent **Dose:** *Anxiety:* Initial, 0.25–0.5 mg tid; ↑ to 4 mg/d max ÷ doses. *Panic:* Initial, 0.5 mg tid; may gradually ↑ to response; ↓ in elderly, debilitated, & hepatic impair **Caution:** [D, –] **CI:** NAG, concomitant itra-/ketoconazole **Disp:** Tabs 0.25, 0.5, 1, 2 mg; Xanax XR 0.5, 1, 2, 3 mg; Niravam (orally disintegrating tablets) 0.25, 0.5, 1, 2 mg; soln 1 mg/mL **SE:** Drowsiness, fatigue, irritability, memory impair, sexual dysfunction, paradoxical Rxns **Notes:** Avoid abrupt D/C after prolonged use

Alprostadil [Prostaglandin E$_1$] (Prostin VR)   **WARNING:** Apnea in up to 12% of neonates especially <2 kg at birth **Uses:** *Conditions ductus arteriosus blood flow must be maintained* sustain pulm/systemic circulation until OR (eg, pulm atresia/stenosis, transposition) **Action:** Vasodilator (ductus arteriosus very sensitive), plt inhibitor **Dose:** 0.05 mcg/kg/min IV; ↓ to lowest that maintains response **Caution:** [X, –] **CI:** Neonatal resp distress syndrome **Disp:** Inj 500 mcg/mL **SE:** Cutaneous vasodilation, Sz-like activity, jitteriness, ↑ temp, ↓ Ca^{2+}, thrombocytopenia, ↓ BP; may cause apnea **Notes:** Keep intubation kit at bedside

Alprostadil, Intracavernosal (Caverject, Edex)   **Uses:** *Erectile dysfunction* **Action:** Relaxes smooth muscles, dilates cavernosal arteries, ↑ lacunar spaces w/ blood entrapment **Dose:** 2.5–60 mcg intracavernosal; titrate in office **Caution:** [X, –] **CI:** ↑ risk of priapism (eg, sickle cell); penile deformities/implants; men in whom sexual activity inadvisable **Disp:** *Caverject:* 5-, 10-, 20-, 40-mcg powder for Inj vials ± diluent syringes 10-, 20-, 40-mcg amp. *Caverject Impulse:* Self-contained syringe (29 gauge) 10 & 20 mcg. *Edex:* 10-, 20-, 40-mcg cartridges **SE:** Local pain w/ Inj **Notes:** Counsel about priapism, penile fibrosis, & hematoma risks, titrate dose in office

Alprostadil, Urethral Suppository (Muse)   **Uses:** *Erectile dysfunction* **Action:** Urethral absorption; vasodilator, relaxes smooth muscle of corpus cavernosa **Dose:** 125–1000-mcg system 5–10 min prior to sex; repeat × 1/24 h; titrate in office **Caution:** [X, –] **CI:** ↑ priapism risk (especially sickle cell, myeloma, leukemia) penile deformities/implants; men in whom sex inadvisable **Disp:** 125, 250, 500, 1000 mcg w/ transurethral system **SE:** ↓ BP, dizziness, syncope, penile/testicular pain, urethral burning/bleeding, priapism **Notes:** Titrate dose in office; duration 30–60 min

Alteplase, Recombinant [tPA] (Activase) **Uses:** *AMI, PE, acute ischemic stroke, & CV cath occlusion* **Action:** Thrombolytic; binds fibrin in thrombus, initiates fibrinolysis **Dose:** *AMI:* 15 mg IV over 1–2 min, then 0.75 mg/kg (max 50 mg) over 30 min, then 0.5 mg/kg over next 60 min (max 35 mg)(*ECC 2005) Stroke:* w/in 3 h of onset $S \times s$: 0.09 mg/kg IV over 1 min, then 0.81 mg/kg; max 90 mg/h Inf over 60 min (*ECC 2005) Cath occlusion:* 10–29 kg 1 mg/mL; ≥30 kg 2 mg/mL **Caution:** [C, ?] **CI:** Active internal bleeding; uncontrolled HTN (SBP = >185 mm Hg/DBP = >110 mm Hg); recent (w/in 3 mo) CVA, GI bleed, trauma; intracranial or intraspinal surgery or Dzs (AVM/aneurysm/subarachnoid hemorrhage); prolonged cardiac massage; intracranial neoplasm, suspected aortic dissection, w/ anticoagulants or INR >1.7, heparin w/in 48 h, plts <100K, Sz at the time of stroke **Disp:** Powder for Inj 2, 50, 100 mg **SE:** Bleeding, bruising (eg, venipuncture sites), ↓ BP **Notes:** Give heparin to prevent reocclusion; in AMI, doses of >150 mg associated w/ intracranial bleeding

Altretamine (Hexalen) **WARNING:** Bone marrow suppression, neurotox common **Uses:** *Epithelial ovarian CA* **Action:** Unknown; cytotoxic agent, unknown alkylating agent; ↓ nucleotide incorporation into DNA/RNA **Dose:** 260 mg/m^2/d in 4 ÷ doses for 14–21 d of a 28-d Rx cycle; dose ↑ to 150 mg/m^2/d for 14 d in multiagent regimens (per protocols); after meals and hs **Caution:** [D, ?/–] **CI:** Preexisting BM depression or neurologic tox **Disp:** Gel caps 50 mg **SE:** N/V/D, cramps; neurotox (neuropathy, CNS depression); minimal myelosuppression **Notes:** ✓ CBC, routine neurologic exams

Aluminum Hydroxide (Amphojel, AlternaGEL, Dermagran) [OTC] **Uses:** *Relief of heartburn, upset or sour stomach, or acid indigestion*; supl to Rx of hyperphosphatemia; *minor cuts, burns (Dermagran)* **Action:** Neutralizes gastric acid; binds PO$_4^{-2}$ **Dose:** *Adults.* 10–30 mL or 300–1200 mg PO q4–6h. *Peds.* 5–15 mL PO q4–6h or 50–150 mg/kg/24 h PO ÷ q4–6h (hyperphosphatemia) **Caution:** [C, ?] **Disp:** Tabs 300, 600 mg; susp 320, 600 mg/5 mL; oint 0.275% (*Dermagran*) **SE:** Constipation **Notes:** OK in renal failure

Aluminum Hydroxide + Magnesium Carbonate (Gaviscon Extra Strength, Liquid) [OTC] **Uses:** *Relief of heartburn, acid indigestion* **Action:** Neutralizes gastric acid **Dose:** *Adults.* 15–30 mL PO pc & hs; 2–4 chew tabs up to qid. *Peds.* 5–15 mL PO qid or PRN; avoid in renal impair **Caution:** [C, ?] ↑ Mg^{2+}, w/ renal Insuff **Disp:** Liq w/ AlOH 95 mg/mg carbonate 358 mg/15 mL; Extra Strength liq AlOH 254 mg/mg carbonate 237 mg/15 mL; chew tabs AlOH 160 mg/mg carbonate 105 mg **SE:** Constipation, D **Notes:** qid doses best pc & hs; may ↓ absorption of some drugs, take 2–3 h apart to ↓ effect

Aluminum Hydroxide + Magnesium Hydroxide (Maalox) [OTC] Uses: *Hyperacidity* (peptic ulcer, hiatal hernia, etc) **Action:** Neutralizes gastric acid **Dose:** *Adults.* 10–20 mL or 2–4 tabs PO qid or PRN. *Peds.* 5–15 mL PO qid or PRN **Caution:** [C, ?] **Disp:** Chew tabs, susp **SE:** May ↑ Mg²⁺ w/ renal Insuff, constipation, D **Notes:** Doses qid best pc & hs

Aluminum Hydroxide + Magnesium Hydroxide & Simethicone (Mylanta, Mylanta II, Maalox Plus) [OTC] Uses: *Hyperacidity w/ bloating* **Action:** Neutralizes gastric acid & defoaming **Dose:** *Adults.* 10–20 mL or 2–4 tabs PO qid or PRN. *Peds.* 5–15 mL PO qid or PRN; avoid in renal impair **Caution:** [C, ?] **Disp:** Tabs, susp, liq **SE:** ↑ Mg²⁺ in renal Insuff, D, constipation **Notes:** Mylanta II contains twice Al & Mg hydroxide of Mylanta; may affect absorption of some drugs

Aluminum Hydroxide + Magnesium Trisilicate (Gaviscon, Regular Strength) [OTC] Uses: *Relief of heartburn, upset or sour stomach, or acid indigestion* **Action:** Neutralizes gastric acid **Dose:** Chew 2–4 tabs qid; avoid in renal impair **Caution:** [C, ?] **Disp:** Mg²⁺; sensitivity **Disp:** AlOH 80 mg/Mg trisilicate 20 mg/tab **SE:** ↑ Mg²⁺ in renal Insuff, constipation, D **Notes:** May affect absorption of some drugs

Amantadine (Symmetrel) Uses: *Rx/prophylaxis influenza A, Parkinsonism, & drug-induced EPS* (Note: Not for influenza, not for use in US due to resistance) **Action:** Prevents infectious viral nucleic acid release into host cell; releases dopamine and blocks reuptake of dopamine in presynaptic nerves **Dose:** *Adults.* *Influenza A:* 200 mg/d PO or 100 mg PO bid w/in 48 h of Sx. *Parkinsonism:* 100 mg PO daily-bid. *Peds 1–9 y:* 4.4–8.8 mg/kg/24 h to 150 mg/24 h max ÷ doses daily-bid. *10–12 y:* 100–200 mg/d in 1–2 ÷ doses; ↓ in renal impair **Caution:** [C, M] **Disp:** Caps 100 mg; tabs 100 mg; soln 50 mg/5 mL **SE:** Orthostatic ↓ BP, edema, insomnia, depression, irritability, hallucinations, dream abnormalities, N/D, dry mouth

Ambrisentan (Letairis)   WARNING: May cause ↑ AST/ALT to >3× ULN, LFTs monthly. CI in PRG; ✓ monthly PRG tests **Uses:** *Pulmonary arterial HTN* **Action:** Endothelin receptor antagonist **Dose:** *Adults.* 5 mg PO/d, max 10 mg/d; not ok w/ hepatic impair **Caution:** [X, –] w/ Cyclosporine, strong CYP3A or 2C19 inhibitor, inducers of P-glycoprotein, CYPs and UGTs **CI:** PRG **Disp:** Tabs 5, 10 mg **SE:** Edema, nasal congestion, sinusitis, dyspnea, flushing, constipation, HA, palpitations, hepatotoxic **Notes:** Available only through the Letairis Education and Access Program (LEAP); D/C AST/ALT >5× ULN or bilirubin >2× ULN or S/Sx of liver dysfunction; childbearing females must use 2 methods of contraception

Amifostine (Ethyol) Uses: *Xerostomia prophylaxis during RT (head, neck, etc) where parotid is in radiation field; ↓ renal tox w/ repeated cisplatin* **Action:** Prodrug, dephosphorylated by alkaline phosphatase to active thiol metabolite; binds cisplatin metabolites **Dose:** 910 mg/m²/d 15-min IV Inf 30 min prechemotherapy **Caution:** [C, +/−] CV Dz **Disp:** 500-mg vials powder, reconstitute in NS **SE:** Transient ↓ BP (>60%), N/V, flushing w/ hot or cold chills, dizziness, ↓ Ca^{2+}, somnolence, sneezing **Notes:** Does not ↓ effectiveness of cyclophosphamide + cisplatin chemotherapy

Amikacin (Amikin) **Uses:** *Serious gram(−) bacterial Infxns* & mycobacteria **Action:** Aminoglycoside; ↓ protein synth *Spectrum:* Good gram(−) bacterial coverage: *Pseudomonas* & *Mycobacterium* sp **Dose:** *Adults & Peds. Conventional:* 5–7.5 mg/kg/dose q8h; once daily; 15–20 mg/kg q24h; ↑ interval w/ renal impair. *Neonates <1200 g, 0–4 wk:* 7.5 mg/kg/dose q18h–24h. *Age <7 d, 1200–2000 g:* 7.5 mg/kg/dose q12h; *>2000 g:* 10 mg/kg/dose q12h. *Age >7 d, 1200–2000 g:* 7 mg/kg/dose q8h; *>2000 g:* 7.5–10 mg/kg/dose q8h **Caution:** [C, +/−] avoid w/ diuretics **Disp:** 50 & 250 mg/mL Inj **SE:** Nephro-/oto-/neurotox, neuromuscular blockage, resp paralysis **Notes:** May be effective in gram(−) resistance to gentamicin & tobramycin; follow Cr; Levels: Peak: 30 min after Inf; Trough <0.5 h before next dose; Therapeutic: Peak 20–30 mcg/mL; Trough: <8 mcg/mL; Toxic Peak >35 mcg/mL; Half-life: 2 h

Amiloride (Midamor) **Uses:** *HTN, CHF, & thiazide-induced ↓ K^+* **Action:** K^+-sparing diuretic; interferes w/ K^+/Na^+ exchange in distal tubule **Dose:** *Adults.* 5–10 mg PO daily. *Peds.* 0.625 mg/kg/d; ↓ w/ renal impair **Caution:** [B, ?] **CI:** ↑ K^+, SCr >1.5, BUN >30, diabetic neuropathy, w/ other K^+-sparing diuretics **Disp:** Tabs 5 mg **SE:** ↑ K^+; HA, dizziness, dehydration, impotence **Notes:** monitor K^+

Aminocaproic Acid (Amicar) **Uses:** *Excessive bleeding from systemic hyperfibrinolysis & urinary fibrinolysis* **Action:** ↓ fibrinolysis; inhibits TPA, inhibits conversion of plasminogen to plasmin **Dose:** *Adults.* 5 g IV or PO (1st h) followed by 1–1.25 g/h IV or PO × 8h or until bleeding controlled; 30 g/d max. *Peds.* 100 mg/kg IV (1st h) then 1 g/m²/h; max 18 g/m²/d; ↓ w/ renal Insuff **Caution:** [C, ?] Upper urinary tract bleeding **CI:** DIC **Disp:** Tabs 500, syrup 250 mg/mL; Inj 250 mg/mL **SE:** ↓ BP, bradycardia, dizziness, HA, fatigue, rash, GI disturbance, ↓ plt Fxn **Notes:** Administer × 8 h or until bleeding controlled; not for upper urinary tract bleeding

Amino-Cerv pH 5.5 Cream **Uses:** *Mild cervicitis,* postpartum cervicitis/cervical tears, postcauterization, postcryosurgery, & postconization **Action:** Hydrating agent; removes excess keratin in hyperkeratotic conditions **Dose:** 1 Applicator-full intravag hs × 2 wk **Caution:** [C, ?] w/ Viral skin Infxn **Disp:** Vaginal cream **SE:** Stinging, local irritation **Notes:** A.K.A. carbamide or urea; contains 8.34% urea, 0.5% sodium propionate, 0.83% methionine, 0.35% cystine, 0.83% inositol, & benzalkonium chloride

Aminoglutethimide (Cytadren) **Uses:** *Cushing syndrome* Adrenocortical carcinoma, breast CA & PCa **Action:** ↓ adrenal steroidogenesis & conversion of androgens to estrogens; 1st gen aromatase inhibitor **Dose:** Initial 250 mg PO 4 × D, titrate q 1–2 wk max 2 g/d; w/ hydrocortisone 20–40 mg/d; ↓ w/ renal

Insuff **Caution:** [D, ?] **Disp:** Tabs 250 mg **SE:** Adrenal Insuff ("medical adrenalectomy"), hypothyroidism, masculinization, ↓ BP, N/V, rare hepatotox, rash, myalgia, fever, drowsiness, lethargy, anorexia **Notes:** give q6h to ↓ N

Aminophylline **Uses:** *Asthma, COPD* & bronchospasm **Action:** Relaxes smooth muscle (bronchi, pulm vessels); stimulates diaphragm **Dose:** *Adults. Acute asthma:* Load 6 mg/kg IV, then 0.4–0.9 mg/kg/h IV cont Inf, not > than 25 mg/min. *Chronic asthma:* 24 mg/kg/24 h PO ÷ q6h. *Peds.* Load 6 mg/kg IV, then 6 wk-6 mo 0.5 mg/kg/h, 6 mo–1 y 0.6–0.7 mg/kg/h, 1–9 y 1 mg/kg/h IV Inf; ↓ w/ hepatic Insuff & w/ some drugs (macrolide & quinolone antibiotics, cimetidine, propranolol) **Caution:** [C, +] Uncontrolled arrhythmias, HTN, Sz disorder, hyperthyroidism, peptic ulcers **Disp:** Tabs 100, 200 mg; PR tabs 100, 200 mg, soln 105 mg/5 mL, Inj 25 mg/mL **SE:** N/V, irritability, tachycardia, ventricular arrhythmias, Szs **Notes:** Individualize dosage; level 10 to 20 mcg/mL, toxic >20 mcg/mL; aminophylline 85% theophylline; erratic rectal absorption

Amiodarone (Cordarone, Pacerone) **WARNING:** Liver tox, exacerbation of arrhythmias and lung damage reported **Uses:** *Recurrent VF or hemodynamically unstable VT,* supraventricular arrhythmias, AF **Action:** Class III antiarrhythmic (Table 10) **Dose:** *Adults. Ventricular arrhythmias:* IV: 15 mg/min for 10 min, then 1 mg/min × 6 h, maint 0.5-mg/min cont Inf or *PO:* Load: 800–1600 mg/d PO × 1–3 wk. Maint: 600–800 mg/d PO for 1 mo, then 200–400 mg/d. *Supraventricular arrhythmias: IV:* 300 mg IV over 1 h, then 20 mg/kg for 24 h, then 600 mg PO daily for 1 wk, maint 100–400 mg daily or *PO:* Load 600–800 mg/d PO for 1–4 wk. *Maint:* Slow ↓ to 100–400 mg daily *(ECC 2005) Cardiac arrest:* 300 mg IV push; 150 mg IV push 3–5 min PRN. *Refractory pulseless VT, VF:* 5 mg/kg rapid IV bolus. *Perfusing arrhythmias:* Load: 5 mg/kg IV/IO over 20–60 min; repeat PRN, max 15 mg/kg/d. *Peds.* 10–15 mg/kg/24 h ÷ q12h PO for 7–10 d, then 5 mg/kg/24 h ÷ q12h or daily (infants require ↑ loading); ↓ w/ liver Insuff **Caution:** [D, –] May require ↓ digoxin/warfarin dose, many drug interactions **CI:** Sinus node dysfunction, 2nd-/3rd-degree AV block, sinus brady (w/o pacemaker), iodine sensitivity **Disp:** Tabs 100, 200, 400 mg; Inj 50 mg/mL **SE:** Pulm fibrosis, exacerbation of arrhythmias, ↑ QT interval; CHF, hypo-/hyperthyroidism, ↑ LFTs, liver failure, corneal microdeposits, optic neuropathy/neuritis, peripheral neuropathy, photosensitivity **Notes:** IV conc >0.2 mg/mL only via central catheter; Levels: *Trough:* just before next dose; *Therapeutic:* 1–2.5 mcg/mL; *Toxic:* >2.5 mcg/mL; *Half-life:* 30–100 h

Amitriptyline (Elavil) **WARNING:** Antidepressants may ↑ suicide risk; consider risks/benefits of use. Monitor pts closely **Uses:** *Depression (not bipolar depression)* peripheral neuropathy, chronic pain, tension HAs **Action:** TCA; ↓ reuptake of serotonin & norepinephrine by presynaptic neurons **Dose:** *Adults. Initial:* 30–50 mg PO hs; may ↑ to 300 mg hs. *Peds.* Not OK <12 y unless for chronic pain. *Initial:* 0.1 mg/kg PO hs, ↑ over 2–3 wk to 0.5–2 mg/kg PO hs; taper to D/C **Caution:** CV Dz, Szs [D,+/–] NAG, hepatic impair **CI:** w/ MAOIs or w/in 14 d of use, during acute MI recovery **Disp:** Tabs 10, 25, 50, 75, 100, 150 mg; Inj 10 mg/mL **SE:** Strong anticholinergic SEs; OD may be fatal; urine retention, sedation, ECG changes, photosensitivity **Notes:** Levels: *Therapeutic:* 120 to 150 ng/mL; *Toxic:* >500 mg/mL; levels may not correlate w/ effectiveness

Amlodipine (Norvasc) Uses: *HTN, stable or unstable angina* **Action:** CCB; relaxes coronary vascular smooth muscle **Dose:** 2.5–10 mg/d PO; ↓ w/ hepatic impair **Caution:** [C, ?] **Disp:** Tabs 2.5, 5, 10 mg **SE:** Peripheral edema, HA, palpitations, flushing, dizziness **Notes:** Take w/o regard to meals

Amlodipine/Atorvastatin (Caduet) Uses: *HTN, chronic stable/ vasospastic angina, control cholesterol & triglycerides* **Action:** CCB & HMG-CoA reductase inhibitor **Dose:** Amlodipine 2.5–10 mg w/ atorvastatin 10–80 mg PO daily **Caution:** [X, –] **CI:** Active liver Dz, ↑ LFTs **Disp:** Tabs amlodipine/ atorvastatin: 2.5/10, 2.5/20, 2.5/40, 5/10, 5/20, 5/40, 5/80, 10/10, 10/20, 10/40, 10/80 mg **SE:** Peripheral edema, HA, palpitations, flushing, myopathy, arthralgia, myalgia, GI upset **Notes:** ✓ LFTs; instruct patient to report muscle pain/weakness

Amlodipine/Olmesartan (Azor) **WARNING: Use of renin- angiotensin agents in PRG can cause injury and death to fetus, D/C immedi- ately when PRG detected** Uses: *Hypertension* **Action:** CCB w/ angiotensin II receptor blocker **Dose:** *Adults.* Initial 2 mg/20 mg, max 10 mg/40 mg q d **Caution:** [C 1st Tri, D 2nd, 3rd Tri, –] w/ K⁺ supl or K⁺ sparing diuretics, renal impair, RAS, severe CAD, AS **CI:** PRG **Disp:** Tab amlodipine/olmesartan 5/20, 10/20, 5/40, 10/40 **SE:** Edema, vertigo, dizziness, ↓ BP

Amlodipine/Valsartan (Exforge) **WARNING: Use of renin- angiotensin agents in PRG can cause injury and death to fetus, D/C immedi- ately when PRG detected** Uses: *Hypertension* **Action:** CCB w/ angiotensin II receptor blocker **Dose:** *Adults.* Initial 5 mg/160 mg, may ↑ after 1–2 wk, max 10 mg/ 320 mg q day, start elderly at ¹/₂ initial dose **Caution:** [C 1st Tri, D 2nd, 3rd Tri, –] w/ K⁺ supl or K⁺-sparing diuretics, renal impair, RAS, severe CAD **CI:** PRG, **Disp:** Tab amlodipine/valsartan mg 5/160, 10/160, 5/320,10/320 **SE:** Edema, vertigo, nasopharyngitis, URI, dizziness, ↓ BP

Ammonium Aluminum Sulfate [Alum] [OTC] Uses: *Hemor- rhagic cystitis when saline bladder irrigation fails* **Action:** Astringent **Dose:** 1–2% soln w/ constant NS bladder irrigation **Caution:** [+/–] **Disp:** Powder for recons **SE:** Encephalopathy possible; ✓ aluminum levels, especially w/ renal Insuff; can precipitate & occlude catheters **Notes:** Safe w/o anesthesia & w/ vesicoureteral reflux

Amoxicillin (Amoxil, Polymox) Uses: *Ear, nose, & throat, lower resp, skin, urinary tract Infxns from susceptible gram(+) bacteria* endocarditis prophylaxis, H. pylori eradication w/ other agents (gastric ulcers)* **Action:** β-Lactam antibiotic; ↓ cell wall synth *Spectrum:* Gram(+) (*Streptococcus* sp, *Enterococcus* sp); some gram(–) (*H. influenzae, E. coli, N. gonorrhoeae, H. pylori, & P. mirabilis*) **Dose:** *Adults.* 250–500 mg PO tid or 500–875 mg bid. *Peds.* 25–100 mg/kg/24 h

PO ÷ q8h, 200–400 mg PO bid (equivalent to 125–250 mg tid); ↓ in renal impair **Caution:** [B, +] **Disp:** Caps 250, 500 mg; chew tabs 125, 200, 250, 400 mg; susp 50 mg/mL, 125, 200, 250, & 400 mg/5 mL; tabs 500, 875 mg **SE:** D; skin rash **Notes:** Cross hypersensitivity w/ PCN; many *E. coli* strains resistant; chew tabs contain phenylalanine

Amoxicillin & Clavulanic Acid (Augmentin, Augmentin 600 ES, Augmentin XR)
Uses: *Ear, lower resp, sinus, urinary tract, skin Infxns caused by β-lactamase–producing *H. influenzae*, *S. aureus*, & *E. coli** **Action:** β-lactam antibiotic w/ β-lactamase inhibitor. *Spectrum:* Gram(+) same as amoxicillin alone, MSSA; gram(−) as w/ amoxicillin alone, β-lactamase–producing *H. influenzae*, *Klebsiella* sp, *M. catarrhalis* **Dose:** *Adults.* 250–500 mg PO q8h or 875 mg q12h; XR 2000 mg PO q12h. *Peds.* 20–40 mg/kg/d as amoxicillin PO ÷ q8h or 45 mg/kg/d ÷ q12h; ↓ in renal impair; take w/ food **Caution:** [B, enters breast milk] **Disp:** Supplied (as amoxicillin/clavulanic): Tabs 250/125, 500/125, 875/125 mg; chew tabs 125/31.25, 200/28.5, 250/62.5, 400/57 mg; susp 125/31.25, 250/62.5, 200/28.5, 400/57 mg/5 mL; susp ES 600/42.9 mg/5 mL; XR tab 1000/62.5 mg **SE:** Abd discomfort, N/V/D, allergic Rxn, vaginitis **Notes:** Do not substitute two 250-mg tabs for one 500-mg tab (OD of clavulanic acid); max clavulanic acid 125 mg/dose

Amphotericin B (Amphocin)
Uses: *Severe, systemic fungal Infxns; oral & cutaneous candidiasis* **Action:** Binds ergosterol in the fungal membrane to alter permeability **Dose:** *Adults & Peds. Test dose:* 1 mg IV adults or 0.1 mg/kg to 1 mg IV in children; then 0.25–1.5 mg/kg/24 h IV over 2–6 h (25–50 mg/d or q other day). Total varies w/ indication. *PO:* 1 mL qid **Caution:** [B, ?] **Disp:** Powder (Inj) 50 mg/vial **SE:** ↓ K⁺/Mg²⁺ from renal wasting; anaphylaxis, HA, fever, chills, nephrotox, ↓ BP, anemia, rigors **Notes:** Monitor Cr/LFTs/K/Mg; ? ↓ in renal impair; pretreatment w/ APAP & antihistamines (Benadryl) ↓ SE

Amphotericin B Cholesteryl (Amphotec)
Uses: *Aspergillosis if intolerant/refractory to conventional amphotericin B,* systemic candidiasis **Action:** Binds ergosterol in fungal membrane, alters permeability **Dose:** *Adults & Peds. Test dose:* 1.6–8.3 mg, over 15–20 min, then 3–4 mg/kg/d IV giving Inf, 7.5 mg/kg/d max; ↓ w/ renal Insuff **Caution:** [B, ?] **Disp:** Powder for Inj 50 mg, 100 mg/vial **SE:** Anaphylaxis; fever, chills, HA, ↓ K⁺, ↓ Mg²⁺, nephrotox, ↓ BP, anemia **Notes:** Do not use in-line filter; ✓ LFTs/lytes

Amphotericin B Lipid Complex (Abelcet)
Uses: *Refractory invasive fungal Infxn in pts intolerant to conventional amphotericin B* **Action:** Binds ergosterol in fungal membrane, alters permeability **Dose:** *Adults & Peds.* 5 mg/kg/d IV single daily dose **Caution:** [B, ?] **Disp:** Inj 5 mg/mL **SE:** Anaphylaxis; fever, chills, HA, ↓ K⁺, ↓ Mg²⁺, nephrotox, ↓ BP, anemia **Notes:** Filter w/ 5-micron needle; do not mix in electrolyte-containing solns; if Inf >2 h, manually mix bag

Amphotericin B Liposomal (AmBisome)
Uses: *Refractory invasive fungal Infxn w/ intolerance to conventional amphotericin B; cryptococcal

meningitis in HIV; empiric for febrile neutropenia; visceral leishmaniasis* **Action:** Binds ergosterol in fungal membrane, alters membrane permeability **Dose:** *Adults & Peds.* 3–6 mg/kg/d, Inf 60–120 min; dose varies by indication; ? ↓ in renal Insuff **Caution:** [B, ?] **Disp:** Powder Inj 50 mg **SE:** Anaphylaxis, fever, chills, HA, ↓ K⁺, ↓ Mg²⁺ nephrotox, ↓ BP, anemia **Notes:** Use no < 1-micron filter

Ampicillin (Amcill, Omnipen) **Uses:** *Resp, GU, or GI tract Infxns; meningitis due to gram(−) & (+) bacteria; SBE prophylaxis* **Action:** β-Lactam antibiotic; ↓ cell wall synth. **Spectrum:** Gram(+) (*Streptococcus* sp, *Staphylococcus* sp, *Listeria*); gram(−) (*Klebsiella* sp, *E. coli, H. influenzae, P. mirabilis, Shigella* sp, *Salmonella* sp) **Dose:** *Adults.* 500 mg–2 g IM or IV q6h or 250–500 mg PO q6h; varies by indication. *Peds Neonates <7 d:* 50–100 mg/kg/24 h IV ÷ q8h. *Term infants:* 75–150 mg/kg/24 h ÷ q6–8h IV or PO. *Children >1 mo:* 100–200 mg/kg/ 24 h ÷ q4–6h IM or IV; 50–100 mg/kg/24 h ÷ q6h PO up to 250 mg/dose. *Meningitis:* 200–400 mg/kg/24 h ÷ q4–6h IV; ↓ w/ renal impair; take on empty stomach **Caution:** [B, M] Cross-hypersensitivity w/ PCN **Disp:** Caps 250, 500 mg; susp 100 mg/mL (reconstituted drops), 125 mg/5 mL, 250 mg/5 mL; powder (Inj) 125, 250, 500, 1, 2, 10 g/vial **SE:** D, rash, allergic Rxn **Notes:** Many *E. coli* resistant

Ampicillin-Sulbactam (Unasyn) **Uses:** *Gynecologic, intra-Abd, skin Infxns due to β-lactamase–producing S. aureus, Enterococcus, H. influenzae, P. mirabilis, & Bacteroides* sp* **Action:** β-lactam antibiotic & β-lactamase inhibitor. **Spectrum:** Gram(+) & (−) as for amp alone; also *Enterobacter, Acinetobacter, Bacteroides* **Dose:** *Adults.* 1.5–3 g IM or IV q6h. *Peds.* 100–400 mg ampicillin/kg/d (150–300 mg Unasyn) q6h; ↓ w/ renal Insuff **Caution:** [B, M] **Disp:** Powder for Inj 1.5, 3 g/vial, 15 g bulk package **SE:** Allergic Rxns, rash, D, Inj site pain **Notes:** A 2:1 ratio ampicillin:sulbactam

Amprenavir (Agenerase) DISCONTINUED replaced by fosamprenavir tid

Anakinra (Kineret) **WARNING:** Associated w/ ↑ incidence of serious Infxn; D/C w/ serious Infxn **Uses:** *Reduce S/Sxs of mod/severe active RA, failed 1 or more DMARD* **Action:** Human IL-1 receptor antagonist **Dose:** 100 mg SQ daily; w/ CrCl <30 mL/min, q other day **Caution:** [B, ?] **CI:** *E. coli*-derived proteins allergy, active Infxn, <18 y **Disp:** 100-mg prefilled syringes; 100 mg (0.67 mL/vial) **SE:** ↓ WBC especially w/ TNF-blockers, Inj site Rxn (may last up to 28 d), Infxn, N/D, Abd pain, flu-like sx, HA

Anastrozole (Arimidex) **Uses:** *Breast CA: postmenopausal w/ metastatic breast CA, adjuvant Rx postmenopausal early hormone-receptor (+) breast CA* **Action:** Selective nonsteroidal aromatase inhibitor, ↓ circulatory estradiol **Dose:** 1 mg/d **Caution:** [D, ?] **CI:** PRG **Disp:** Tabs 1 mg **SE:** May ↑ cholesterol; N/V/D, HTN, flushing, ↑ bone/tumor pain, HA, somnolence, mood disturbance, depression, rash **Notes:** No effect on adrenal steroids or aldosterone

Anidulafungin (Eraxis)   Uses: *Candidemia, esophageal candidiasis, other *Candida* Infxn (peritonitis, intra-Abd abscess)* **Action:** Echinocandin; ↓ cell wall synth **Spectrum:** *C. albicans, C. glabrata, C. parapsilosis, C. tropicalis* **Dose:** Candidemia, others: 200 mg IV × 1, then 100 mg IV daily (Tx ≥14 d after last + culture); Esophageal candidiasis: 100 mg IV × 1, then 50 mg IV daily (Tx >14 d and 7 d after resolution of Sx); 1.1 mg/min max Inf rate **Caution:** [C, ?/–] **CI:** Echinocandin hypersensitivity **Disp:** Powder 50 mg/vial, 100 mg/vial **SE:** Histamine-mediated Inf Rxns (urticaria, flushing, ↓ BP, dyspnea, etc), fever, N/V/D, ↓ K⁺, HA, ↑ LFTs, hep, worsening hepatic failure **Notes:** ↓ Inf rate to <1.1 mg/min w/ Inf Rxns

Anistreplase (Eminase)   Uses: *AMI* **Action:** Thrombolytic; activates conversion of plasminogen to plasmin, ↑ thrombolysis **Dose:** 30 units IV over 2–5 min *(ECC 2005)* **Caution:** [C, ?] **CI:** Active internal bleeding, Hx CVA, recent (<2 mo) intracranial or intraspinal surgery/trauma/neoplasm, AVM, aneurysm, bleeding diathesis, severe HTN **Disp:** 30 units/vial **SE:** Bleeding, ↓ BP, hematoma **Notes:** Ineffective if readministered >5 d after the previous dose of anistreplase or streptokinase, or streptococcal Infxn (production of antistreptokinase Ab)

Anthralin (Anthra-Derm)   Uses: *Psoriasis* **Action:** Keratolytic **Dose:** Apply daily **Caution:** [C, ?] **CI:** Acutely inflamed psoriatic eruptions, erythroderma **Disp:** Cream, oint 0.1, 0.25, 0.4, 0.5, 1% **SE:** Irritation; hair/fingernails/skin discoloration

Antihemophilic Factor [AHF, Factor VIII] (Monoclate)   Uses: *Classic hemophilia A, von Willebrand Dz* **Action:** Antihemophilic factor VIII needed to convert prothrombin to thrombin **Dose:** *Adults & Peds.* 1 AHF unit/kg ↑ factor VIII level by 2 Int Unit/dL; units required = (wgt in kg) (desired factor VIII ↑ as % nl) × (0.5); prevent spontaneous hemorrhage = 5% nl; hemostasis after trauma/surgery = 30% nl; head injuries, major surgery, or bleeding = 80–100% nl **Caution:** [C, ?] **Disp:** ✓ each vial for units contained, powder for recons **SE:** Rash, fever, HA, chills, N/V **Notes:** Determine % nl factor VIII before dosing

Antihemophilic Factor (Recombinant) (Xyntha)   Uses: *Control/ prevent bleeding & surgical prophylaxis in hemophilia A* **Action:** ↑ levels of factor VIII **Dose:** *Adults.* Required units = body wgt (kg) × desired factor VIII rise (Int Units/dL or % of normal) × 0.5 (Int Units/kg per Int Units/dL); frequency/duration determined by type of bleed (see insert) **Caution:** [C, ?/–] severe hypersensitivity Rxn possible **CI:** None **Disp:** Inj powder: 250, 500, 1000, 2000 Int Units **SE:** HA, fever, N/V/D, weakness, allergic Rxn **Notes:** Monitor for the development of factor VIII neutralizing antibodies

Antithymocyte Globulin (See Lymphocyte Immune Globulin, page 151)

Apomorphine (Apokyn)   WARNING: Do not administer IV Uses: *Acute, intermittent hypomobility ("off") episodes of Parkinson Dz* **Action:** Dopamine agonist **Dose:** *Adults.* 0.2 mL SQ supervised test dose; if BP OK, initial 0.2 mL (2 mg) SQ during "off" periods; only 1 dose per "off" period; titrate dose;

0.6 mL (6 mg) max single doses; use w/ antiemetic; ↓ in renal impair **Caution:** [C, +/–] Avoid EtOH; antihypertensives, vasodilators, cardio- or cerebrovascular Dz, hepatic impair **CI:** 5-HT$_3$ antagonists, sulfite allergy **Disp:** Inj 10 mg/mL, 3-mL pen cartridges; 2-mL amp **SE:** Emesis, syncope, ↑ QT, orthostatic ↓ BP, somnolence, ischemia, Inj site Rxn, abuse potential, dyskinesia, fibrotic conditions, priapism, chest pain/angina, yawning, rhinorrhea **Notes:** Daytime somnolence may limit activities; trimethobenzamide 300 mg tid PO or other non–5-HT$_3$ antagonist antiemetic given 3 d prior to & up to 2 mo following initiation

Apraclonidine (Iopidine) Uses: *Glaucoma, intraocular HTN* **Action:** α$_2$-Adrenergic agonist **Dose:** 1–2 gtt of 0.5% tid; 1 gtt of 1% before and after surgical procedure **Caution:** [C, ?] **CI:** w/in 14 d of or w/ MAOI **Disp:** 0.5, 1% soln **SE:** Ocular irritation, lethargy, xerostomia

Aprepitant (Emend) Uses: *Prevents N/V associated w/ emetogenic CA chemotherapy (eg, cisplatin) (use in combo w/ other antiemetics)*, post OP N/V **Action:** Substance P/neurokinin 1(NK$_1$) receptor antagonist **Dose:** 125 mg PO day 1, 1 h before chemotherapy, then 80 mg PO days 2 & 3; post-op N/V: 40 mg w/in 3 h of induction **Caution:** [B, ?/–]; substrate & mod CYP3A4 inhibitor; CYP2C9 inducer (Table 11) **CI:** Use w/ pimozide, **Disp:** Caps 40, 80, 125 mg **SE:** Fatigue, asthenia, hiccups **Notes:** ↓ effect OCP and warfarin

Aprotinin (Trasylol) Withdrawn from US market 2008

Arformoterol (Brovana) **WARNING:** Long-acting β$_2$-adrenergic agonists may increase the risk of asthma-related death. Use only for pts not adequately controlled on other asthma-controller meds Uses: *Maint in COPD* **Action:** Selective LA β$_2$-adrenergic agonist **Dose:** *Adults.* 15 mcg bid nebulization **Caution:** [C, ?] **CI:** Hypersensitivity **Disp:** Soln: 15 mcg/2 mL **SE:** Pain, back pain, CP, D, sinusitis, nervousness, palpitations, allergic Rxn **Notes:** Not for acute bronchospasm. Refrigerate, use immediately after opening

Argatroban (Acova) Uses: *Prevent/Tx thrombosis in HIT, PCI in pts w/ HIT risk* **Action:** Anticoagulant, direct thrombin inhibitor **Dose:** 2 mcg/kg/min IV; adjust until aPTT 1.5–3 × baseline not to exceed 100 s; 10 mcg/kg/min max; ↓ w/ hepatic impair **Caution:** [B, ?] Avoid PO anticoagulants, ↑ bleeding risk; avoid use w/ thrombolytics **CI:** Overt major bleed **Disp:** Inj 100 mg/mL **SE:** AF, cardiac arrest, cerebrovascular disorder, ↓ BP, VT, N/V/D, sepsis, cough, renal tox, ↓ Hgb **Note:** Steady state in 1–3 h; ✓ aPTT w/ Inf start and after each dose change

Aripiprazole (Abilify, Abilify Discmelt) **WARNING:** Increased mortality in elderly with dementia-related psychosis; ↑ suicidal thinking in children, adolescents, and young adults w/ major depressive disorder (MDD) Uses: *Schizophrenia adults and peds 13–17 y, mania or mixed episodes associated w/ bipolar disorder, MDD in adults, agitation w/ schizophrenia* **Action:** Dopamine & serotonin antagonist **Dose:** *Adults. Schizophrenia:* 10–15 mg PO/d; *Acute agitation:* 9.75 mg/1.3 mL IM; *Bipolar:* 15 mg/d; *MDD adjunct* w/ other antidepressants initial 2 mg/d, 10 mg/d ok. **Peds.** *Schizophrenia: 13–17 y:* start 2 mg/d, usual 10 mg/d; max 30 mg/d for all adult and peds uses; ↓ dose w/ CYP3A4/ CYP2D6 inhibitors (Table 11); ↑ dose w/ CYP3A4 inducer **Caution:** [C, –] **Disp:** Tabs 2, 5, 10, 15, 20, 30 mg; Discmelt (disintegrating tabs 10, 15, 20, 30 mg), soln 1 mg/mL, Inj 7.5 mg/mL **SE:** Neuroleptic malignant syndrome, tardive dyskinesia, orthostatic ↓ BP, cognitive & motor impair, ↑ glucose **Notes:** Discmelt contains phenylalanine

Artificial Tears (Tears Naturale) [OTC]
Uses: *Dry eyes* **Action:** Ocular lubricant **Dose:** 1–2 gtt tid-qid **Disp:** OTC soln **SE:** mild stinging, temp blurred vision

Armodafinil (Nuvigil)
Uses: *Narcolepsy, shift work sleep disorder (SWSD), and obstructive sleep apnea/hypopnea syndrome (OSAHS)* **Action:** ?; binds dopamine receptor, ↓ dopamine reuptake **Dose:** *Adults.* OSAHS/Narcolepsy: 150 or 250 mg PO daily in A.M.; SWSD: 150 mg PO q day 1 h prior to start of shift; ↓ w/ hepatic impair; adjust w/ substrates for CYP3A4/5, CYP2C19 **Caution:** [C, ?] **CI:** Hypersensitivity to modafinil/armodafinil **Disp:** Tabs 50, 150, 200 mg **SE:** HA, nausea, dizziness, insomnia, xerostomia, rash including SJS, angioedema, anaphylactoid Rxns, multiorgan hypersensitivity Rxns

L-Asparaginase (Elspar, Oncaspar)
Uses: *ALL* (in combo w/ other agents) **Action:** Protein synth inhibitor **Dose:** 500–20,000 Int Units/m²/d for 1–14 d (per protocols) **Caution:** [C, ?] **CI:** Active/Hx pancreatitis; history of allergic Rxn, thrombosis or hemorrhagic event w/ prior Rx w/ asparaginase **Disp:** Powder (Inj) 10,000 units/vial **SE:** Allergy 20–35% (urticaria to anaphylaxis); fever, chills, N/V, anorexia, Abd cramps, depression, agitation, Sz, pancreatiti, ↑ glucose or LFTs, coagulopathy **Notes:** Test dose ok, ✓ glucose, coagulation studies, LFTs

Aspirin (Bayer, Ecotrin, St. Joseph's) [OTC]
Uses: *Angina, CABG, PTCA, carotid endarterectomy, ischemic stroke, TIA, MI, arthritis, pain,* HA, *fever,* inflammation, Kawasaki Dz **Action:** Prostaglandin inhibitor **Dose:** *Adults. Pain, fever:* 325–650 mg q4–6h PO or PR (4g/d max). *RA:* 3–6 g/d PO in ÷ doses. *Plt inhibitor:* 81–325 mg PO daily. *Prevent MI:* 81 (preferred)–325 mg PO daily. *Acute Coronary Syndrome:* 160–325 mg PO ASAP, chewing preferred at onset *(ECC 2005).* *Peds. Antipyretic:* 10–15 mg/kg/dose PO or PR q4–6h up to 80 mg/kg/24 h. *RA:* 60–100 mg/kg/24 h PO ÷ q4–6h (keep levels 15–30 mg/dL); *Kawasaki Dz:* 80–100 mg/kg/d ÷ q6h, 3–5 mg/kg/d after fever resolves; for all uses 4 g/d max; avoid w/ CrCl <10 mL/min, severe liver Dz **Caution:** [C, M] Linked to Reye syndrome; avoid w/ viral illness in peds <16 y **CI:** Allergy to ASA, chickenpox/ flu Sxs, syndrome of nasal polyps, angioedema, & bronchospasm to NSAIDs **Disp:** Tabs 325, 500 mg; chew tabs 81 mg; EC tabs 81, 162, 325, 500, 650, 975 mg; SR tabs 650, 800 mg; effervescent tabs 325, 500 mg; supp 125, 200, 300, 600 mg **SE:** GI upset, erosion, & bleeding **Notes:** D/C 1 wk prior to surgery; avoid/limit EtOH; Salicylate Levels: *Therapeutic:* 100 to 250 mcg/mL; *Toxic:* >300 mcg/mL

Aspirin & Butalbital Compound (Fiorinal) [C-III] Uses: *Tension HA,* pain **Action:** barbiturate w/ analgesic **Dose:** 1–2 PO q4h PRN, max 6 tabs/d; avoid w/ CrCl <10 mL/min or severe liver Dz **Caution:** [C (D w/ prolonged use or high doses at term), ?] **CI:** ASA allergy, GI ulceration, bleeding disorder, porphyria, syndrome of nasal polyps, angioedema, & bronchospasm to NSAIDs **Disp:** Caps (*Fiorgen PF, Lanorinal*), Tabs (*Lanorinal*) ASA 325 mg/butalbital 50 mg/caffeine 40 mg **SE:** Drowsiness, dizziness, GI upset, ulceration, bleeding **Notes:** Butalbital habit-forming; D/C 1 wk prior to surgery, avoid or limit EtOH

Aspirin + Butalbital, Caffeine, & Codeine (Fiorinal + Codeine) [C-III] Uses: Mild *pain,* HA, especially tension HA w/ stress **Action:** Sedative and narcotic analgesic **Dose:** 1–2 tabs/caps PO q4–6h PRN max 6/d **Caution:** [C, ?] **CI:** Allergy to ASA and codeine; syndrome of nasal polyps, angioedema, & bronchospasm to NSAIDs, bleeding diathesis, peptic ulcer or significant GI lesions, porphyria **Disp:** Caps/tab contains 325-mg ASA, 40-mg caffeine, 50 mg of butalbital, 30 mg of codeine **SE:** Drowsiness, dizziness, GI upset, ulceration, bleeding **Notes:** D/C 1 wk prior to surgery, avoid/limit EtOH

Aspirin + Codeine (Empirin No. 3, 4) [C-III] Uses: Mild to *mod pain,* symptomatic nonproductive cough **Action:** Combined effects of ASA & codeine **Dose:** *Adults.* 1–2 tabs PO q4–6h PRN. *Peds.* ASA 10 mg/kg/dose; codeine 0.5–1 mg/kg/dose q4h **Caution:** [D, M] **CI:** Allergy to ASA/codeine, PUD, bleeding, anticoagulant Rx, children w/ chickenpox or flu Sxs, syndrome of nasal polyps, angioedema, & bronchospasm to NSAIDs **Disp:** Tabs 325 mg of ASA & codeine (Codeine in No. 3 = 30 mg, No. 4 = 60 mg) **SE:** Drowsiness, dizziness, GI upset, ulceration, bleeding **Notes:** D/C 1 wk prior to surgery; avoid/limit EtOH

Atazanavir (Reyataz) WARNING: Hyperbilirubinemia may require drug D/C Uses: *HIV-1 Infxn* **Action:** Protease inhibitor **Dose:** Antiretroviral naïve 400 mg PO daily w/ food; experienced pts 300 mg w/ ritonavir 100 mg; when given w/ efavirenz 600 mg, administer atazanavir 300 mg + ritonavir 100 mg once/d; separate doses from buffered didanosine administration; ↓ w/ hepatic impair **Caution:** CDC recommends HIV-infected mothers not breast-feed [B, –]; ↑ levels of statins (avoid use) sildenafil, antiarrhythmics, warfarin, cyclosporine, TCAs; ↓ w/ St. John's wort, H₂-receptor antagonists **CI:** w/ midazolam, triazolam, ergots, pimozide **Disp:** Caps 100, 150, 200, 300 mg **SE:** HA, N/V/D, rash, Abd pain, DM, photosensitivity, ↑ PR interval **Notes:** May have less-adverse effect on cholesterol; if given w/ H₂ blocker, give together or at least 10 h after H₂; if given w/ proton pump inhibitor, separate by 12 h; concurrent use not ok in experienced pts

Atenolol (Tenormin) Uses: *HTN, angina, MI* **Action:** selective β-adrenergic receptor blocker **Dose:** 25–50 q day up to 100 mg/d; *HTN & angina:* 50–100 mg PO. *AMI:* 5 mg IV slowly over 5 min, may repeat in 10 min then 50 mg PO bid if tolerated; 5 mg IV over 5 min; in 10 min, 5 mg slow IV; if tolerated in 10 min, start 50 mg PO, then 50 mg PO bid *(ECC 2005);* ↓ in renal impair

Caution: [D, M] DM, bronchospasm; abrupt D/C can exacerbate angina & ↑ MI risk **CI:** Bradycardia, cardiogenic shock, cardiac failure, 2nd-/3rd-degree AV block, sinus node dysfunction, pulm edema **Disp:** Tabs 25, 50, 100 mg; Inj 5 mg/10 mL **SE:** Bradycardia, ↓ BP, 2nd-/3rd-degree AV block, dizziness, fatigue

Atenolol & Chlorthalidone (Tenoretic)   **Uses:** *HTN* **Action:** β-Adrenergic blockade w/ diuretic **Dose:** 50–100 mg/d PO based on atenolol; ↓ dose w/ CrCL <35 mL/min **Caution:** [D, M] DM, bronchospasm **CI:** See atenolol; anuria, sulfonamide cross-sensitivity **Disp:** Tenoretic 50: Atenolol 50 mg/chlorthalidone 25 mg; Tenoretic 100: Atenolol 100 mg/chlorthalidone 25 mg **SE:** Bradycardia, ↓ BP, 2nd- or 3rd-degree AV block, dizziness, fatigue, wt ↓ K⁺, photosensitivity

Atomoxetine (Strattera)   WARNING: Severe liver injury may rarely occur; DC w/ jaundice or ↑ LFTs, ↑ frequency of suicidal thinking; monitor closely **Uses:** *ADHD* **Action:** Selective norepinephrine reuptake inhibitor **Dose:** *Adults & children >70 kg:* 40 mg PO/d, after 3 d minimum, ↑ to 80–100 mg ÷ daily-bid. *Peds <70 kg:* 0.5 mg/kg × 3 d, then ↑ 1.2 mg/kg daily or bid (max 1.4 mg/kg or 100 mg); ↓ dose w/ hepatic Insuff or in combo w/ CYP2D6 inhibitors (Table 11) [C, ?/–] **Caution:** w/ known structural cardiac anomalies, cardiac history **CI:** NAG, w/ or w/in 2 wk of D/C an MAOI; **Disp:** Caps 5, 10, 18, 25, 40, 60, 80, 100 mg **SE:** HA, insomnia, dry mouth, Abd pain, N/V, anorexia ↑ BP, tachycardia, wgt loss, sexual dysfunction, jaundice, ↑ LFTs **Notes:** AHA recommends all children receiving stimulants for ADHD receive CV assessment before therapy initiated; D/C immediately w/ jaundice

Atorvastatin (Lipitor)   **Uses:** *↑ Cholesterol & triglycerides* **Action:** HMG-CoA reductase inhibitor **Dose:** Initial 10 mg/d, may ↑ to 80 mg/d **Caution:** [X, –] **CI:** Active liver Dz, unexplained ↑ LFTs **Disp:** Tabs 10, 20, 40, 80 mg **SE:** Myopathy, HA, arthralgia, myalgia, GI upset, chest pain, edema, insomnia dizziness **Notes:** Monitor LFTs, instruct patient to report unusual muscle pain or weakness

Atovaquone (Mepron)   **Uses:** *Rx & prevention PCP and Toxoplasma gondii encephalitis* **Action:** ↓ nucleic acid & ATP synth **Dose:** Rx: 750 mg PO bid for 21 d. *Prevention:* 1500 mg PO once/d (w/ meals) **Caution:** [C, ?] **Disp:** Susp 750 mg/5 mL **SE:** Fever, HA, anxiety, insomnia, rash, N/V, cough

Atovaquone/Proguanil (Malarone)   **Uses:** *Prevention or Rx Plasmodium falciparum malaria* **Action:** Antimalarial **Dose:** *Adults.* Prevention: 1 tab PO 2 d before, during, & 7 d after leaving endemic region; Rx: 4 tabs PO single dose daily × 3 d. *Peds.* See insert **Caution:** [C, ?] **CI:** prophylactic use when CrCl <30 mL/min **Disp:** Tab atovaquone 250 mg/proguanil 100 mg; peds 62.5/25 mg **SE:** HA, fever, myalgia, N/V, ↑ LFTs

Atracurium (Tracrium)   **Uses:** *Anesthesia adjunct to facilitate ET intubation* **Action:** Nondepolarizing neuromuscular blocker **Dose:** *Adults & Peds >2 y.* 0.4–0.5 mg/kg IV bolus, then 0.08–0.1 mg/kg q20–45min PRN **Caution:** [C, ?] **Disp:** Inj 10 mg/mL **SE:** Flushing **Notes:** Pt must be intubated & on controlled ventilation; use adequate amounts of sedation & analgesia

Atropine, systemic (AtroPen Auto-injector) **WARNING:** Primary protection against exposure to chemical nerve agent and insecticide poisoning is the wearing of specially designed protective garments **Uses:** *Preanesthetic; symptomatic bradycardia & asystole, AV block, organophosphate (insecticide) and acetylcholinesterase (nerve gas) inhibitor antidote; cycloplegic* **Action:** Antimuscarinic; blocks acetylcholine at parasympathetic sites, cycloplegic **Dose:** *Adults.* *(2005 ECC)*: *Asystole or PEA:* 1 mg IV/IO push. Repeat PRN q3–5min to 0.03–0.04 mg/kg max. *Bradycardia:* 0.5–1.0 mg IV q3–5min as needed; max 0.03–0.04 mg/kg: ET 2–3 mg in 10 mL NS. *Preanesthetic:* 0.3–0.6 mg IM. *Poisoning:* 1–2 mg IV bolus, repeat q3–5min PRN to reverse effects. *Peds. (ECC 2005):* 0.01–0.03 mg/kg IV q2–5min, max 1 mg, min dose 0.1 mg. *Preanesthetic:* 0.01 mg/kg/dose SQ/IV (max 0.4 mg). *Poisoning:* 0.05 mg/kg IV, repeat q3–5min PRN to reverse effects **Caution:** [C, +] **CI:** NAG, adhesions between iris and lens, tachycardia, GI obst, ileus, severe ulcerative colitis, obstructive uropathy, Mobitz II block **Disp:** Inj 0.05, 0.1, 0.3, 0.4, 0.5, 0.8, 1 mg/mL; AtroPen Auto-injector: 0.25, 0.5, 1, 2 mg/dose; tabs 0.4 mg, MDI 0.36 mg/Inh **SE:** Flushing, mydriasis, tachycardia, dry mouth & nose, blurred vision, urinary retention, constipation psychosis **Notes:** SLUDGE (Salivation, Lacrimation, Urination, Diaphoresis, GI motility, Emesis) are Sx of organophosphate poisoning; Auto-injector limited distribution; see also ophthal forms below

Atropine, Benzoic Acid, Hyoscyamine Sulfate, Methenamine, Methylene Blue, Phenyl Salicylate (Urised) **Uses:** *lower urinary tract discomfort* **Action:** Methenamine in acid urine releases formaldehyde (antiseptic), methylene blue/benzoic acid mild antiseptic, phenyl salicylate mild analgesic, hyoscyamine and atropine parasympatholytic ↓ muscle spasm **Dose:** *Adults.* 2 tabs PO qid *Peds >6 y:* Individualize **Caution:** [C, ?/–] avoid w/ sulfonamides **CI:** NAG, pyloric/duodenal obst, BOO, coronary artery spasm **Disp:** Tab: atropine 0.03 mg/benzoic acid 4.5 mg/hyoscyamine 0.03 mg/methenamine 40.8 mg/methylene blue 5.4 mg/phenyl salicylate 18.1 mg **SE:** Rash, dry mouth, flushing, ↑ pulse, dizziness, blurred vision, urine/feces discoloration, voiding difficulty **Notes:** Take w/ plenty of fluid, can cause crystalluria

Atropine, ophthalmic (Isopto Atropine, generic) **Uses:** *cycloplegic refraction, uveitis, amblyopia* **Action:** Antimuscarinic; cycloplegic, dilates pupils **Dose:** *Adults.* *Refraction:* 1–2 gtt 1 h before; *Uveitis:* 1–2 gtt daily-qid *Peds.* 1 gtt in nonamblyopic eye daily **Caution:** [C, +] NAG, adhesions between iris and lens **Disp:** 2.5 & 15-mL bottle 1% ophthal soln, 1% oint **SE:** Local irritation, burning, blurred vision, light sensitivity **Notes:** Compress lacrimal sac 2–3 min after instillation; effects can last 1–2 wk

Atropine/pralidoxime (DuoDote) **WARNING:** For use by personnel with appropriate training; wear protective garments; do not rely solely on medication; evacuation and decontamination ASAP **Uses:** *Nerve agent (tabun, sarin, others) and insecticide poisoning* **Action:** Atropine blocks effects of excess acetylcholine;

pralidoxime reactivates acetylcholinesterase inactivated by organophosphorus poisoning **Dose:** 1 Inj in midlateral thigh; wait 10–15 min for effect; if Sx are severe, give 2 additional Inj; if alert & oriented no additional doses **Caution:** [C, ?] **Disp:** Auto-injector 2.1 mg atropine/600 mg pralidoxime **SE:** Dry mouth, blurred vision, dry eyes, photophobia, confusion, HA, tachycardia, ↑ BP, flushing, urinary retention, constipation, Abd pain N, V, emesis **Notes:** Severe sx of poisoning: confusion, dyspnea w/ copious secretions, weakness, twitching, involuntary urination and defecation, convulsions, unconsciousness; limited distribution

Azathioprine (Imuran)   WARNING: May ↑ neoplasia w/ chronic use; mutagenic and hematologic tox possible

Uses: *Adjunct to prevent renal transplant rejection, RA,* SLE, Crohn Dz, ulcerative colitis **Action:** Immunosuppressive; antagonizes purine metabolism **Dose:** *Adults. Crohn and ulcerative colitis,* start 50 mg/d, ↑ 25 mg q1–2wk, target dose 2–3 mg/kg/d **Adults & Peds.** *Renal transplant:* 3–5 mg/kg/d IV/PO single daily dose, taper by 0.5 mg/kg q4wk to lowest effective dose. RA 1 mg/kg/d once daily or ÷ bid × 6–8 wk, ↑ 0.5 mg/kg/d q4wk to 2.5 mg/kg/d; ↓ w/ renal Insuff **Caution:** [D, ?] **CI:** PRG **Disp:** Tabs, 50, 75, 100 mg; powder for Inj 100 mg **SE:** GI intolerance, fever, chills, leukopenia, thrombocytopenia **Notes:** Handle Inj w/ cytotoxic precautions; interaction w/ allopurinol; do not administer live vaccines on therapy; ✓ CBC and LFTs; dose per local transplant protocol, usually start 1–3 d pretransplant

Azelastine (Astelin, Optivar)

Uses: *Allergic rhinitis (rhinorrhea, sneezing, nasal pruritus); allergic conjunctivitis* **Action:** Histamine H_1-receptor antagonist **Dose:** *Nasal:* 2 sprays/nostril bid. *Ophth:* 1 gtt in each affected eye bid **Caution:** [C, ?/–] **CI:** Component sensitivity **Disp:** Nasal 137 mcg/spray; ophthal soln 0.05% **SE:** Somnolence, bitter taste, HA, colds Sx (rhinitis, cough)

Azithromycin (Zithromax)

Uses: *Community-acquired pneumonia, pharyngitis, otitis media, skin Infxns, nongonococcal (chlamydial) urethritis, chancroid & PID; Rx & prevention of MAC in HIV* **Action:** Macrolide antibiotic; bacteriostatic; ↓ protein synth. **Spectrum:** *Chlamydia, H. ducreyi, H. influenzae, Legionella, M. catarrhalis, M. pneumoniae, M. hominis, N. gonorrhoeae, S. aureus, S. agalactiae, S. pneumoniae, S. pyogenes* **Dose:** *Adults. Resp tract Infxns:* PO: Caps 500 mg day 1, then 250 mg/d PO × 4 d; *sinusitis* 500 mg PO × 3 d; *IV:* 500 mg × 2 d, then 500 mg PO × 7–10 d or 500 mg IV daily × 2 d, then 500 mg/d PO × 7–10 d. *Nongonococcal urethritis:* 1 g PO × 1. *Gonorrhea, uncomplicated:* 2 g PO × 1. *Prevent MAC:* 1200 mg PO once/wk. **Peds.** *Otitis media:* 10 mg/kg PO day 1, then 5 mg/kg/d days 2–5. *Pharyngitis:* 12 mg/kg/d PO × 5 d; take susp on empty stomach; tabs OK w/ or w/o food; ↓ w/ CrCl <10 mL/mg **Caution:** [B, +] **Disp:** Tabs 250, 500, 600 mg; Z-Pack (5-d); Tri-Pak (500-mg tabs × 3); susp 1 g; single-dose packet (ZMAX) ER susp (2 g); susp 100, 200 mg/5 mL; Inj powder 500 mg; 2.5 mL ophthal soln 1% **SE:** GI upset, metallic taste

Azithromycin Ophthalmic 1% (AzaSite)

Uses: *Bacterial conjunctivitis* **Action:** bacteriostatic **Dose:** *Adults.* 1 gtt bid, q8–12 h × 2 d, then 1 gtt q day × 5 d. **Peds ≥1 y:** 1 gtt bid, q8–12h × 2d then, then 1 gtt q day × 5 d **Caution:** [B, +/–] **CI:** None **Disp:** 1% in 2.5 mL bottle **SE:** Irritation, burning, stinging, contact dermatitis, corneal erosion, dry eye, dysgeusia, nasal congestion, sinusitis, ocular discharge, keratitis **Notes:** Avoid contact w/use

Aztreonam (Azactam) Uses: *Aerobic gram(–) UTIs, lower resp, intra-Abd, skin, gynecologic Infxns & septicemia* **Action:** *Monobactam:* ↓ cell wall synth. *Spectrum:* Gram(–) (*Pseudomonas, E. coli, Klebsiella, H. influenzae, Serratia, Proteus, Enterobacter, Citrobacter*) **Dose:** *Adults.* 1–2 g IV/IM q6–12h. *UTI 500–1 g IV q8–12h. Meningitis 2 g IV q6–8h* **Peds.** *Premature:* 30 mg/kg/dose IV q12h. *Term & children:* 30 mg/kg/dose q6–8h; ↓ in renal impair **Caution:** [B, +] **Disp:** Inj (soln), 1 g, 2 g/50 mL Inj powder for recons 500 mg 1 g, 2 g **SE:** N/V/D, rash, pain at Inj site **Notes:** No gram(+) or anaerobic activity; OK in PCN-allergic pts

Bacitracin, ophthalmic (AK-Tracin Ophthalmic); Bacitracin & Polymyxin B, ophthalmic (AK Poly Bac Ophthalmic, Polysporin Ophthalmic); Bacitracin, Neomycin, & Polymyxin B, ophthalmic (AK Spore Ophthalmic, Neosporin Ophthalmic); Bacitracin, Neomycin, Polymyxin B, & Hydrocortisone, Ophthalmic (AK Spore HC Ophthalmic, Cortisporin Ophthalmic) Uses: *Steroid-responsive inflammatory ocular conditions* **Action:** Topical antibiotic w/ anti-inflammatory **Dose:** Apply q3–4h into conjunctival sac **Caution:** [C, ?] **CI:** Viral, mycobacterial, fungal eye Infxn **Disp:** See Bacitracin, topical equivalents, below

Bacitracin, topical (Baciguent); Bacitracin & Polymyxin B, Topical (Polysporin); Bacitracin, Neomycin, & Polymyxin B, Topical (Neosporin); Bacitracin, Neomycin, Polymyxin B, & Hydrocortisone, topical (Cortisporin); Bacitracin, Neomycin, Polymyxin B, & Lidocaine, topical (Clomycin) Uses: *Prevent/Rx of *minor skin Infxns** **Action:** Topical antibiotic w/ added components (anti-inflammatory & analgesic) **Dose:** Apply sparingly bid-qid **Caution:** [C, ?] not for deep wounds, puncture, or animal bites **Disp:** Bacitracin 500 units/g oint; Bacitracin 500 units/polymyxin B sulfate 10,000 units/g oint & powder; Bacitracin 400 units/neomycin 3.5 mg/polymyxin B 5000 U/g oint; Bacitracin 400 units/neomycin 3.5 mg/polymyxin B 5000 units/hydrocortisone 10 mg/g oint; Bacitracin 500 units/neomycin 3.5 mg/polymyxin B 5000 units/lidocaine 40 mg/g oint **Notes:** Ophthal, systemic, & irrigation forms available, not generally used due to potential tox

Baclofen (Lioresal Intrathecal, generic) **WARNING:** IT abrupt discontinuation can lead to organ failure, rhabdomyolysis, and death **Uses:** *Spasticity due to severe chronic disorders (eg, MS, amyotrophic lateral sclerosis, or spinal cord lesions),* trigeminal neuralgia, intractable hiccups **Action:** Centrally acting skeletal muscle relaxant; ↓ transmission of monosynaptic & polysynaptic cord reflexes **Dose:** *Adults.* Initial, 5 mg PO tid; ↑ q3d to effect; max 80 mg/d. *Intrathecal:* via implantable pump (see insert) *Peds 2–7 y:* 10–15 mg/d ÷ q8h; titrate, max 40 mg/d. *>8 y:* Max 60 mg/d. *IT:* via implantable pump (see insert); ↓ in renal impair; take w/ food or milk **Caution:** [C, +] Epilepsy, neuropsychological disturbances; **Disp:** Tabs 10, 20 mg; IT Inj 50 mcg/mL, 10 mg/20 mL, 10 mg/5 mL **SE:** Dizziness, drowsiness, insomnia, ataxia, weakness; ↓ BP

Balsalazide (Colazal)   **Uses:** *Ulcerative colitis* **Action:** 5-ASA derivative, anti-inflammatory, ↓ leukotriene synth **Dose:** 2.25 g (3 caps) tid × 8–12 wk **Caution:** [B, ?] Severe renal failure **CI:** Mesalamine or salicylate hypersensitivity **Disp:** Caps 750 mg **SE:** Dizziness, HA, N, Abd pain, agranulocytosis, renal impair, allergic Rxns **Notes:** Daily dose of 6.75 g = to 2.4 g mesalamine

Basiliximab (Simulect)   **WARNING:** Administer only under the supervision of a physician experienced in immunosuppression therapy in an appropriate facility **Uses:** *Prevent acute transplant rejection* **Action:** IL-2 receptor antagonists **Dose:** *Adults & Peds >35 kg:* 20 mg IV 2 h before transplant, then 20 mg IV 4 d posttransplant. *Peds <35 kg:* 12 mg/m² (max 20 mg) IV 2 h prior to transplant; same dose IV 4 d posttransplant **Caution:** [B, ?/–] **CI:** Hypersensitivity to murine proteins **Disp:** Inj powder 10, 20 mg **SE:** Edema, HTN, HA, dizziness, fever, pain, Infxn, GI effects, electrolyte disturbances **Notes:** A murine/human MoAb

BCG [Bacillus Calmette-Guérin] (TheraCys, Tice BCG)   **WARNING:** Contains live, attenuated mycobacteria; risk for transmission; handle as a biohazard; nosocomial Infxns reported in immunosuppressed; fatal Rxns reported **Uses:** *Bladder CA (superficial),* *TB prophylaxis* **Action:** Attenuated live BCG culture, immunomodulator **Dose:** *Bladder CA,* 1 vial prepared & instilled in bladder for 2 h. Repeat once/wk × 6 wk; then 1 treatment at 3, 6, 12, 18, & 24 mo after **Caution:** [C, ?] Asthma **CI:** Immunocompromised, steroid use, febrile illness, UTI, gross hematuria, w/ traumatic catheterization or UTI **Disp:** Powder for recons 81 mg (10.5 ± 8.7 × 10⁸ CFU/vial) (TheraCys), 50 mg (1–8 × 10⁸ CFU/vial) (Tice BCG) **SE:** *Intravesical:* Hematuria, urinary frequency, dysuria, bacterial UTI, rare BCG sepsis **Notes:** Routine US adult BCG immunization not ok; occasionally used in high-risk children who are PPD(–) & cannot take INH; intravesical use, dispose/void in toilet with chlorine bleach

Becaplermin (Regranex Gel)   **WARNING:** Increased mortality due to malignancy reported; use w/ caution in known malignancy **Uses:** *Local wound care adjunct w/ *diabetic foot ulcers* **Action:** Recombinant PDGF, enhances granulation tissue **Dose:** *Adults.* Based on lesion; 4/3-in ribbon 2-g tube, 2/3-in ribbon 15-g tube/in × in² of ulcer; cover w/moist gauze; rinse after 12 h; do not reapply; repeat in 12 h. See insert **Caution:** [C, ?] **CI:** Neoplasmatic site **Disp:** 0.01% gel in 2-, 15-g tubes **SE:** Rash **Notes:** Use w/ good wound care; wound must be vascularized; reassess after 10 wk if ulcer not ↓ by 30% or not healed by 20 wk

Beclomethasone (Beconase)   **Uses:** *Allergic rhinitis* refractory to antihistamines & decongestants; *nasal polyps* **Action:** Inhaled steroid **Dose:**

Adults & Peds. Aqueous inhaler: 1–2 sprays/nostril bid **Caution:** [C, ?] **Disp:** Nasal metered-dose inhaler **SE:** Local irritation, burning, epistaxis **Notes:** Nasal spray delivers 42 mcg/dose

Beclomethasone (QVAR)
Uses: Chronic *asthma* **Action:** Inhaled corticosteroid **Dose:** *Adults & Peds 5–11 y:* 40–160 mcg 1–4 Inhs bid; initial 40–80 mcg Inh bid if on bronchodilators alone; 40–160 mcg w/ other inhaled steroids; 320 mcg bid max; taper to lowest effective dose bid; rinse mouth/throat after **Caution:** [C, ?] **CI:** Acute asthma **Disp:** PO metered-dose inhaler; 40, 80 mcg/Inh **SE:** HA, cough, hoarseness, oral candidiasis **Notes:** Not effective for acute asthma

Belladonna & Opium Suppositories (B&O Supprettes) [C-II]
Uses: *Bladder spasms; mod/severe pain* **Action:** Antispasmodic, analgesic **Dose:** 1 supp PR q6h PRN; **Caution:** [C, ?] **CI:** Glaucoma, resp depression **Disp:** 15A = 30 mg opium/16.2 mg belladonna extract; 16A = 60 mg opium/16.2 mg belladonna extract **SE:** Anticholinergic (eg, sedation, urinary retention, constipation)

Benazepril (Lotensin)
Uses: *HTN,* DN, CHF **Action:** ACE inhibitor **Dose:** 10–80 mg/d PO **Caution:** [C (1st tri), D (2nd & 3rd tri), +] **CI:** Angioedema, Hx edema, bilateral RAS **Disp:** Tabs 5, 10, 20, 40 mg **SE:** Symptomatic ↓ BP w/ diuretics; dizziness, HA, ↑ K+, nonproductive cough

Bendamustine (Treanda)
Uses: *CLL* **Action:** Mechlorethamine derivative; alkylating agent **Dose:** *Adults.* 100 mg/m² IV over 30 min days 1 & 2 of 28-d cycle, up to 6 cycles (w/ tox see insert for dose changes; do not use w/ CrCl <40 mL/min, severe hepatic impair) **Caution:** [D, ?/–] **CI:** Hypersensitivity to bendamustine or mannitol **Disp:** Inj powder 100 mg **SE:** Pyrexia, N/V, dry mouth, fatigue, cough, stomatitis, rash, myelosuppression, Infxn, Inf Rxns & anaphylaxis, tumor lysis syndrome, skin Rxns **Notes:** Consider use of allopurinol to prevent tumor lysis syndrome

Benzocaine & Antipyrine (Auralgan)
Uses: *Analgesia in severe otitis media* **Action:** Anesthetic w/ local decongestant **Dose:** Fill ear & insert a moist cotton plug; repeat 1–2 h PRN **Caution:** [C, ?] **CI:** w/ perforated eardrum **Disp:** Soln 5.4% antipyrine, 1.4% benzocaine **SE:** Local irritation

Benzonatate (Tessalon Perles)
Uses: Symptomatic relief of *cough* **Action:** Anesthetizes the stretch receptors in the resp passages **Dose:** *Adults & Peds >10 y:* 100 mg PO tid (max 600 mg/d) **Caution:** [C, ?] **Disp:** Caps 100, 200 mg **SE:** Sedation, dizziness, GI upset **Notes:** Do not chew or puncture the caps

Benztropine (Cogentin)
Uses: *Parkinsonism & drug-induced extrapyramidal disorders* **Action:** Partially blocks striatal cholinergic receptors **Dose:** *Adults. Parkinsonism:* initial 0.5–1 mg PO/IM/IV qhs, ↑ q 5–6 d PRN by 0.5 mg, usual dose 1–2 mg, 6 mg/d max. *Extrapyramidal:* 1–4 mg PO/IV/IM q day-bid. *Acute Dystonia:* 1–2 mg IM/IV, then 1–2 mg PO bid. *Peds >3 y:* 0.02–0.05 mg/kg/dose 1–2/d **Caution:** [C, ?] w/ Urinary Sxs, NAG, hot environments, CNS or mental disorders, other phenothiazines or TCA **CI:** <3 y **Disp:** Tabs 0.5, 1,

2 mg; Inj 1 mg/mL **SE:** Anticholinergic(tachycardia, ileus, N/V, etc), anhydrosis, heat stroke **Notes:** Physostigmine 1–2 mg SQ/IV to reverse severe Sxs

Beractant (Survanta) **Uses:** *Prevention & Rx of RDS in premature infants* **Action:** Replaces pulm surfactant **Dose:** 100 mg/kg via ET tube; repeat 3 × q6h PRN; max 4 doses/48 h **Disp:** Susp 25 mg of phospholipid/mL **SE:** Transient bradycardia, desaturation, apnea **Notes:** Administer via 4-quadrant method

Betaxolol (Kerlone) **Uses:** *HTN* **Action:** Competitively blocks β-adrenergic receptors, β_1 **Caution:** [C (1st tri), D (2nd or 3rd tri), +/–] **CI:** Sinus bradycardia, AV conduction abnormalities, uncompensated cardiac failure **Dose:** 5–20 mg/d **Disp:** Tabs 10, 20 mg **SE:** Dizziness, HA, bradycardia, edema, CHF

Betaxolol, ophthalmic (Betoptic) **Uses:** Open-angle glaucoma **Action:** Competitively blocks β_1-adrenergic receptors, **Dose:** 1–2 gtt bid **Caution:** [C (1st tri), D (2nd or 3rd tri), ?/–] **Disp:** Soln 0.5%; susp 0.25% **SE:** Local irritation, photophobia

Bethanechol (Urecholine, Duvoid, others) **Uses:** *Acute post-op/postpartum nonobstructive urinary retention; neurogenic bladder with retention* **Action:** Stimulates cholinergic smooth muscle in bladder & GI tract **Dose:** *Adults.* Initial 5–10 mg then repeat qh until response or 50 mg; typical 10–50 mg tid-qid, 200 mg/d max tid-qid; 2.5–5 mg SQ tid-qid & PRN. *Peds.* 0.3–0.6 mg/kg/24 h PO ÷ tid-qid or 0.15–2 mg/kg/d SQ ÷ 3–4 doses; take on empty stomach **Caution:** [C, –] **CI:** BOO, PUD, epilepsy, hyperthyroidism, bradycardia, COPD, AV conduction defects, Parkinsonism, ↓ BP, vasomotor instability **Disp:** Tabs 5, 10, 25, 50 mg; Inj 5 mg/mL **SE:** Abd cramps, D, salivation, ↓ BP **Notes:** Do not use IM/IV

Bevacizumab (Avastin) **WARNING:** Associated w/ GI perforation, wound dehiscence, & fatal hemoptysis **Uses:** *Met colorectal CA w/5-FU, NSCLC w/paclitaxel and carboplatin* **Action:** Vascular endothelial GF inhibitor **Dose:** *Adults. Colon:* 5 mg/kg or 10 mg/kg IV q14d; *NSCLC:* 15 mg/kg q21d; 1st dose over 90 min; 2nd over 60 min, 3rd over 30 min if tolerated **Caution:** [C, –] Do not use w/in 28 d of surgery if time for separation of drug & anticipated surgical procedures is unknown; D/C w/serious adverse effects **Disp:** 100 mg/4 mL, 400 mg/16 mL vials **SE:** Wound dehiscence, GI perforation, tracheoesophageal fistula, arterial thrombosis, hemoptysis, hemorrhage, HTN, proteinuria, CHF, Inf Rxns, D, leukopenia **Notes:** Monitor for ↑ BP & proteinuria

Bicalutamide (Casodex) **Uses:** *Advanced PCa w/ GnRH agonists [eg, leuprolide, goserelin]* **Action:** Nonsteroidal antiandrogen **Dose:** 50 mg/d **Caution:** [X, ?] **CI:** Women **Disp:** Caps 50 mg **SE:** Hot flashes, loss of libido, impotence, D/N/V, gynecomastia, & LFTs elevation

Bicarbonate (See Sodium Bicarbonate, page XXX) Bisacodyl (Dulcolax) [OTC] **Uses:** *Constipation; pre-op bowel preparation* **Action:** Stimulates peristalsis **Dose:** *Adults.* 5–15 mg PO or 10 mg PR PRN.

Peds <2 y: 5 mg PR PRN. *>2 y:* 5 mg PO or 10 mg PR PRN (do not chew tabs or give w/in 1 h of antacids or milk) **Caution:** [C, ?] **CI:** Acute abdomen or bowel obst, appendicitis, gastroenteritis **Disp:** EC tabs 5 mg; tab 5 mg; supp 10 mg; enema soln 10 mg/30 mL **SE:** Abd cramps, proctitis, & inflammation w/ supps

Bismuth Subcitrate/Metronidazole/Tetracycline (Pylera)

WARNING: Metronidazole possibly carcinogenic based on animal studies **Uses:** *H. pylori* infxn w/ omeprazole* **Action:** Eradicates *H. pylori*, see agents **Dose:** 3 caps qid w/ omeprazole 20 mg bid for 10 d **Caution:** [D, –] **CI:** Pregnancy, childhood to 8 y (tetracycline during tooth development causes teeth discoloration), w/ renal/hepatic impair, component hypersensitivity **Disp:** Caps w/ 140-mg bismuth subcitrate potassium, 125-mg metronidazole, & 125-mg tetracycline hydrochloride **SE:** Stool abnormality, D, dyspepsia, Abd pain, HA, flu-like syndrome, taste perversion, vaginitis, dizziness; see SE for each component

Bismuth Subsalicylate (Pepto-Bismol) [OTC]

Uses: Indigestion, N, & *D*; combo for Rx of *H. pylori* infxn* **Action:** Antisecretory & antiinflammatory **Dose:** *Adults.* 2 tabs or 30 mL PO PRN (max 8 doses/24 h). *Peds.* (For all max 8 doses/24 h). *3–6 y:* 1/3 tab or 5 mL PO PRN. *6–9 y* 2/3 tab or 10 mL PO PRN. *9–12 y:* 1 tab or 15 mL PO PRN **Caution:** [C, D (3rd tri), –] Avoid w/ renal failure; hx severe GI bleed **CI:** Influenza or chickenpox (↑ risk of Reye syndrome), ASA allergy (see aspirin) **Disp:** Chew tabs; caplets 262 mg; liq 262, 525 mg/15 mL; susp 262 mg/15 mL **SE:** May turn tongue & stools black

Bisoprolol (Zebeta)

Uses: *HTN* **Action:** Competitively blocks β_1-adrenergic receptors **Dose:** 2.5–10 mg/d (max dose 20 mg/d); ↓ w/ renal impair **Caution:** [C (D 2nd & 3rd tri), +/–] **CI:** Sinus bradycardia, AV conduction abnormalities, uncompensated cardiac failure **Disp:** Tabs 5, 10 mg **SE:** Fatigue, lethargy, HA, bradycardia, edema, CHF **Notes:** Not dialyzed

Bivalirudin (Angiomax)

Uses: *Anticoagulant w/ ASA in unstable angina undergoing PTCA, PCI, or in pts undergoing PCI w/ or at risk of HIT/HITTS* **Action:** Anticoagulant, thrombin inhibitor **Dose:** 0.75 mg/kg IV bolus, then 1.75 mg/kg/h for duration of procedure and up to 4 h postprocedure; ✓ ACT 5 min after bolus, may repeat 0.3 mg/kg bolus if necessary (give w/ aspirin 300–325 mg/d) start pre-PTCA) **Caution:** [B, ?] **CI:** Major bleeding **Disp:** Powder 250 mg for Inj **SE:** Bleeding, back pain, N, HA

Bleomycin Sulfate (Blenoxane)

Uses: *Testis CA; Hodgkin Dz & NHLs; cutaneous lymphomas; & squamous cell CA (head & neck, larynx, cervix, skin, penis); malignant pleural effusion sclerosing agent* **Action:** Induces DNA breakage (scission) **Dose:** (per protocols); ↓ w/ renal impair **Caution:** [D, ?] **CI:** Severe pulm Dz (pulm fibrosis) **Disp:** Powder (Inj) 15, 30 units **SE:** Hyperpigmentation & allergy (rash to anaphylaxis); fever in 50%; lung tox (idiosyncratic & dose related); pneumonitis w/ fibrosis; Raynaud phenomenon, N/V **Notes:** Test dose 1 unit, especially in lymphoma pts; lung tox w/ total dose >400 units or single dose >30 units; avoid high FiO_2 in general anesthesia to ↓ tox

Bortezomib (Velcade)   WARNING: May worsen preexisting neuropathy
Uses: *Rx multiple myeloma or mantel cell lymphoma w/ one failed previous Rx*
Action: Proteasome inhibitor **Dose:** 1.3 mg/m^2 bolus IV 2 ×/wk for 2 wk (days 1, 2, 8, 11), w/ 10-d rest period (=1 cycle); ↓ dose w/ hematologic tox, neuropathy
Caution: [D, ?/–] w/ Drugs CYP450 metabolized (Table 11) **Disp:** 3.5-mg vial
SE: Asthenia, GI upset, anorexia, dyspnea, HA, orthostatic ↓ BP, edema, insomnia, dizziness, rash, pyrexia, arthralgia, neuropathy

Botulinum Toxin Type A (Botox, Botox Cosmetic)   **Uses:** *Glabellar lines (cosmetic), blepharospasm, cervical dystonia, axillary hyperhidrosis, strabismus* **Action:** Neurotoxin, ↓ acetylcholine release from nerve endings, ↓ neuromuscular transmission; denervates sweat glands and muscles **Dose:** *Adults. Glabellar lines (cosmetic):* 0.1 mL IM × 5 sites q3–4mo; *Blepharospasm:* 1.25–2.5 units IM/site q3mo; max 200 units/30 d cum dose; *Cervical dystonia* 198–300 units IM divided <100 units into sternocleidomastoid; *Hyperhidrosis, axillary:* 50 units intradermal/axilla divided; *Strabismus:* 1.25–2.5 units IM/site q3mo; inject extraocular muscles w/EMG guidance **Peds.** *Blepharospasm: >12 y:* See Adults. *Cervical dystonia: >16 y:* 198–300 units IM ÷ among affected muscles; use <100 units in sternocleidomastoid; *Strabismus: >12 y:* 1.25–2.5 units IM/site q3mo; 25 units/site max; inject extraocular muscles w/ EMG guidance **Caution:** [C, ?] Do not exceed dosing ok; w/ neurologic Dz; caution sedentary patient to resume activity slowly after Inj; aminoglycosides and nondepolarizing muscle blockers may ↑ effects **CI:** hypersensitivity to components, infect at Inj site **Disp:** Inj powder **SE:** Anaphylaxis, erythema multiforme, dysphagia, dyspnea, syncope, HA, NAG, Inj site pain

Brimonidine (Alphagan P)   **Uses:** *Open-angle glaucoma, ocular HTN* **Action:** α$_2$-Adrenergic agonist **Dose:** 1 gtt in eye(s) tid (wait 15 min to insert contacts) **Caution:** [B, ?] **CI:** MAOI therapy **Disp:** 0.15, 0.1% soln **SE:** Local irritation, HA, fatigue

Brimonidine/Timolol (Combigan)   **Uses:** *↓ IOP in glaucoma or ocular HTN* **Action:** Selective α$_2$-adrenergic agonist and nonselective β-adrenergic antagonist **Dose:** *Adults & Peds ≥2 y:* 1 gtt bid ~ q12h **Caution:** [C, –] **CI:** Asthma, severe COPD, sinus brady, 2nd-/3rd-degree AV block, CHF cardiac failure, cardiogenic shock, component hypersensitivity **Disp:** Soln: (2 mg/mL brimonidine, 5 mg/mL timolol) 5, 10, 15 mL **SE:** Allergic conjunctivitis, conjunctival folliculosis, conjunctival hyperemia, eye pruritus, ocular burning & stinging **Notes:** Instill other ophthal products 5 min apart

Brinzolamide (Azopt)   **Uses:** *Open-angle glaucoma, ocular HTN* **Action:** Carbonic anhydrase inhibitor **Dose:** 1 gtt in eye(s) tid **Caution:** [C, ?] **CI:** Sulfonamide allergy **Disp:** 1% susp **SE:** Blurred vision, dry eye, blepharitis, taste disturbance

Bromocriptine (Parlodel)   **Uses:** *Parkinson Dz, hyperprolactinemia, acromegaly, pituitary tumors* **Action:** Agonist to striatal dopamine receptors; ↓

prolactin secretion **Dose:** Initial, 1.25 mg PO bid; titrate to effect, w/ food **Caution:** [B, ?] **CI:** Severe ischemic heart Dz or PVD **Disp:** Tabs 2.5 mg; caps 5 mg **SE:** ↓ BP, Raynaud phenomenon, dizziness, N, GI upset, hallucinations

Budesonide (Rhinocort Aqua, Pulmicort)
Uses: *Allergic & non-allergic rhinitis, asthma* **Action:** Steroid **Dose:** *Adults.* Rhinocort Aqua 1–4 sprays/nostril/d; Turbuhaler 1–4 Inh bid; Pulmicort Flexhaler 1–2 Inh bid *Peds.* *Rhinocort Aqua* intranasal: 1–2 sprays/nostril/d; *Pulmicort Turbuhaler:* 1–2 Inh bid; *Respules:* 0.25–0.5 mg daily or bid (rinse mouth after PO use) **Caution:** [B, ?/–] **CI:** w/ acute asthma **Disp:** Metered-dose *Turbuhaler* 200 mcg/Inh; *Flexhaler* 90, 180 mcg/Inh; *Respules* 0.25, 0.5,1 mg/2 mL; *Rhinocort Aqua* 32 mcg/spray **SE:** HA, N, cough, hoarseness, *Candida* Infxn, epistaxis

Budesonide, oral (Entocort EC)
Uses: *Mild-mod Crohn Dz* **Action:** Steroid, anti-inflammatory **Dose:** *Adults.* initial, 9 mg PO q A.M. to 8 wk max: maint 6 mg PO q A.M. taper by 3 mo; avoid grapefruit juice **CI:** Active TB and fungal Infxn **Caution:** [C, ?/–] DM, glaucoma, cataracts, HTN, CHF **Disp:** Caps 3 mg ER **SE:** HA, N, ↑ wgt, mood change, *Candida* Infxn, epistaxis **Notes:** Do not cut/crush/chew; taper on D/C

Budesonide/Formoterol (Symbicort)
WARNING: Long-acting β₂-adrenergic agonists may ↑ risk of asthma-related death. Use only for pts not adequately controlled on other meds **Uses:** *Maint Rx of asthma* **Action:** Steroid w/ LA selective β₂-adrenergic agonist **Dose:** *Adults & Peds >12 y:* 2 Inh bid (use lowest effective dose), 640/18 mcg/d max **Caution:** [C, ?/–] **CI:** Status asthmaticus/ acute episodes **Disp:** Inh (budesonide/formoterol): 80/4.5 mcg, 160/4.5 mcg **SE:** HA, GI discomfort, nasopharyngitis, palpitations, tremor, nervousness, URI, paradoxical bronchospasm, hypokalemia, cataracts, glaucoma **Notes:** Not for acute bronchospasm; not for transferring pt from chronic systemic steroids; rinse & spit w/ water after each dose

Bumetanide (Bumex)
Uses: *Edema from CHF, hepatic cirrhosis, & renal Dz* **Action:** Loop diuretic; ↓ reabsorption of Na⁺ & Cl⁻, in ascending loop of Henle & the distal tubule **Dose:** *Adults.* 0.5–2 mg/d PO; 0.5–1 mg IV/IM q8–24h (max 10 mg/d). *Peds.* 0.015–0.1 mg/kg PO q6h-24h (max 10 mg/d) **Caution:** [D,?] **CI:** Anuria, hepatic coma, severe electrolyte depletion **Disp:** Tabs 0.5, 1, 2 mg; Inj 0.25 mg/mL **SE:** ↓ K⁺, ↓ Na⁺, ↑ Cr, ↑ uric acid, dizziness, ototox **Notes:** Monitor fluid & lytes

Bupivacaine (Marcaine)
WARNING: Administration only by clinicians experienced in local anesthesia due to potential tox; avoid 0.75% for OB anesthesia due to reports of cardiac arrest and death **Uses:** *Local, regional, & spinal anesthesia, local & regional analgesia* **Action:** Local anesthetic **Dose:** *Adults & Peds.* Dose dependent on procedure (tissue vascularity, depth of anesthesia, etc) (Table 2) **Caution:** [C, ?] **CI:** Severe bleeding, ↓ BP, shock & arrhythmias, local Infxns at site, septicemia **Disp:** Inj 0.25, 0.5, 0.75% **SE:** ↓ BP, bradycardia, dizziness, anxiety

Buprenorphine (Buprenex) [C-III] Uses: *Mod/severe pain* **Action:** Opiate agonist-antagonist **Dose:** 0.3–0.6 mg IM or slow IV push q6h PRN **Caution:** [C, ?/–] **Disp:** 0.3 mg/mL **SE:** Sedation, ↓ BP, resp depression **Notes:** Withdrawal if opioid-dependent

Bupropion hydrobromide (Aplenzin) **WARNING:** ↑ suicide risk in pts <24 y w/ major depressive/other psychiatric disorders; not for ped use **Uses:** *Depression* **Action:** Aminoketone, ? action **Dose:** *Adults.* 174 mg PO, q day q A.M., ↑ PRN to 348 mg q day on day 4 if tolerated, max 522 mg/d; see insert if switching from Wellbutrin; mild–mod hepatic/renal impair ↓ frequency/dose; severe hepatic impair 174 mg max q other day **Caution:** [C, –] w/ Drugs that ↓ Sz threshold, ↑ w/ stimulants, CYP2D6-metabolized meds (Table 11) **CI:** Sz disorder, bulimia, anorexia nervosa, w/in 14 d of MAOIs, other forms of bupropion, abrupt D/C of EtOH, or sedatives **Disp:** ER Tab 174, 348, 522 mg **SE:** Dry mouth, N, Abd pain, insomnia, dizziness, pharyngitis, agitation, anxiety, tremor, palpitation, tremor, sweating, tinnitus, myalgia, anorexia, urinary frequency, rash **Notes:** Do not cut/crush/chew, avoid EtOH

Bupropion hydrochloride (Wellbutrin, Wellbutrin SR, Wellbutrin XL, Zyban) **WARNING:** Closely monitor for worsening depression or emergence of suicidality, increased suicidal behavior in young adults **Uses:** *Depression, smoking cessation adjunct,* ADHD **Action:** Weak inhibitor of neuronal uptake of serotonin & norepinephrine; ↓ neuronal dopamine reuptake **Dose:** *Depression:* 100–450 mg/d ÷ bid-tid; SR 150–200 mg bid; XL 150–450 mg daily. *Smoking cessation (Zyban, Wellbutrin XR):* 150 mg/d × 3 d, then 150 mg bid × 8–12 wk, last dose before 6 P.M.; ↓ dose w/ renal/hepatic impair **Caution:** [C, ?/–] **CI:** Sz disorder, Hx anorexia nervosa or bulimia, MAOI, w/in 14 d, abrupt D/C of EtOH or sedatives **Disp:** Tabs 75, 100 mg; SR tabs100, 150, 200 mg; XL tabs 150, 300 mg; Zyban 150 mg tabs **SE:** Szs, agitation, insomnia, HA, tachycardia, ↓ wgt **Notes:** Avoid EtOH & other CNS depressants, SR & XR do not cut/chew/crush

Buspirone (BuSpar) **WARNING:** Closely monitor for worsening depression or emergence of suicidality **Uses:** *Short-term relief of *anxiety* **Action:** Antianxiety; antagonizes CNS serotonin and dopamine receptors **Dose:** Initial: 7.5 mg PO bid; ↑ by 5 mg q2–3d to effect; usual 20–30 mg/d; max 60 mg/d **CI:** w/ MAOI **Caution:** [B, ?/–] Avoid w/ severe hepatic/renal Insuff **Disp:** Tabs ÷ dose 5, 10, 15, 30 mg **SE:** Drowsiness, dizziness, HA, N, EPS, serotonial syndrome, hostility, depression **Notes:** No abuse potential or physical/psychological dependence

Busulfan (Myleran, Busulfex) **WARNING:** Can cause severe bone marrow suppression **Uses:** *CML,* preparative regimens for allogeneic & ABMT in high doses **Action:** Alkylating agent **Dose:** (per protocol) **Caution:** [D, ?] **Disp:** Tabs 2 mg, Inj 60 mg/10 mL **SE:** Bone marrow suppression, ↑ BP, pulm fibrosis, N (w/ highdose), gynecomastia, adrenal Insuff, skin hyperpigmentation

Butabarbital, Hyoscyamine Hydrobromide, Phenazopyridine (Pyridium Plus) Uses: *Relieve urinary tract pain w/ UTI, procedures, trauma* **Action:** Phenazopyridine (topical anesthetic), hyoscyamine (parasympatholytic, ↓ spasm) & butabarbital (sedative) **Dose:** 1 PO qid, pc & hs; w/ antibiotic for UTI, 2 d max **Caution:** [C, ?] **Disp:** Tab butabarbital/hyoscyamine/phenazopyridine 15 mg/0.3 mg/150 mg **SE:** HA, rash, itching, GI distress, methemoglobinemia, hemolytic anemia, anaphylactoid-like Rxns, dry mouth, dizziness, drowsiness, blurred vision **Notes:** Colors urine orange, may tint skin, sclera; stains clothing/contacts

Butorphanol (Stadol) [C-IV]
Uses: *Anesthesia adjunct, pain* & migraine HA **Action:** Opiate agonist-antagonist w/ central analgesic actions **Dose:** 1–4 mg IM or IV q3–4h PRN. *Migraine:* 1 spray in 1 nostril, repeat × 1 60–90 min, then q3–4h. ↓ in renal impair **Caution:** [C (D if high dose or prolonged use at term), +] **Disp:** Inj 1, 2 mg/mL; nasal 1 mg/spray (10 mg/mL) **SE:** Drowsiness, dizziness, nasal congestion **Notes:** May induce withdrawal in opioid dependency

Calcipotriene (Dovonex)
Uses: *Plaque psoriasis* **Action:** Keratolytic **Dose:** Apply bid **Caution:** [C, ?] **CI:** ↑ Ca^{2+}; vit D tox; do not apply to face **Disp:** Cream; oint; soln 0.005% **SE:** Skin irritation, dermatitis

Calcitonin (Fortical, Miacalcin)
Uses: *Miacalcin:* *Paget Dz, emergent Rx hypercalcemia, postmenopausal osteoporosis* *Fortical:* *postmenopausal osteoporosis; osteogenesis imperfecta* **Action:** Polypeptide hormone (salmon derived), inhibits osteoclasts **Dose:** *Paget Dz:* 100 units/d IM/SQ initial, 50 units/d or 50–100 units q1–3d maint. *Hypercalcemia:* 4 units/kg IM/SQ q12h; ↑ to 8 units/kg q12h, max q6h. *Osteoporosis:* 100 units q other day IM/SQ; intranasal 200 units = 1 nasal spray/d **Caution:** [C, ?] **Disp:** *Fortical, Miacalcin* nasal spray 200 Int Units/activation; Inj, *Miacalcin* 200 units/mL (2 mL) **SE:** Facial flushing, N, Inj site edema, nasal irritation, polyuria, may ↑ granular casts in urine **Notes:** For nasal spray alternate nostrils daily; insure adequate calcium and vit D intake; *Fortical* is rDNA derived from salmon

Calcitriol (Rocaltrol, Calcijex)
Uses: *Predialysis reduction of ↑ PTH levels to treat bone Dz; ↑ Ca^{2+} on dialysis* **Action:** 1,25-Dihydroxycholecalci-ferol (vit D analog); ↑ Ca^{2+} and phosphorus absorption; ↑ bone mineralization **Dose:** *Adults. Renal failure:* 0.25 mcg/d PO, ↑ 0.25 mcg/d q4–6wk PRN; 0.5 mcg 3 ×/wk IV, ↑ PRN. *Hypoparathyroidism:* 0.5–2 mcg/d. *Peds. Renal failure:* 15 ng/kg/d, ↑ PRN; maint 30–60 ng/kg/d. *Hypoparathyroidism:* *<5 y:* 0.25–0.75 mcg/d. *>6 y:* 0.5–2 mcg/d **Caution:** [C, ?] **↑ Mg^{2+}** possible w/antacids **CI:** ↑ Ca^{2+}; vit D tox **Disp:** Inj 1 mcg/mL (in 1 mL); caps 0.25, 0.5 mcg; soln 1 mcg/mL **SE:** ↑ Ca^{2+} possible **Notes:** Monitor to keep Ca^{2+} WNL; Use nonaluminum phosphate binders and low-phosphate diet to control serum phosphate

Calcium Acetate (PhosLo)
Uses: *ESRD-associated hyperphosphatemia* **Action:** Ca^{2+} supl w/o aluminum to ↓ PO_4^{-2} absorption **Dose:** 2–4 tabs PO w/ meals **Caution:** [C, ?] **CI:** ↑ Ca^{2+} **Disp:** Gelcap 667 mg **SE:** Can ↑ Ca^{2+}, hypophosphatemia, constipation **Notes:** Monitor Ca^{2+}

Calcium Carbonate (Tums, Alka-Mints) [OTC] Uses: *Hyper-acidity-associated w/ peptic ulcer Dz, hiatal hernia, etc* Action: Neutralizes gastric acid Dose: 500 mg–2 g PO PRN, 7 g/d max; ↓ w/ renal impair Caution: [C, ?] Disp: Chew tabs 350, 420, 500, 550, 750, 850 mg; susp SE: ↑ Ca²⁺, ↓ PO⁻⁴, constipation

Calcium Glubionate (Neo-Calglucon) [OTC] Uses: *Rx & pre-vent calcium deficiency* Action: Ca²⁺ supl Dose: *Adults.* 6–18 g/d ÷ doses. *Peds.* 600–2000 mg/kg/d ÷ qid (9 g/d max); ↓ in renal impair Caution: [C, ?] CI: ↑ Ca²⁺ Disp: OTC syrup 1.8 g/5 mL = elemental Ca 115 mg/5 mL SE: ↑ Ca²⁺, ↓ PO⁻⁴, constipation

Calcium Salts (Chloride, Gluconate, Gluceptate) Uses: *Ca²⁺ replacement,* VF, Ca²⁺ blocker tox, Mg²⁺ intoxication, tetany, *hyperphosphatemia in ESRD* Action: Ca²⁺ supl/replacement Dose: *Adults.* Replacement: 1–2 g/d PO. *Tetany:* 1 g CaCl over 10–30 min; repeat in 6 h PRN; *Hyperkalemia/calcium chan-nel blocker OD:* 8–16 mg/kg (usually 5–10 mL) IV; 2–4 mg/kg (usually 2 mL) IV before IV calcium blockers *(ECC 2005)* Peds. Replacement: 200–500 mg/kg/d PO or IV ÷ qid. *Cardiac emergency:* 100 mg/kg/dose IV gluconate salt q10min. *Tetany:* 10 mg/kg CaCl over 5–10 min; repeat in 6 h or use Inf (200 mg/kg/d max). *Adults & Peds.* ↓ Ca²⁺ due to citrated blood Inf: 0.45 mEq Ca/100 mL citrated blood Inf (↓ in renal impair) Caution: [C, ?] CI: ↑ Ca²⁺ Disp: CaCl Inj 10% = 100 mg/mL = Ca 27.2 mg/mL = 10-mL amp; Ca gluconate Inj 10% = 100 mg/mL = Ca 9 mg/mL; tabs 500 mg = 45-mg Ca, 650 mg = 58.5-mg Ca, 975 mg = 87.75-mg Ca, 1 g = 90-mg Ca; Ca gluceptate Inj 220 mg/mL = 18-mg/mL Ca SE: Bradycardia, cardiac arrhythmias, ↑ Ca²⁺, constipation Notes: CaCl 270 mg (13.6 mEq) elemental Ca/g, & calcium gluconate 90 mg (4.5 mEq) Ca/g. RDA for Ca: *Peds <6 mo:* 210 mg/d; *6 mo–1 y:* 270 mg/d; *1–3 y:* 500 mg/d; *4–9 y:* 800 mg/d; *10–18 y:* 1200 mg/d. *Adults.* 1000 mg/d; *>50 y:* 1200 mg/d

Calfactant (Infasurf) Uses: *Prevention & Rx of RSD in infants* Action: Exogenous pulm surfactant Dose: 3 mL/kg instilled into lungs. Can repeat 3 total doses given 12 h apart Caution: [?, ?] Disp: Intratracheal susp 35 mg/mL SE: Monitor for cyanosis, airway obst, bradycardia during administration

Candesartan (Atacand) Uses: *HTN,* DN, CHF Action: Angiotensin II receptor antagonist Dose: 4–32 mg/d (usual 16 mg) d Caution: [C (1st tri, D (2nd & 3rd tri), –] CI: Primary hyperaldosteronism; bilateral RAS Disp: Tabs 4, 8, 16, 32 mg SE: Dizziness, HA, flushing, angioedema

Capsaicin (Capsin, Zostrix, others) [OTC] Uses: Pain due to *postherpetic neuralgia,* chronic neuralgia, *arthritis, diabetic neuropathy,* post-op pain, psoriasis, intractable pruritus Action: Topical analgesic Dose: Apply tid-qid Caution: [C, ?] Disp: OTC creams; gel; lotions; roll-ons SE: Local irritation, neurotox, cough Note: Wk to onset of action

Captopril (Capoten, others) Uses: *HTN, CHF, MI,* LVD, DN Action: ACE inhibitor Dose: *Adults.* HTN: Initial, 25 mg PO bid-tid; ↑ to maint q1–2wk by 25-mg increments/dose (max 450 mg/d) to effect. *CHF:* Initial, 6.25–12.5 mg PO tid; titrate PRN LVD: 50 mg PO tid. *DN:* 25 mg PO tid. **Peds Infants <2 mo:** 0.05–0.5 mg/kg/dose PO q8–24h. **Children:** Initial, 0.3–0.5 mg/kg/dose PO; ↑ to 6 mg/kg/d max in 2–4 divided doses; 1 h ac **Caution:** [C (1st tri); D (2nd & 3rd tri) +]; unknown effects in renal impair **CI:** Hx angioedema, bilateral RAS **Disp:** Tabs 12.5, 25, 50, 100 mg **SE:** Rash, proteinuria, cough, ↑ K+

Carbamazepine (Tegretol XR, Carbatrol, Epitol, Equetro)
WARNING: Aplastic anemia & agranulocytosis have been reported w/ carbamazepine; pts w/ Asian ancestry should be tested to determine potential for skin Rxns **Uses:** *Epilepsy, trigeminal neuralgia, acute mania w/ bipolar disorder (Equetro)* EtOH withdrawal **Action:** Anticonvulsant **Dose: Adults.** *Initial:* 200 mg PO bid or 100 mg 4 times/d as susp; ↑ by 200 mg/d; usual 800–1200 mg/d ÷ doses. *Acute Mania (Equetro):* 400 mg/d, divided bid, adjust by 200 mg/d to response 1600 mg/d max. **Peds <6 y:** 5 mg/kg/d, ↑ to 10–20 mg/kg/d in 2–4 doses. **6–12 y:** *Initial:* 100 mg PO bid or 10 mg/kg/24 h PO ÷ daily-bid; ↑ to maint 20–30 mg/kg/24 h ÷ tid-qid; ↓ in renal impair; take w/ food **Caution:** [D, +] **CI:** MAOI use, Hx BM suppression **Disp:** Tabs 100, 200, 400; chew tabs 100 mg, 200 mg; XR tabs 100, 200, 400 mg; *Equetro* Caps ER 100, 200, 300 mg; susp 100 mg/5 mL **SE:** Drowsiness, dizziness, blurred vision, N/V, rash, Stevens-Johnson syndrome (SJS)/toxic epidermal necrolysis (TEN), ↓ Na+, leukopenia, agranulocytosis **Notes:** Monitor CBC & levels; *Trough:* Just before next dose; *Therapeutic: Peak* 8–12 mcg/mL (monotherapy), 4–8 (polytherapy); *Toxic Trough:* >15 mcg/mL; *Half-life:* 15–20 h; generic products not interchangeable, many drug interactions, administer susp in 3–4 ÷ doses daily; skin tox (SJS/TEN) ↑ w/ HLA-B*1502 allele

Carbidopa/Levodopa (Sinemet, Parcopa) Uses: *Parkinson Dz* Action: ↑ CNS dopamine levels Dose: 25/100 mg bid-qid; ↑ as needed (max 200/2000 mg/d) Caution: [C, ?] CI: NAG, suspicious skin lesion (may activate melanoma), melanoma, MAOI use Disp: Tabs (mg carbidopa/mg levodopa) 10/100, 25/100, 25/250; tabs SR (mg carbidopa/mg levodopa) 25/100, 50/200; ODT (oral disintegrating tab) 10/100, 25/100, 25/250 SE: Psych disturbances, orthostatic ↓ BP, dyskinesias, cardiac arrhythmias

Carboplatin (Paraplatin) WARNING: Administration only by physician experienced in cancer chemotherapy; BM suppression possible; anaphylaxis may occur Uses: *Ovarian,* lung, head & neck, testicular, urothelial, & brain *CA, NHL*, & allogeneic & ABMT in high doses Action: DNA cross-linker; forms DNA-platinum adducts Dose: 360 mg/m² (ovarian carcinoma); AUC dosing 4–8 mg/mL (Culvert formula: mg = AUC × [25 + calculated GFR]); adjust based on plt count, CrCl, & BSA (Egorin formula); up to 1500 mg/m² used in ABMT setting (per protocols) Caution: [D, ?] CI: Severe BM suppression, excessive bleeding Disp: Inj 50, 150, 450 mg vial (10 mg/mL) SE: Anaphylaxis, ↓ BM, N/V/D,

nephrotox, hematuria, neurotox, ↑ LFTs **Notes:** Physiologic dosing based on Culvert or Egorin formula allows ↑ doses w/ ↓ tox

Carisoprodol (Soma) **Uses:** *Adjunct to sleep & physical therapy to relieve painful musculoskeletal conditions* **Action:** Centrally acting muscle relaxant **Dose:** 250–350 mg PO tid-qid **Caution:** [C, M] Tolerance may result; w/ renal/hepatic impair **CI:** Allergy to meprobamate; acute intermittent porphyria **Disp:** Tabs 250, 350 mg **SE:** CNS depression, drowsiness, dizziness, HA, tachycardia **Notes:** Avoid EtOH & other CNS depressants; available in combo w/ ASA or codeine.

Carmustine [BCNU] (BiCNU, Gliadel) **WARNING:** BM suppression, dose-related pulm tox possible; administer under direct supervision of experienced physician **Uses:** *Primary or adjunct brain tumors, multiple myeloma, Hodgkin and non-Hodgkin lymphomas* multiple myeloma, induction for allogeneic & ABMT (high dose)* surgery & RT adjunct high-grade glioma and recurrent glioblastoma *(Gliadel* implant)* **Action:** Alkylating agent; nitrosourea forms DNA cross-links to inhibit DNA **Dose:** 150–200 mg/m² q6–8wk single or ÷ dose daily Inj over 2 d; 20–65 mg/m² q4–6wk; 300–900 mg/m² in BMT (per protocols); up to 8 implants in CNS op site; ↓ w/ hepatic & renal impair **Caution:** [D, ?] ↓ WBC, RBC, plt counts, renal/hepatic impair **CI:** ↓ BM, PRG **Disp:** Inj 100 mg/vial; *Gliadel* wafer 7.7 mg **SE:** ↓ BP, N/V, ↓ WBC & plt, phlebitis, facial flushing, hepatic/renal dysfunction, pulm fibrosis (may occur years after), optic neuroretinitis; heme tox may persist 4–6 wk after dose **Notes:** Do not give course more frequently than q6wk (cumulative tox); ✓ baseline PFTs, monitor pulm status

Carteolol (Ocupress, Carteolol Ophthalmic) **Uses:** *HTN, ↑ intraocular pressure, chronic open-angle glaucoma* **Action:** Blocks β-adrenergic receptors (β₁, β₂), mild ISA **Dose:** Ophthal 1 gtt in eye(s) bid **Caution:** [C, ?/–] Cardiac failure, asthma **CI:** Sinus bradycardia; heart block >1st degree; bronchospasm **Disp:** Ophthal soln 1% **SE:** conjunctival hyperemia, anisocoria, keratitis, eye pain **Notes:** Oral forms no longer available in US

Carvedilol (Coreg, Coreg CR) **Uses:** *HTN, Mild to severe CHF, LVD post-MI* **Action:** Blocks adrenergic receptors, β₁, β₂, α₁ **Dose:** *HTN:* 6.25–12.5 mg bid or CR 20–80 mg PO daily. *CHF:* 3.125–25 mg bid; w/ food to minimize ↓ BP **Caution:** [C (1st tri); D (2nd & 3rd tri), ?/–] asthma, DM **CI:** Decompensated CHF, 2nd-/3rd-degree heart block, SSS, severe bradycardia w/o pacemaker, asthma, severe hepatic impair **Disp:** Tabs 3.125, 6.25, 12.5, 25 mg; CR Tabs 10, 20, 40, 80 mg **SE:** Dizziness, fatigue, hyperglycemia, may mask/potentiate hypoglycemia, bradycardia, edema, hypercholesterolemia **Notes:** Do not D/C abruptly; ↑ digoxin levels

Caspofungin (Cancidas) **Uses:** *Invasive aspergillosis refractory/intolerant to standard therapy, esophageal candidiasis* **Action:** Echinocandin; ↓ fungal cell wall synth; highest activity in regions of active cell growth **Dose:** 70 mg IV load day 1, 50 mg/d IV; slow Inf; ↓ in hepatic impair **Caution:** [C, ?/–] Do not use w/ cyclosporine; not studied as initial therapy **CI:** Allergy to any component **Disp:**

Inj 50, 70 mg powder for recons **SE:** Fever, HA, N/V, thrombophlebitis at site, ↑ LFTs **Notes:** Monitor during Inf; limited experience beyond 2 wk of therapy

Cefaclor (Raniclor) **Uses:** *Bacterial Infxns of the upper & lower resp tract, skin, bone, urinary tract, abdomen* **Action:** 2nd-gen cephalosporin; ↓ cell wall synth. *Spectrum:* More gram(–) activity than 1st-gen cephalosporins; effective against gram(+) (*Streptococcus* sp, *S. aureus*); good gram(–) against *H. influenzae*, *E. coli*, *Klebsiella*, *Proteus* **Dose:** *Adults.* 250–500 mg PO tid; ER 375–500 mg bid. *Peds.* 20–40 mg/kg/d PO ÷ 8–12 h; ↓ renal impair **Caution:** [B, +] antacids ↓ absorption ER + Cephalosporin/PCN allergy **Disp:** Caps 250, 500 mg; Tabs ER 375, 500 mg; chew tabs *(Raniclor)* 250, 375 mg; susp 125, 187, 250, 375 mg/5 mL **SE:** N/D, rash, eosinophilia, ↑ LFTs, HA, rhinitis, vaginitis

Cefadroxil (Duricef) **Uses:** *Infxns of skin, bone, upper & lower resp tract, urinary tract* **Action:** 1st-gen cephalosporin; ↓ cell wall synth. *Spectrum:* Good gram(+)(group A β-hemolytic *Streptococcus*, *Staphylococcus*); gram(–) (*E. coli*, *Proteus*, *Klebsiella*) **Dose:** *Adults.* 1–2 g/d PO, 2 ÷ doses *Peds.* 30 mg/kg/d ÷ bid; ↓ in renal impair **Caution:** [B, +] **CI:** Cephalosporin/PCN allergy **Disp:** Caps 500 mg; tabs 1 g; susp, 250, 500 mg/5 mL **SE:** N/V/D, rash, eosinophilia, ↑ LFTs

Cefazolin (Ancef, Kefzol) **Uses:** *Infxns of skin, bone, upper & lower resp tract, urinary tract* **Action:** 1st-gen cephalosporin; β-lactam ↓ cell wall synth. *Spectrum:* Good gram(+) bacilli & cocci, (*Streptococcus*, *Staphylococcus* [except *Enterococcus*]); some gram(–) (*E. coli*, *Proteus*, *Klebsiella*) **Dose:** *Adults.* 1–2 g IV q8h **Peds.** 25–100 mg/kg/d IV ÷ q6–8h; ↓ in renal impair **Caution:** [B, +] **CI:** Cephalosporin/PCN allergy **Disp:** Inj: 500 mg, 1, 10, 20 g **SE:** D, rash, eosinophilia, ↑ LFTs, Inj site pain **Notes:** Widely used for surgical prophylaxis

Cefdinir (Omnicef) **Uses:** *Infxns of the resp system, skin, bone, & urinary tract* **Action:** 3rd-gen cephalosporin; ↓ cell wall synth *Spectrum:* Many gram (+) & (–) organisms; more active than cefaclor & cephalexin against *Streptococcus*, *Staphylococcus*; some anaerobes **Dose:** *Adults.* 300 mg PO bid or 600 mg/d PO. **Peds.** 7 mg/kg PO bid or 14 mg/kg/d PO; ↓ in renal impair **Caution:** [B, +] w/ PCN-sensitive pts, serum sickness-like Rxns reported **CI:** Hypersensitivity to cephalosporins **Disp:** Caps 300 mg; susp 125, 250 mg/5 mL **SE:** Anaphylaxis, D, rare pseudomembranous colitis

Cefditoren (Spectracef) **Uses:** *Acute exacerbations of chronic bronchitis, pharyngitis, tonsillitis; skin Infxns* **Action:** 3rd-gen cephalosporin; ↓ cell wall synth. *Spectrum:* Good gram(+) (*Streptococcus & Staphylococcus*); gram (–) (*H. influenzae & M. catarrhalis*) **Dose:** *Adults & Peds >12 y: Skin:* 200 mg PO bid × 10 d. *Chronic bronchitis, pharyngitis, tonsillitis:* 400 mg PO bid × 10 d; avoid antacids w/ in 2 h; take w/ meals; ↓ in renal impair **Caution:** [B, ?] Renal/hepatic impair **CI:** Cephalosporin/PCN allergy, milk protein, or carnitine deficiency **Disp:** 200 mg tabs **SE:** HA, N/V/D, colitis, nephrotox, hepatic dysfunction, Stevens-Johnson syndrome, toxic epidermal necrolysis, allergic Rxns **Notes:** Causes renal excretion of carnitine; tabs contain milk protein

Cefepime (Maxipime) **Uses:** *comp/uncomp UTI, pneumonia, empiric febrile neutropenia, skin/soft-tissue Infxns, comp intra-Abd Infxns* **Action:** 4th-gen cephalosporin; ↓ cell wall synth. *Spectrum:* gram(+) *S. pneumoniae, S. aureus,* gram(–) *K. pneumoniae, E. coli, P. aeruginosa, & Enterobacter* sp **Dose:** *Adults.* 1–2 g IV q8–12h. *Peds.* 50 mg/kg q8h for febrile neutropenia; 50 mg/kg bid for skin/soft-tissue Infxns; ↓ in renal impair **Caution:** [B, +] CI: Cephalosporin/PCN allergy **Disp:** Inj 500 mg, 1, 2 g **SE:** Rash, pruritus, N/V/D, fever, HA, (+) Coombs test w/o hemolysis **Notes: Can** give IM or IV

Cefixime (Suprax) **Uses:** *Resp tract, skin, bone, & urinary tract Infxns* **Action:** 3rd-gen cephalosporin; ↓ cell wall synth. *Spectrum: S. pneumoniae, S. pyogenes, H. influenzae, & enterobacteria* **Dose:** *Adults.* 400 mg PO ÷ daily-bid. *Peds.* 8–20 mg/kg/d PO ÷ daily-bid; ↓ w/ renal impair **Caution:** [B, +] CI: Cephalosporin/PCN allergy **Disp:** Susp 100, 200 mg/5 mL **SE:** N/V/D, flatulence, & Abd pain **Notes:** Monitor renal & hepatic Fxn; use susp for otitis media

Cefoperazone (Cefobid) **Uses:** *Rx Infxns of the resp, skin, urinary tract, sepsis* **Action:** 3rd-gen cephalosporin; ↓ bacterial cell wall synth. *Spectrum:* gram(–) (eg, *E. coli, Klebsiella*), *P. aeruginosa* but < ceftazidime; gram(+) variable against *Streptococcus & Staphylococcus* sp **Dose:** *Adults.* 2–4 g/d IM/IV ÷ q 8–12h (16 g/d max). *Peds.* (Not approved) 100–150 mg/kg/d IM/IV ÷ bid-tid (12 g/d max); ↓ in renal/hepatic impair **Caution:** [B, +] May ↑ bleeding risk CI: Cephalosporin/PCN allergy **Disp:** Powder for Inj 1, 2, 10 g **SE:** D, rash, eosinophilia, ↑ LFTs, hypoprothrombinemia, & bleeding (due to MTT side chain) **Notes:** May interfere w/ warfarin; disulfiram-like Rxn

Cefotaxime (Claforan) **Uses:** *Infxns of lower resp tract, skin, bone & joint, urinary tract, meningitis, sepsis, PID, GC* **Action:** 3rd-gen cephalosporin; ↓ cell wall synth. *Spectrum:* Most gram(–) (not *Pseudomonas*), some gram(+) cocci *S. pneumoniae, S. aureus* (penicillinase/nonpenicillinase producing), *H. influenzae* (including ampicillin-resistant), not *Enterococcus;* many PCN-resistant pneumococci **Dose:** *Adults. Uncomplicated Infxn:* 2 g IV/IM q12h; *Mod–severe Infxn* 1–2 g IV/IM q 8–12 h; Severe/septicemia 2 g IV/IM q4–8h; *GC urethritis, cervicitis, rectal in female:* 0.5 g IM × 1; rectal GC men 1 g IM × 1; *Peds.* 50–200 mg/kg/d IV ÷ q6–8h; ↓ w/ renal/hepatic impair **Caution:** [B, +] Arrhythmia w/ rapid Inj; w/colitis CI: Cephalosporin/PCN allergy **Disp:** Powder for Inj 500 mg, 1, 2, 10, 20 g, pre-mixed Infs 20 mg/mL, 40 mg/mL **SE:** D, rash, pruritus, colitis, eosinophilia, ↑ transaminases

Cefotetan (Cefotan) **Uses:** *Infxns of the upper & lower resp tract, skin, bone, urinary tract, abdomen, & gynecologic system* **Action:** 2nd-gen cephalosporin; ↓ cell wall synth **Spectrum:** Less active against gram(+) anaerobes including *B. fragilis;* gram(–), including *E. coli, Klebsiella, & Proteus* **Dose:** *Adults.* 1–3 g IV q12h. *Peds.* 20–40 mg/kg/d IV ÷ q12h (6 g/d max) ↓ w/ renal impair **Caution:** [B, +] May ↑ bleeding risk; w/ Hx of PCN allergies; w/ other nephrotoxic drugs CI: Cephalosporin/PCN allergy **Disp:** Powder for Inj 1, 2,

10 g **SE:** D, rash, eosinophilia, ↑ transaminases, hypoprothrombinemia, & bleeding (due to MTT side chain) **Notes:** May interfere w/ warfarin

Cefoxitin (Mefoxin) **Uses:** *Infxns of the upper & lower resp tract, skin, bone, urinary tract, abdomen, & gynecologic system* **Action:** 2nd-gen cephalosporin; ↓ cell wall synth. *Spectrum:* Good gram(–) against enteric bacilli (ie, *E. coli, Klebsiella,* & *Proteus*); anaerobic *B. fragilis* **Dose:** *Adults.* 1–2 g IV q6–8h. **Peds.** 80–160 mg/kg/d ÷ q4–6h (12 g/d max); ↓ w/ renal impair **Caution:** [B, +] **CI:** Cephalosporin/PCN allergy **Disp:** Powder for Inj 1, 2, 10 g **SE:** D, rash, eosinophilia, ↑ transaminases

Cefpodoxime (Vantin) **Uses:** *Rx resp, skin, & urinary tract Infxns* **Action:** 3rd-gen cephalosporin; ↓ cell wall synth. *Spectrum:* S. pneumoniae or non-β-lactamase-producing *H. influenzae*; acute uncomplicated *N. gonorrhoeae*; some uncomplicated gram(–) (*E. coli, Klebsiella, Proteus*) **Dose:** *Adults.* 100–400 mg PO q12h. **Peds.** 10 mg/kg/d PO ÷ bid; ↓ in renal impair, w/ food **Caution:** [B, +] **CI:** Cephalosporin/PCN allergy **Disp:** Tabs 100, 200 mg; susp 50, 100 mg/5 mL **SE:** D, rash, HA, eosinophilia, ↑ transaminases **Notes:** Drug interactions w/ agents that ↑ gastric pH

Cefprozil (Cefzil) **Uses:** *Rx resp tract, skin, & urinary tract Infxns* **Action:** 2nd-gen cephalosporin; ↓ cell wall synth. *Spectrum:* Active against MSSA, *Streptococcus,* & gram(–) bacilli (*E. coli, Klebsiella, P. mirabilis, H. influenzae, Moraxella*) **Dose:** *Adults.* 250–500 mg PO daily-bid. **Peds.** 7.5–15 mg/kg/d PO ÷ bid; ↓ in renal impair **Caution:** [B, +] **CI:** Cephalosporin/PCN allergy **Disp:** Tabs 250, 500 mg; susp 125, 250 mg/5 mL **SE:** D, dizziness, rash, eosinophilia, ↑ transaminases **Notes:** Use higher doses for otitis & pneumonia

Ceftazidime (Fortaz, Tazicef) **Uses:** *Rx resp tract, skin, bone, urinary tract Infxns, meningitis, & septicemia* **Action:** 3rd-gen cephalosporin; ↓ cell wall synth. *Spectrum:* P. aeruginosa sp, good gram(–) activity **Dose:** *Adults.* 500–2 g IV/IM q8–12h. **Peds.** 30–50 mg/kg/dose IV q8h; ↓ in renal impair **Caution:** [B, +] PCN sensitivity **CI:** Cephalosporin/PCN allergy **Disp:** Powder for Inj 500 mg, 1, 2, 6 g **SE:** D, rash, eosinophilia, ↑ transaminases **Notes:** Use only for proven or strongly suspected Infxn to ↓ development of drug resistance

Ceftibuten (Cedax) **Uses:** *Rx resp tract, skin, urinary tract Infxns & otitis media* **Action:** 3rd-gen cephalosporin; ↓ cell wall synth. *Spectrum:* H. influenzae & M. catarrhalis; weak against S. pneumoniae **Dose:** *Adults.* 400 mg/d PO. **Peds.** 9 mg/kg/d PO; ↓ in renal impair; take on empty stomach (susp) **Caution:** [B, +] **CI:** Cephalosporin/PCN allergy **Disp:** Caps 400 mg; susp 90 mg/5 mL **SE:** D, rash, eosinophilia, ↑ transaminases

Ceftizoxime (Cefizox) **Uses:** *Rx resp tract, skin, bone, & urinary tract Infxns, meningitis, septicemia* **Action:** 3rd-gen cephalosporin; ↓ cell wall synth. *Spectrum:* Good gram(–) bacilli (not *Pseudomonas*), some gram(+) cocci (not *Enterococcus*), & some anaerobes **Dose:** *Adults.* 1–4 g IV q8–12h. **Peds.** 150–200 mg/kg/d IV ÷ q6–8h; ↓ in renal impair **Caution:** [B, +] **CI:** Cephalosporin/PCN allergy **Disp:** Inj 1, 2, 10 g **SE:** D, fever, rash, eosinophilia, thrombocytosis, ↑ transaminases

Ceftriaxone (Rocephin) **WARNING:** Avoid in hyperbilirubinemic neonates or coinfused w/ calcium-containing products **Uses:** *Resp tract (pneumonia), skin, bone, Abd, urinary tract Infxns, meningitis, & septicemia* **Action:** 3rd-gen cephalosporin; ↓ cell wall synth. *Spectrum:* Mod gram(+); excellent β-lactamase producers **Dose:** *Adults.* 1–2 g IV/IM q12–24h. *Peds.* 50–100 mg/kg/d IV/IM ÷ q12–24h; ↓ w/ renal impair **Caution:** [B, +] **CI:** Cephalosporin allergy; hyperbilirubinemic neonates **Disp:** Powder for Inj 250 mg, 1, 2, 10 g; premixed 20, 40 mg/mL **SE:** D, rash, leukopenia, thrombocytosis, eosinophilia, ↑ LFTs

Cefuroxime (Ceftin [PO], Zinacef [parenteral]) **Uses:** *Upper & lower resp tract, skin, bone, urinary tract, abdomen, gynecologic Infxns* **Action:** 2nd-gen cephalosporin; ↓ cell wall synth *Spectrum:* Staphylococci, group B streptococci, *H. influenzae*, *E. coli*, *Enterobacter*, *Salmonella*, & *Klebsiella* **Dose:** *Adults.* 750 mg–1.5 g IV q6h or 250–500 mg PO bid. *Peds.* 75–150 mg/kg/d IV ÷ q8h or 20–30 mg/kg/d PO ÷ bid; ↓ w/ renal impair; take PO w/ food **Caution:** [B, +] **CI:** Cephalosporin/PCN allergy **Disp:** Tabs 250, 500 mg; susp 125, 250 mg/5 mL; powder for Inj 750 mg, 1.5, 7.5 g **SE:** D, rash, eosinophilia, ↑ LFTs **Notes:** Cefuroxime film-coated tabs & susp not bioequivalent; do not substitute on a mg/mg basis; IV crosses blood–brain barrier

Celecoxib (Celebrex) **WARNING:** ↑ Risk of serious CV thrombotic events, MI, & stroke, can be fatal; ↑ risk of serious GI adverse events including bleeding, ulceration, & perforation of the stomach or intestines; can be fatal **Uses:** *Osteoarthritis, RA, ankylosing spondylitis acute pain, primary dysmenorrhea preventive in FAP* **Action:** NSAID; ↓ COX-2 pathway **Dose:** 100–200 mg/d or bid; FAP: 400 mg PO bid; ↓ w/ hepatic impair; take w/ food/milk **Caution:** [C/D (3rd tri), ?] **CI:** Renal impair **CI:** Sulfonamide allergy, perioperative coronary artery bypass graft **Disp:** Caps 100, 200 400 mg **SE:** See Warning; GI upset, HTN, edema, renal failure, HA **Notes:** Watch for Sxs of GI bleed; no effect on plt/bleeding time; can affect drugs metabolized by P-450 pathway

Cephalexin (Keflex, Panixine DisperDose) **Uses:** *Skin, bone, upper/lower resp tract (streptococcal pharyngitis), otitis media, uncomp cystitis Infxns* **Action:** 1st-gen cephalosporin; ↓ cell wall synth. *Spectrum: Streptococcus (including β-hemolytic), Staphylococcus, E. coli, Proteus, & Klebsiella* **Dose:** *Adults & Peds ≥15 y:* 250–1000 mg PO qid; Rx cystitis 7–14 d (4 g/d max). *Peds <15 y.* 25–100 mg/kg/d PO ÷ bid-qid; ↓ w/ renal impair; on empty stomach **Caution:** [B, +] **CI:** Cephalosporin/PCN allergy **Disp:** Caps 250, 500 mg; *(Panixine DisperDose)* tabs for oral susp 100, 125, 250 mg; susp 125, 250 mg/5 mL **SE:** D, rash, eosinophilia, gastritis, dyspepsia, ↑ LFTs, *C. difficile* colitis, vaginitis

Cephradine (Velosef) **Uses:** *Resp, GU, GI, skin, soft-tissue, bone, & joint Infxns* **Action:** 1st-gen cephalosporin; ↓ cell wall synth. *Spectrum:* Gram(+)

bacilli & cocci (not *Enterococcus*); some gram(–) (*E. coli, Proteus, & Klebsiella*) **Dose:** *Adults.* 250–500 mg q6–12h (8 g/d max). *Peds >9 mo:* 25–100 mg/kg/d ÷ bid-qid (4 g/d max); ↓ in renal impair **Caution:** [B, +] **CI:** Cephalosporin/PCN allergy **Disp:** Caps: 250, 500 mg; powder for susp 125, 250 mg/5 mL **SE:** Rash, eosinophilia, ↑ LFTs, N/V/D

Certolizumab (Cimzia)   **WARNING:** TB, invasive fungal infxns, and other opportunistic infxns, some fatal, reported. Evaluate for TB risk factors, test for latent TB prior to and during therapy **Uses:** *Tx of Crohn Dz* **Action:** TNF α-blocker **Dose:** *Adults.* 400 mg SQ initially and wk 2 & 4; w/ response then 400 mg SQ q4wk **Caution:** [B, ?]; w/ predisposition to Infxn; do not start therapy during active Infxn; D/C w/ serious Infxn **CI:** None **Disp:** Inj powder 200 mg **SE:** HA, N, nasopharyngitis, UTI, URI, arthralgia, hypersensitivity Rxn, serious Infxns, TB, opportunistic Infxns, malignancies, demyelinating Dz, CHF, pancytopenia, lupus-like syndrome **Notes:** Do not give live/attenuated vaccines during therapy; avoid use with anakinra

Cetirizine (Zyrtec, Zyrtec D) [OTC]   **Uses:** *Allergic rhinitis & other allergic Sxs including urticaria* **Action:** Nonsedating antihistamine; *Zyrtec D* contains decongestant **Dose:** *Adults & Children ≥6 y:* 5–10 mg/d. Zyrtec D 5/120 mg PO bid while **Peds 6–11 mo:** 2.5 mg daily. *12 mo-5 y:* 2.5 mg daily-bid; ↓ to q day in renal/hepatic impair **Caution:** [C, ?/–] w/ HTN, BPH, rare CNS stimulation, DM, heart Dz **CI:** Allergy to cetirizine, hydroxyzine **Disp:** Tabs 5, 10 mg; chew tabs 5, 10 mg; syrup 1 mg/5 mL; *Zyrtec D:* Tabs 5/120 mg (cetirizine/pseudoephedrine) **SE:** HA, drowsiness, xerostomia **Notes:** Can cause sedation; swallow ER tabs whole

Cetuximab (Erbitux)   **WARNING:** Severe Inf Rxns including rapid onset of airway obst (bronchospasm, stridor, hoarseness), urticaria, & ↓ BP; permanent D/C required; ↑ risk sudden death and cardiopulmonary arrest **Uses:** *EGFR + metastatic colorectal CA w/wo irinotecan, unresectable head/neck small cell carcinoma w/ RT; monotherapy in metastatic head/neck cancer* **Action:** Human/mouse recombinant MoAb; binds EGFR, ↓ tumor cell growth **Dose:** Per protocol; load 400 mg/m² IV over 2 h; 250 mg/m² given over 1h × 1 wk **Caution:** [C, –] **Disp:** Inj 100 mg/50 mL **SE:** Acneform rash, asthenia/malaise, N/V/D, Abd pain, alopecia, Inf Rxn, derm tox, interstitial lung Dz, fever, sepsis, dehydration, kidney failure, PE **Notes:** Assess tumor for EGFR before Rx; pretreat w/ diphenhydramine; w/ mild SE ↓ Inf rate by 50%; limit sun exposure

Charcoal, activated (Supterchar, Actidose, Liqui-Char)   **Uses:** *Emergency poisoning by most drugs & chemicals (see CI)* **Action:** Adsorbent detoxicant **Dose:** Give w/ 70% sorbitol (2 mL/kg); repeated use of sorbitol not OK *Adults. Acute intoxication:* 25–100 g/dose. *GI dialysis:* 20–50 g q6h for 1–2 d. *Peds 1–12 y: Acute intoxication:* 1–2 g/kg/dose. *GI dialysis:* 5–10 g/dose q4–8h **Caution:** [C,?] May cause V (hazardous w/ petroleum & caustic ingestions); do not mix w/ dairy **CI:** Not effective for cyanide, mineral acids, caustic alkalis,

organic solvents, iron, EtOH, methanol poisoning, Li; do not use sorbitol in pts w/ fructose intolerance, intestinal obst, nonintact GI tracts **Disp:** Powder, liq, caps **SE:** Some liq soln forms in sorbitol base (a cathartic); V/D, black stools, constipation **Notes:** Charcoal w/ sorbitol not OK in children <1 y; monitor for ↓ K^+ & Mg^{2+}; protect airway in lethargic/comatose pts

Chloral Hydrate (Aquachloral, Supprettes) [C-IV]   **Uses:** *Short-term nocturnal & pre-op sedation* **Action:** Sedative hypnotic; active metabolite trichloroethanol **Dose:** *Adults. Hypnotic:* 500 mg–1 g PO or PR 30 min hs or before procedure. *Sedative:* 250 mg PO or PR tid. *Peds. Hypnotic:* 20–50 mg/kg/24 h PO or PR 30 min hs or before procedure. *Sedative:* 5–15 mg/kg/dose q8h; avoid w/ CrCl <50 mL/min or severe hepatic impair **Caution:** [C, +] Porphyria & in neonates, long-term care facility residents **CI:** Allergy to components; severe renal, hepatic or cardiac Dz **Disp:** Caps 500 mg; syrup 500 mg/5 mL; supp 325, 500 mg **SE:** GI irritation, drowsiness, ataxia, dizziness, nightmares, rash **Notes:** May accumulate; tolerance may develop >2 wk; taper dose; mix syrup in H_2O or fruit juice; do not crush caps; avoid EtOH & CNS depressants

Chlorambucil (Leukeran)   **WARNING:** Myelosuppressive, carcinogenic, teratogenic, associated with infertility **Uses:** *CLL, Hodgkin Dz,* Waldenström macroglobulinemia **Action:** Alkylating agent (nitrogen mustard) **Dose:** (per protocol) 0.1–0.2 mg/kg/d for 3–6 wk or 0.4 mg/kg/dose q2wk; ↓ w/ renal impair **Caution:** [D,?] Sz disorder & BM suppression; affects human fertility **CI:** Previous resistance; alkylating agent allergy; w/ live vaccines **Disp:** Tabs 2 mg **SE:** ↓ BM, CNS stimulation, N/V, drug fever, rash, secondary leukemias, alveolar dysplasia, pulm fibrosis, hepatotoxic **Notes:** Monitor LFTs, CBC, plts, serum uric acid; ↓ dose if pt has received radiation

Chlordiazepoxide (Librium, Mitran, Libritabs) [C-IV]   **Uses:** *Anxiety, tension, EtOH withdrawal,* & pre-op apprehension **Action:** Benzodiazepine; antianxiety agent **Dose:** *Adults. Mild anxiety:* 5–10 mg PO tid-qid or PRN. *Severe anxiety:* 25–50 mg IM, IV, or PO q6–8h or PRN *Peds >6 y:* 0.5 mg/kg/24 h PO or IM ÷ q6–8h; ↓ in renal impair, elderly **Caution:** [D, ?] Resp depression, CNS impair, Hx of drug dependence; avoid in hepatic impair **CI:** Preexisting CNS depression, NAG **Disp:** Caps 5, 10, 25 mg; Inj 100 mg **SE:** Drowsiness, CP, rash, fatigue, memory impair, xerostomia, wgt gain **Notes:** Erratic IM absorption

Chlorothiazide (Diuril)   **Uses:** *HTN, edema* **Action:** Thiazide diuretic **Dose:** *Adults.* 500 mg–1 g PO daily-bid; 100–1000 mg/d IV (for edema only). *Peds >6 mo:* 10–20 mg/kg/24 h PO ÷ bid; 4 mg/kg/d IV; OK w/ food **Caution:** [D,+] **CI:** Sensitivity to thiazides/sulfonamides, anuria **Disp:** Tabs 250, 500 mg; susp 250 mg/5 mL; Inj 500 mg/vial **SE:** ↓ K^+, Na^+, dizziness, hyperglycemia, hyperuricemia, hyperlipidemia, photosensitivity **Notes:** Do not use IM/SQ; take early in the day to avoid nocturia; use sunblock; monitor lytes

Chlorpheniramine (Chlor-Trimeton, others) [OTC]   **WARNING:** OTC meds w/ chlorpheniramine should not be used in peds <2 y **Uses:** *Allergic rhinitis,* common cold **Action:** Antihistamine **Dose:** *Adults.* 4 mg PO q4–6h or 8–12 mg PO bid of ER **Peds.** 0.35 mg/kg/24 h PO ÷ q4–6h or 0.2 mg/kg/24 h SR **Caution:** [C, ?/–] BOO; NAG; hepatic Insuff **CI:** Allergy **Disp:** Tabs 4 mg; chew tabs 2 mg; SR tabs 8, 12 mg **SE:** Anticholinergic SE & sedation common, postural ↓ BP, QT changes, extrapyramidal Rxns, photosensitivity **Notes:** Do not cut/crush/chew ER forms; deaths in pts <2 y; associated w/ cough and cold meds (MMWR 2007;56(01):1–4)

Chlorpromazine (Thorazine) **Uses:** *Psychotic disorders, N/V,* apprehension, intractable hiccups **Action:** Phenothiazine antipsychotic; antiemetic **Dose:** *Adults. Psychosis:* 10–25 mg PO bid-tid (usual 30–2000 mg/d in ÷ doses). *Severe Sxs:* 25 mg IM/IV initial; may repeat in 1–4 h; then 25–50 mg PO or PR tid. *Hiccups:* 25–50 mg PO tid-qid. *Children >6 mo: Psychosis & N/V:* 0.5–1 mg/kg/dose PO q4–6h or IM/IV q6–8h; **Caution:** [C, ?/–] Safety in children <6 mo not established; Szs, avoid w/ hepatic impair; BM suppression **CI:** Sensitivity w/ phenothiazines; NAG **Disp:** Tabs 10, 25, 50, 100, 200 mg; soln 100 mg/mL; Inj 25 mg/mL **SE:** Extrapyramidal SE & sedation; α-adrenergic blocking properties; ↓ BP; ↑ QT interval **Notes:** Do not D/C abruptly; dilute PO conc in 2–4 oz of liq

Chlorpropamide (Diabinese) **Uses:** *Type 2 DM* **Action:** Sulfonylurea; ↑ pancreatic insulin release; ↑ peripheral insulin sensitivity; ↓ hepatic glucose output **Dose:** 100–500 mg/d; w/ food, ↓ hepatic impair **Caution:** [C, ?/–] CrCl < 50 mL/min; ↓ in hepatic impair **CI:** Cross-sensitivity w/ sulfonamides **Disp:** Tabs 100, 250 mg **SE:** HA, dizziness, rash, photosensitivity, hypoglycemia, SIADH **Notes:** Avoid EtOH (disulfiram-like Rxn)

Chlorthalidone (Hygroton, others) **Uses:** *HTN* **Action:** Thiazide diuretic **Dose:** *Adults.* 25–100 mg PO daily. **Peds.** (Not approved) 2 mg/kg/dose PO 3×/wk or 1–2 mg/kg/d PO; ↓ in renal impair; OK w/ food, milk **Caution:** [D, +] **CI:** Cross-sensitivity w/ thiazides or sulfonamides; anuria **Disp:** Tabs 15, 25, 50 mg **SE:** ↓ K+, dizziness, photosensitivity, hyperglycemia, hyperuricemia, sexual dysfunction

Chlorzoxazone (Paraflex, Parafon Forte DSC, others) **Uses:** *Adjunct to rest & physical therapy to relieve discomfort associated w/ acute, painful musculoskeletal conditions* **Action:** Centrally acting skeletal muscle relaxant **Dose:** *Adults.* 250–500 mg PO tid-qid. **Peds.** 20 mg/kg/d in 3–4 ÷ doses **Caution:** [C, ?] Avoid EtOH & CNS depressants **CI:** Severe liver Dz **Disp:** Tabs 250, 500 mg **SE:** Drowsiness, tachycardia, dizziness, hepatotox, angioedema

Cholecalciferol [Vitamin D₃] (Delta D) **Uses:** Dietary supl to Rx vit D deficiency **Action:** ↑ intestinal Ca^{2+} absorption **Dose:** 400–1000 Int Units/d PO **Caution:** [A (D doses above the RDA), +] **CI:** ↑ Ca^{2+}, hypervitaminosis, allergy **Disp:** Tabs 400, 1000 Int Units **SE:** Vit D tox (renal failure, HTN, psychosis) **Notes:** 1 mg cholecalciferol = 40,000 Int Units vit D activity

Cholestyramine (Questran, Questran Light, Prevalite) **Uses:** *Hypercholesterolemia;* hyperlipidemia, pruritus associated w/ partial biliary

obst; D associated w/ excess fecal bile acids* pseudomembranous colitis, dig tox, hyperoxaluria **Action:** Binds intestinal bile acids, forms insoluble complexes **Dose:** A*dults.* Titrate: 4 g/d-bid ↑ to max 24 g/d ÷ 1–6 doses/d. *Peds.* 240 mg/kg/d in 3 ÷ doses **Caution:** [C, ?] Constipation, phenylketonuria, may interfere with other drug absorption; consider supl w/ fat-soluble vits **CI:** Complete biliary or bowel obst; w/ mycophenolate hyperlipoproteinemia types III, IV, V **Disp:** (*Questran*) 4 g cholestyramine resin/9 g powder; (*Prevalite*) w/ aspartame: 4 g resin/5.5 g powder (*Questran Light*) 4 g resin/6.4 g powder **SE:** Constipation, Abd pain, bloating, HA, rash, vit K deficiency **Notes:** OD may cause GI obst; mix 4 g in 2–6 oz of noncarbonated beverage; take other meds 1–2 h before or 6 h after; ✓ lipids

Ciclesonide, Inhalation (Alvesco) **Uses:** *Asthma maint* **Action:** Inhaled steroid **Dose:** *Adults & Peds >12 y:* On bronchodilators alone: 80 mcg bid (320 mcg/d max). *Inhaled corticosteroids:* 80 mcg bid (640 mcg/d max). *On oral corticosteroids:* 320 mcg bid, 640 mcg/d max **Caution:** [C, ?] **CI:** Status asthmaticus or other acute episodes of asthma, hypersensitivity **Disp:** Inh 80, 160 mcg/ actuation **SE:** HA, nasopharyngitis, sinusitis, pharyngolaryngeal pain, URI, arthralgia, nasal congestion **Notes:** Oral *Candida* risk, rinse mouth and spit after, taper systemic steroids slowly when transferring to ciclesonide, monitor growth in pediatric pts, counsel on use of device, clean mouthpiece weekly

Ciclesonide, nasal (Omnaris) **Uses:** Allergic rhinitis **Action:** Nasal corticosteroid **Dose:** *Adults & Peds >12 y.* 2 sprays each nostril 1×/d **Caution:** [C,?/–]w/ Ketoconazole **CI:** Component allergy **Disp:** Intranasal spray susp, 50 mcg/ spray, 120 doses **SE:** adrenal suppression, delayed nasal wound healing, URI, HA, ear pain, epistaxis ↑ risk viral Dz (eg, chickenpox), delayed growth in children

Ciclopirox (Loprox, Penlac) **Uses:** *Tinea pedis, tinea cruris, tinea corporis, cutaneous candidiasis, tinea versicolor, tinea rubrum* **Action:** Antifungal antibiotic; cellular depletion of essential substrates &/or ions **Dose:** *Adults & Peds >10 y:* Massage into affected area bid. *Onychomycosis:* apply to nails daily, w/ removal q7d **Caution:** [B, ?] **CI:** Component sensitivity **Disp:** Cream 0.77%, gel 0.77%, topical susp 0.77%, shampoo 1%, nail lacquer 8% **SE:** Pruritus, local irritation, burning **Notes:** D/C w/ irritation; avoid dressings; gel best for athlete's foot

Cidofovir (Vistide) **WARNING:** Renal impair is the major tox. Follow administration instructions; possible carcinogenic, teratogenic **Uses:** *CMV retinitis w/ HIV* **Action:** Selective inhibition of viral DNA synth **Dose:** *Rx:* 5 mg/kg IV over 1 h once/wk for 2 wk w/ probenecid. *Maint:* 5 mg/kg IV once/2 wk w/ probenecid (2 g PO 3 h prior to cidofovir, then 1 g PO at 2 h & 8 h after cidofovir); ↓ in renal impair **Caution:** [C, –] SCr >1.5 mg/dL or CrCl <55 mL/min or urine protein >100 mg/dL; w/ other nephrotoxic drugs **CI:** Probenecid or sulfa allergy **Disp:** Inj 75 mg/mL **SE:** Renal tox, chills, fever, HA, N/V/D, thrombocytopenia, neutropenia **Notes:** Hydrate w/ NS prior to each Inf

Cilostazol (Pletal) **Uses:** *Reduce Sxs of intermittent claudication* **Action:** Phosphodiesterase III inhibitor; ↑ s cAMP in plts & blood vessels, vasodilate & inhibit plt aggregation **Dose:** 100 mg PO bid, 1/2 h before or 2 h after breakfast & dinner **Caution:** [C, +/–] ↓ dose w/ drugs that inhibit CYP3A4 & CYP2C19 (Table 11) **CI:** CHF, hemostatic disorders, active pathologic bleeding **Disp:** Tabs 50, 100 mg **SE:** HA, palpitation, D

Cimetidine (Tagamet) (Tagamet HB, Tagamet DS OTC) **Uses:** *Duodenal ulcer; ulcer prophylaxis in hypersecretory states (eg, trauma, burns); & GERD* **Action:** H_2-receptor antagonist **Dose:** *Adults. Active ulcer:* 2400 mg/d IV cont Inf or 300 mg IV q6h; 400 mg PO bid or 800 mg hs. *Maint:* 400 mg PO hs. *GERD:* 300–600 mg PO q6h; maint 800 mg PO hs. *Peds. Infants:* 10–20 mg/kg/24 h PO or IV ÷ q6–12h. *Children:* 20–40 mg/kg/24 h IV or PO ÷ q6h; ↓ w/ renal Insuff & in elderly **Caution:** [B, +] Many drug interactions (P-450 system) **CI:** Component sensitivity **Disp:** Tabs 200, 300, 400, 800 mg; liq 300 mg/5 mL; Inj 300 mg/2 mL **SE:** Dizziness, HA, agitation, thrombocytopenia, gynecomastia **Notes:** 1 h before or 2 h after antacids; avoid EtOH

Cinacalcet (Sensipar) **Uses:** *Secondary hyperparathyroidism in CRF; ↑ Ca^{2+} in parathyroid carcinoma* **Action:** ↓ PTH by ↑ calcium-sensing receptor sensitivity **Dose:** *Secondary hyperparathyroidism:* 30 mg PO daily. *Parathyroid carcinoma:* 30 mg PO bid, titrate q2–4wk based on calcium & PTH levels; swallow whole; take w/ food **Caution:** [C, ?/–] w/ Szs, adjust w/ CYP3A4 inhibitors (Table 11) **Disp:** Tabs 30, 60, 90 mg **SE:** N/V/D, myalgia, dizziness, ↓ Ca^{2+} **Notes:** Monitor Ca^{2+}, PO_4^{-2}, PTH

Ciprofloxacin (Cipro, Cipro XR, Proquin XR) **WARNING:** ↑ risk of tendonitis and tendon rupture **Uses:** *Rx lower resp tract, sinuses, skin & skin structure, bone/joints, & UT Infxns, including prostatitis* **Action:** Quinolone antibiotic; ↓ DNA gyrase. **Spectrum:** Broad gram(+) & (–) aerobics; few *Streptococcus*; good *Pseudomonas, E. coli, B. fragilis, P. mirabilis, K. pneumoniae, C. jejuni,* or *Shigella* **Dose:** *Adults.* 250–750 mg PO q12h; XR 500–1000 mg PO q24h; or 200–400 mg IV q12h; ↓ in renal impair **Caution:** [C, ?/–] *Children <18 y* **CI:** Component sensitivity **Disp:** Tabs 100, 250, 500, 750 mg; Tabs XR 500, 1000 mg; susp 5 g/100 mL, 10 g/100 mL; Inj 200, 400 mg; premixed piggyback 200, 400 mg/100 mL **SE:** Restlessness, N/V/D, rash, ruptured tendons, ↑ LFTs **Notes:** Avoid antacids; reduce/restrict caffeine intake; interactions w/ theophylline, caffeine, sucralfate, warfarin, antacids, most tendon problems in Achilles, rare shoulder and hand

Ciprofloxacin, ophthalmic (Ciloxan) **Uses:** *Rx & prevention of ocular Infxns (conjunctivitis, blepharitis, corneal abrasions)* **Action:** Quinolone antibiotic; ↓ DNA gyrase **Dose:** 1–2 gtt in eye(s) q2h while awake for 2 d, then 1–2 gtt q4h while awake for 5 d, oint 1/2-inch ribbon in eye tid × 2 d, then bid × 5 d **Caution:** [C, ?/–] **CI:** Component sensitivity **Disp:** Soln 3.5 mg/mL; oint 0.3%, 35 g **SE:** Local irritation

Ciprofloxacin & Dexamethasone, otic (Ciprodex Otic) **Uses:** *Otitis externa, otitis media peds* **Action:** Quinolone antibiotic; ↓ DNA gyrase;

w/ steroid **Dose:** *Adults.* 4 gtt in ear(s) bid × 7 d. *Peds >6 mo:* *4* gtt in ear(s) bid for 7 d **Caution:** [C, ?/–] **CI:** viral ear Infxns **Disp:** Susp ciprofloxacin 0.3% & dexamethasone 1% **SE:** ear discomfort **Notes:** OK w/ tympanostomy tubes

Ciprofloxacin and Hydrocortisone, otic (Cipro HC Otic)
Uses: *Otitis externa* **Action:** Quinolone antibiotic; ↓ DNA gyrase; w/ steroid **Dose:** *Adults & Peds >1 mo.* 1–2 gtt in ear(s) bid × 7 d **Caution:** [C, ?/–] **CI:** Perforated tympanic membrane, viral Infxns of the external canal **Disp:** Susp ciprofloxacin 0.2% & hydrocortisone 1% **SE:** HA, pruritus

Cisplatin (Platinol, Platinol AQ)   **WARNING:** Anaphylactic-like Rxn, ototox, cumulative renal tox; doses >100 mg/m² q3–4wk rarely used, do not confuse w/ carboplatin **Uses:** *Testicular, bladder, ovarian,* SCLC, NSCLC, breast, head & neck, & penile CAs; osteosarcoma; ped brain tumors **Action:** DNA-binding; denatures double helix; intrastrand cross-linking **Dose:** 10–20 mg/m²/d for 5 d q3wk; 50–120 mg/m² q3–4wk (per protocols); ↓ w/ renal impair **Caution:** [D, –] Cumulative renal tox may be severe; ↓ BM, hearing impair, preexisting renal Insuff **CI:** w/ anthrax or live vaccines, platinum-containing compound allergy; w/ cidofovir **Disp:** Inj 1 mg/mL **SE:** Allergic Rxns, N/V, nephrotox (↑ w/ administration of other nephrotoxic drugs; minimize by NS Inf & mannitol diuresis), high-frequency hearing loss in 30%, peripheral "stocking glove"-type neuropathy, cardiotox (ST, T-wave changes), ↓ Mg²⁺, mild ↓ BM, hepatotox; renal impair dose-related & cumulative **Notes:** Give taxanes before platinum derivatives; ✓ Mg²⁺, lytes before & w/in 48 h after cisplatin

Citalopram (Celexa)   **WARNING:** Closely monitor for worsening depression or emergence of suicidality, particularly in pts <24 y **Uses:** *Depression* **Action:** SSRI **Dose:** Initial 20 mg/d, may ↑ to 40 mg/d; ↓ in elderly & hepatic/renal Insuff **Caution:** [C, +/–] Hx of mania, Szs & pts at risk for suicide **CI:** MAOI or w/in 14 d of MAOI use **Disp:** Tabs 10, 20, 40 mg; soln 10 mg/5 mL **SE:** Somnolence, insomnia, anxiety, xerostomia, N, diaphoresis, sexual dysfunction **Notes:** May cause ↓ Na⁺/SIADH

Cladribine (Leustatin)   **WARNING:** Dose-dependent reversible myelo-suppression; neurotox, nephrotox, administer by physician with experience in chemotherapy regimens **Uses:** *HCL, CLL, NHLs, progressive MS* **Action:** Induces DNA strand breakage; interferes w/ DNA repair/synth; purine nucleoside analog **Dose:** 0.09–0.1 mg/kg/d cont IV Inf for 1–7 d (per protocols); ↓ w/ renal impair **Caution:** [D, ?/–] Causes neutropenia & Infxn **CI:** Component sensitivity **Disp:** Inj 1 mg/mL **SE:** ↓ BM, T-lymphocyte ↓ may be prolonged (26–34 wk), fever in 46%, tumor lysis syndrome, Infxns (especially lung & IV sites), rash (50%), HA, fatigue, N/V **Notes:** Consider prophylactic allopurinol; monitor CBC

Clarithromycin (Biaxin, Biaxin XL)   **Uses:** *Upper/lower resp tract, skin/skin structure Infxns, H. pylori Infxns, & Infxns caused by nontuberculosis (atypical) Mycobacterium; prevention of MAC Infxns in HIV-Infxn*

Action: Macrolide antibiotic, ↓ protein synth. *Spectrum: H. influenzae, M. catarrhalis, S. pneumoniae, M. pneumoniae, & H. pylori* **Dose: Adults.** 250–500 mg PO bid or 1000 mg (2 × 500 mg XL tab)/d. *Mycobacterium:* 500 mg PO bid. *Peds >6 mo:* 7.5 mg/kg/dose PO bid; ↓ w/ renal impair **Caution:** [C, ?] Antibiotic-associated colitis; rare QT prolongation & ventricular arrhythmias, including torsade de pointes **CI:** Macrolide allergy; w/ ranitidine in pts w/ Hx of porphyria or CrCl <25 mL/min **Disp:** Tabs 250, 500 mg; susp 125, 250 mg/5 mL; 500 mg XL tab **SE:** ↑ QT interval, causes metallic taste, N/D, Abd pain, HA, rash **Notes:** Multiple drug interactions, ↑ theophylline & carbamazepine levels; do not refrigerate susp

Clemastine Fumarate (Tavist, Dayhist, Antihist-1) [OTC]

Uses: *Allergic rhinitis & Sxs of urticaria* **Action:** Antihistamine **Dose: Adults & Peds >12 y:** 1.34 mg bid-2.68 mg tid; max 8.04 mg/d *<6 y:* 0.335–0.670 mg/d ÷ into 2–3 doses (max 1.34 mg/d), *6–12 y:* 0.67–1.34 mg bid (max 4.02 /d) **Caution:** [B, M] BOO; Do not take w/ MAOI **CI:** NAG **Disp:** Tabs 1.34, 2.68 mg; syrup 0.67 mg/5 mL **SE:** Drowsiness, dyscoordination, epigastric distress, urinary retention **Notes:** Avoid EtOH

Clindamycin (Cleocin, Cleocin-T, others)

WARNING: Pseudomembranous colitis may range from mild to life-threatening **Uses:** *Rx aerobic & anaerobic Infxns; topical for severe acne & vaginal Infxns* **Action:** Bacteriostatic; interferes w/ protein synth. *Spectrum:* Streptococci, pneumococci, staphylococci, & gram(+) & (–) anaerobes; no activity against gram(–) aerobes **Dose: Adults.** PO: 150–450 mg PO q6–8h. *IV:* 300–600 mg IV q6h or 900 mg IV q8h. *Vaginal:* 1 applicator hs for 7 d. **Topical:** Apply 1% gel, lotion, or soln bid. *Peds Neonates:* (Avoid use; contains benzyl alcohol) 10–15 mg/kg/24 h ÷ q8–12h. *Children >1 mo:* 10–30 mg/kg/24 h ÷ q6–8h, to a max of 1.8 g/d PO or 4.8 g/d IV. *Topical:* Apply 1%, gel, lotion, or soln bid; ↓ in severe hepatic impair **Caution:** [B, +] Can cause fatal colitis **CI:** Hx pseudomembranous colitis **Disp:** Caps 75, 150, 300 mg; susp 75 mg/5 mL; Inj 300 mg/2 mL; vaginal cream 2%, topical soln 1%, gel 1%, lotion 1%, vaginal supp 100 mg **SE:** D may be C. difficile pseudomembranous colitis, rash, ↑ LFTs **Notes:** D/C drug w/ D, evaluate for C. difficile

Clofarabine (Clolar)

Uses: *Rx relapsed/refractory ALL after at least 2 regimens in children 1–21 y* **Action:** Antimetabolite; ↓ ribonucleotide reductase w/ false nucleotide base-inhibiting DNA synth **Dose:** 52 mg/m^2 IV over 2 h daily × 5 d (repeat q2–6wk); per protocol **Caution:** [D, –] **Disp:** Inj 20 mg/20 mL **SE:** N/V/D, anemia, leukopenia, thrombocytopenia, neutropenia, Infxn, ↑ AST/ALT **Notes:** Monitor for tumor lysis syndrome & systemic inflammatory response syndrome (SIRS)/capillary leak syndrome; hydrate well

Clonazepam (Klonopin) [C-IV]

Uses: *Lennox-Gastaut syndrome, akinetic & myoclonic Szs, absence Szs, panic attacks,* restless legs syndrome, neuralgia, parkinsonian dysarthria, bipolar disorder **Action:** Benzodiazepine; anticonvulsant **Dose: Adults.** 1.5 mg/d PO in 3 ÷ doses; ↑ by 0.5–1 mg/d q3d PRN up to 20 mg/d. *Peds.* 0.01–0.03 mg/kg/24 h PO ÷ tid; ↑ to 0.1–0.2 mg/kg/24 h ÷ tid;

avoid abrupt D/C **Caution:** [D, M] Elderly pts, resp Dz, CNS depression, severe hepatic impair, NAG **CI:** Severe liver Dz, acute NAG **Disp:** Tabs 0.5, 1, 2 mg, oral disintegrating tabs 0.125, 0.25, 0.5, 1, 2 mg **SE:** CNS side effects, including drowsiness, dizziness, ataxia, memory impair **Notes:** Can cause retrograde amnesia; a CYP3A4 substrate

Clonidine, oral (Catapres)
Uses: *HTN*; opioid, EtOH, & tobacco withdrawal, ADHD **Action:** Centrally acting α-adrenergic stimulant **Dose:** *Adults.* 0.1 mg PO bid, adjust daily by 0.1- to 0.2-mg increments (max 2.4 mg/d). *Peds.* 5–10 mcg/kg/d ÷ q8–12h (max 0.9 mg/d); ↓ in renal impair **Caution:** [C, +/–] Avoid w/ β-blocker, elderly, severe CV Dz, renal impair **CI:** Component sensitivity **Disp:** Tabs 0.1, 0.2, 0.3 mg **SE:** drowsiness, orthostatic ↓ BP, xerostomia, constipation, bradycardia, dizziness **Notes:** More effective for HTN if combined w/ diuretics; withdraw slowly, rebound HTN w/ abrupt D/C of doses >0.2 mg bid; ADHD use in peds needs CV assessment before starting epidural clonidine (Duraclon) used for chronic CA pain

Clonidine, transdermal (Catapres TTS)
Uses: *HTN* **Action:** Centrally acting α-adrenergic stimulant **Dose:** 1 patch q7d to hairless area (upper arm/torso); titrate to effect; ↓ w/ severe renal impair; **Caution:** [C, +/–] Avoid w/ β-blocker, withdraw slowly, in elderly, severe CV Dz and w/ renal impair **CI:** Component sensitivity **Disp:** TTS-1, TTS-2, TTS-3 (delivers 0.1, 0.2, 0.3 mg, respectively, of clonidine/d for 1 wk) **SE:** Drowsiness, orthostatic ↓ BP, xerostomia, constipation, bradycardia **Notes:** Do not D/C abruptly (rebound HTN) Doses >2 TTS-3 usually not associated w/ ↑ efficacy; steady state in 2–3 d

Clopidogrel (Plavix)
Uses: *Reduce atherosclerotic events,* administer ASAP in ECC setting w/ high-risk ST depression or T-wave inversion **Action:** ↓ Plt aggregation **Dose:** 75 mg/d; 300–600 mg PO × 1 dose can be used to load pts; 300 mg PO, then 75 mg/d 1–9 mo *(ECC 2005)* **Caution:** [B, ?] Active bleeding; risk of bleeding from trauma & other; TTP; liver Dz **CI:** Coagulation disorders, active/ intracranial bleeding; CABG planned w/in 5–7 d **Disp:** Tabs 75, 300 mg **SE:** ↑ bleeding time, GI intolerance, HA, dizziness, rash, thrombocytopenia, ↓ WBC **Notes:** Plt aggregation to baseline ~ 5 d after D/C, plt transfusion to reverse acutely

Clorazepate (Tranxene) [C-IV]
Uses: *Acute anxiety disorders, acute EtOH withdrawal Sxs, adjunctive therapy in partial Szs* **Action:** Benzodiazepine; antianxiety agent **Dose:** *Adults.* 15–60 mg/d PO single or ÷ doses. *Elderly & debilitated pts:* Initial 7.5–15 mg/d in ÷ doses. *EtOH withdrawal:* Day 1: Initial 30 mg; then 30–60 mg ÷ doses; Day 2: 45–90 mg ÷ doses; Day 3: 22.5–45 mg ÷ doses; Day 4: 15–30 mg ÷ doses. *Peds.* 3.75–7.5 mg/dose bid to 60 mg/d max ÷ bid-tid **Caution:** [D, ?/–] Elderly, Hx depression **CI:** NAG; Not OK <9 y of age **Disp:** Tabs 3.75, 7.5, 15 mg; Tabs-SD (daily) 11.25, 22.5 mg **SE:** CNS depressant effects (drowsiness, dizziness, ataxia, memory impair), ↓ BP **Notes:** Monitor pts w/ renal/ hepatic impair (drug may accumulate); avoid abrupt D/C; may cause dependence

Clotrimazole (Lotrimin, Mycelex, others) [OTC] Uses: *Candidiasis & tinea Infxns* **Action:** Antifungal; alters cell wall permeability. *Spectrum:* Oropharyngeal candidiasis, dermatophytoses, superficial mycoses, cutaneous candidiasis, & vulvovaginal candidiasis **Dose:** *PO: Prophylaxis:* 1 troche dissolved in mouth tid *Rx:* 1 troche dissolved in mouth 5×/d for 14 d. *Vaginal 1% Cream:* 1 applicator-full hs for 7 d. *2% Cream:* 1 applicator-full hs for 3 d *Tabs:* 100 mg vaginally hs for 7 d or 200 mg (2 tabs) vaginally hs for 3 d or 500-mg tabs vaginally hs once. *Topical:* Apply bid 10–14 d **Caution:** [B (C if PO), ?] Not for systemic fungal Infxn; safety in children <3 y not established **CI:** Component allergy **Disp:** 1% cream; soln; lotion; troche 10 mg; vaginal tabs 100, 200, 500 mg; vaginal cream 1%, 2% **SE:** *Topical:* Local irritation; *PO:* N/V, ↑ LFTs **Notes:** PO prophylaxis immunosuppressed pts

Clotrimazole & Betamethasone (Lotrisone) Uses: *Fungal skin Infxns* **Action:** Imidazole antifungal & anti-inflammatory. *Spectrum:* Tinea pedis, cruris, & corpora **Dose:** ≥17 y. Apply & massage into area bid for 2–4 wk **Caution:** [C, ?] Varicella Infxn <12 y **Disp:** Cream 1/0.05% 15, 45 g; lotion 1/0.05% 30 mL **SE:** Local irritation, rash **Notes:** Not for diaper dermatitis or under occlusive dressings

Clozapine (Clozaril & FazaClo) WARNING: Myocarditis, agranulocytosis, Szs, & orthostatic ↓ BP associated w/ clozapine; ↑ mortality in elderly w/ dementia-related psychosis Uses: *Refractory severe schizophrenia*; childhood psychosis; obsessive-compulsive disorder (OCD), bipolar disorder **Action:** "Atypical" TCA **Dose:** 25 mg daily-bid initial; ↑ to 300–450 mg/d over 2 wk; maintain lowest dose possible; do not D/C abruptly **Caution:** [B, +/–] Monitor for psychosis & cholinergic rebound **CI:** Uncontrolled epilepsy; comatose state; WBC <3500 cells/mm³ and ANC <2000 cells/mm³ before Rx or <3000 cells/mm³ during Rx **Disp:** Orally disintegrating tabs 12.5, 25, 100 mg; tabs 25, 100 mg **SE:** Sialorrhea, tachycardia, drowsiness, ↑ wgt, constipation, incontinence, rash, Szs, CNS stimulation, hyperglycemia **Notes:** Avoid activities where sudden loss of consciousness could cause harm; benign temperature ↑ may occur during the 1st 3 wk of Rx, weekly CBC mandatory 1st 6 mo, then q other wk

Cocaine [C-II] Uses: *Topical anesthetic for mucous membranes* **Action:** Narcotic analgesic, local vasoconstrictor **Dose:** Lowest topical amount that provides relief; 1 mg/kg max **Caution:** [C, ?] **CI:** PRG, ocular anesthesia **Disp:** Topical soln & viscous preparations 4–10%; powder **SE:** CNS stimulation, nervousness, loss of taste/smell, chronic rhinitis, CV tox, abuse potential **Notes:** Use only on PO, laryngeal, & nasal mucosa; do not use on extensive areas of broken skin

Codeine [C-II] Uses: *Mild-mod pain; symptomatic relief of cough* **Action:** Narcotic analgesic; ↓ cough reflex **Dose:** *Adults. Analgesic:* 15–20 mg PO or IM qid PRN. *Antitussive:* 10–20 mg PO q4h PRN; max 120 mg/d. *Peds. Analgesic:* 0.5–1 mg/kg/dose PO q4–6h PRN. *Antitussive:* 1–1.5 mg/kg/24 h PO ÷ q4h; max 30 mg/24 h; ↓ in renal/hepatic impair **Caution:** [C (D if prolonged use or high dose at term), +] CNS depression, Hx drug abuse, severe hepatic impair **CI:** Component sensitivity **Disp:** Tabs 15, 30, 60 mg; soln 15 mg/5 mL; Inj 15, 30 mg/mL **SE:** Drowsiness, constipation, ↓ BP **Notes:** Usually combined w/ APAP for pain or w/ agents (eg, terpin hydrate) as an antitussive; 120 mg IM = 10 mg IM morphine

Colchicine
Uses: *Acute gouty arthritis & prevention of recurrences; familial Mediterranean fever*; primary biliary cirrhosis **Action:** ↓ migration of leukocytes; ↓ leukocyte lactic acid production **Dose:** *Initial:* 0.6–1.2 mg PO, then 0.6 mg q1–2h until relief or GI SE develop (max 8 mg/d); do not repeat for 3 d. *Prophylaxis:* PO: 0.6 mg/d or 3–4 d/wk; ↓ renal impair **Caution:** [D, +] Elderly **CI:** Serious renal, GI, hepatic, or cardiac disorders; blood dyscrasias **Disp:** Tabs 0.6 mg **SE:** N/V/D, Abd pain, BM suppression, hepatotox; local Rxn w/ SQ/IM **Notes:** IV no longer available

Colesevelam (WelChol)
Uses: *Reduction of LDL & total cholesterol alone or in combo w/ an HMG-CoA reductase inhibitor* **Action:** Bile acid sequestrant **Dose:** 3 tabs PO bid or 6 tabs daily w/ meals **Caution:** [B, ?] Severe GI motility disorders; in pts w/ triglycerides >300 mg/dL (may ↑ levels); use not established in peds **CI:** Bowel obst, serum triglycerides >500; hx hypertriglyceridemia-pancreatitis **Disp:** Tabs 625 mg **SE:** Constipation, dyspepsia, myalgia, weakness **Notes:** May ↓ absorption of fat-soluble vits

Colestipol (Colestid)
Uses: *Adjunct to ↓ serum cholesterol in primary hypercholesterolemia, relieve pruritus associated w/ ↑ bile acids* **Action:** Binds intestinal bile acids to form insoluble complex **Dose:** *Granules:* 5–30 g/d ÷ 2–4 doses; tabs: 2–16 g/d ÷ daily-bid **Caution:** [C, ?] Avoid w/ high triglycerides, GI dysfunction **CI:** Bowel obst **Disp:** Tabs 1 g; granules 5, 7.5, 300, 450, 500 g **SE:** Constipation, Abd pain, bloating, HA, GI irritation & bleeding **Notes:** Do not use dry powder; mix w/ beverages, cereals, etc; may ↓ absorption of other meds and fat-soluble vits

Conivaptan HCL (Vaprisol)
Uses: Euvolemic & hypervolemic hyponatremia **Action:** Dual arginine vasopressin V_{1A}/V_2 receptor antagonist **Dose:** 20 mg IV × 1 over 30 min, then 20 mg cont IV Inf over 24 h; 20 mg/d cont IV Inf for 1–3 more d; may ↑ to 40 mg/d if Na^+ not responding; 4 d max use; use large vein, change site q24h **Caution:** [C; ?/–] Rapid ↑ Na^+ (>12 mEq/L/24 h) may cause osmotic demyelination syndrome; impaired renal/hepatic Fxn; may ↑ digoxin levels; CYP3A4 inhibitor (Table 11) **CI:** Hypovolemic hyponatremia; w/ CYP3A4 inhibitors **Disp:** Amp 20 mg/4 mL **SE:** Inf site Rxns, HA, N/V/D, constipation, ↓ K^+, orthostatic ↓ BP, thirst, dry mouth, pyrexia, pollakiuria, polyuria, Infxn **Notes:** Monitor Na^+, vol and neurologic status; D/C w/ very rapid ↑ Na^+; mix only w/ 5% dextrose

Copper IUD Contraceptive (ParaGard T 380A)
Uses: *Contraception, long-term (up to 10 y)* **Action:** ?, interfere w/ sperm survival/transport **Dose:** Insert any time during menstrual cycle; replace at 10 y max **Caution:** [C, ?]

Remove w/ intrauterine PRG, increased risk of comps w/ PRG and device in place **CI:** Acute PID or in high-risk behavior, postpartum endometritis, cervicitis **Disp:** 52 mg IUD **SE:** PRG, ectopic PRG, pelvic Infxn immunocompromise, embedment, perforation expulsion, Wilson Dz, fainting w/ insert, vag bleeding, expulsion **Notes:** Counsel patient does not protect against STD/HIV; see insert for detailed instructions; 99% effective

Cortisone See Steroids (page 214) and Tables 3 & 4

Cromolyn Sodium (Intal, NasalCrom, Opticrom, others)
Uses: *Adjunct to the Rx of asthma; prevent exercise-induced asthma; allergic rhinitis; ophthal allergic manifestations*; food allergy, systemic mastocytosis, IBD **Action:** Antiasthmatic; mast cell stabilizer **Dose:** *Adults & Children >12 y: Inh:* 20 mg (as powder in caps) inhaled qid or metered-dose inhaler 2 puffs qid. *PO:* 200 mg qid 15–20 min ac, up to 400 mg qid. *Nasal instillation:* Spray once in each nostril 2–6 ×/d. *Ophthal:* 1–2 gtt in each eye 4–6 × d. *Peds. Inh:* 2 puffs qid of metered-dose inhaler. *PO:* **Infants <2 y:** (not OK) 20 mg/kg/d in 4 ÷ doses. **2–12 y:** 100 mg qid ac feeding **Caution:** [B, ?] w/ Renal/hepatic impair **CI:** Acute asthmatic attacks **Disp:** PO conc 100 mg/5 mL; soln for nebulizer 20 mg/2 mL; metered-dose inhaler; nasal soln 40 mg/mL; ophthal soln 4% **SE:** Unpleasant taste, hoarseness, coughing **Notes:** No benefit in acute Rx; 2–4 wk for maximal effect in perennial allergic disorders

Cyanocobalamin [Vitamin B₁₂] (Nascobal) **Uses:** *Pernicious anemia & other vit B₁₂ deficiency states; ↑ requirements due to PRG; thyrotoxicosis; liver or kidney Dz* **Action:** Dietary vit B₁₂ supl **Dose:** *Adults.* 30 mcg/d × 5–10 d; 100 mcg IM or SQ daily; intranasal: 500 mcg once/wk for pts in remission, for 5–10 d, then 100 mcg IM 2 ×/wk for 1 mo, then 100 mcg IM monthly. *Peds.* Use 0.2 mcg/kg × 2 d test dose; if OK 30–50 mcg/d for 2 or more wk (total 10 mcg) then maint: 100 mg/mo. **Caution:** [A (C if dose exceeds RDA), +] **CI:** Allergy to cobalt; hereditary optic nerve atrophy; Leber Dz **Disp:** Tabs 50, 100, 250, 500, 1000, 2500, 5000 mcg; Inj 100, 1000 mcg/mL; intranasal (Nascobal) gel 500 mcg/0.1 mL **SE:** Itching, D, HA, anxiety **Notes:** PO absorption erratic and not; ok for use w/ hyperalimentation

Cyclobenzaprine (Flexeril) **Uses:** *Relief of muscle spasm* **Action:** Centrally acting skeletal muscle relaxant; reduces tonic somatic motor activity **Dose:** 5–10 mg PO bid-qid (2–3 wk max) **Caution:** [B, ?] Shares the toxic potential of the TCAs; urinary hesitancy, NAG **CI:** Do not use concomitantly or w/in 14 d of MAOIs; hyperthyroidism; heart failure; arrhythmias **Disp:** Tabs 5, 10 mg **SE:** Sedation & anticholinergic effects **Notes:** May inhibit mental alertness or physical coordination

Cyclobenzaprine, extended release (Amrix) **Uses:** *Muscle spasm* **Action:** ? Centrally acting long-term muscle relaxant **Dose:** 15–30 mg PO daily 2–3 wk; 30 mg/d max **Caution:** [B, ?/–] w/ Urinary retention, NAG, w/ EtOH/CNS depressant **CI:** MAOI w/in 14 d, elderly, arrhythmias, heart block,

CHF, MI recovery phase, ↑ thyroid **Disp:** Caps 15, 30 ER **SE:** Dry mouth, drowsiness, dizziness, HA, N, blurred vision, dysgeusia **Notes:** Avoid abrupt D/C w/ long-term use

Cyclopentolate, ophthalmic (Cyclogyl, Cylate)
Uses: *Cycloplegia, mydriasis* **Action:** Cycloplegic mydriatic, anticholinergic inhibits iris sphincter and ciliary body **Dose:** *Adults.* 1 gtt in eye 40–50 min preprocedure, may repeat × 1 in 5–10 min **Peds.** As adult, children 0.5%; infants use 0.5% **Caution:** (C [may cause late-term fetal anoxia/bradycardia, +/–], premature infants HTN, Down syndrome, elderly, **CI:** NAG Glaucoma **Disp:** Ophthal soln 0.5, 1, 2% **SE:** Tearing, HA, irritation, eye pain, photophobia, arrhythmia, tremor, ↑ IOP, confusion **Notes:** Compress lacrimal sac for several min after dose; heavily pigmented irises may require ↑ strength; peak 25–75 min, cycloplegia 6–24 h, mydriasis up to 24 h; 2% soln may result in psychotic Rxns and behavioral disturbances in peds

Cyclopentolate with Phenylephrine (Cyclomydril)
Uses: *Mydriasis greater than cyclopentolate alone* **Action:** Cycloplegic mydriatic, α-adrenergic agonist w/ anticholinergic to inhibit iris sphincter **Dose:** 1 gtt in eye q 5–10 min (max 3 doses) 40–50 min preprocedure **Caution:** (C [may cause late-term fetal anoxia/bradycardia, +/–] HTN, elderly w/ CAD **CI:** NAG Glaucoma **Disp:** Ophthal soln cyclopentolate 0.2%/phenlephrine 1% (2, 5 mL) **SE:** Tearing, HA, irritation, eye pain, photophobia, arrhythmia, tremor **Notes:** Compress lacrimal sac for several min after dose; heavily pigmented irises may require ↑ strength; peak 25–75 min, cycloplegia 6–24 h, mydriasis up to 24 h

Cyclophosphamide (Cytoxan, Neosar)
Uses: *Hodgkin Dz & NHLs; multiple myeloma; small cell lung, breast, & ovarian Ca; mycosis fungoides; neuroblastoma; retinoblastoma; acute leukemias; allogeneic & ABMT in high doses; severe rheumatologic disorders (SLE, JRA)* **Action:** Alkylating agent **Dose:** *Adults.* (per protocol) 500–1500 mg/m^2; single dose 2- to 4-wk intervals; 1.8 g/m^2 to 160 mg/kg (at 12 g/m^2 in 75-kg individual) in the BMT setting (per protocols). *Peds. SLE:* 500–750 mg/m^2 q mo. *JRA:* 10 mg/kg q 2 wk; ↓ w/ renal impair **Caution:** [D, ?] w/ BM suppression, hepatic Insuff **CI:** Component sensitivity **Disp:** Tabs 25, 50 mg; Inj 500 mg, 1 g, 2 g **SE:** ↓ BM; hemorrhagic cystitis, SIADH, alopecia, anorexia; N/V; hepatotox; rare interstitial pneumonitis; irreversible testicular atrophy possible; cardiotox rare; 2nd malignancies (bladder, ALL), risk 3.5% at 8 y, 10.7% at 12 y **Notes:** Hemorrhagic cystitis prophylaxis: cont bladder irrigation & mesna uroprotection; encourage hydration, long-term bladder Ca screening

Cyclosporine (Sandimmune, Neoral, Gengraf)
WARNING: ↑ risk neoplasm, ↑ risk skin malignancies, ↑ risk HTN and nephrotox **Uses:** *Organ rejection in kidney, liver, heart, & BMT w/ steroids; RA; psoriasis* **Action:** Immunosuppressant; reversible inhibition of immunocompetent lymphocytes **Dose:** *Adults & Peds. PO:* 15 mg/kg/d12h pretransplant; after 2 wk, taper by

5 mg/wk to 5–10 mg/kg/d. *IV:* If NPO, give 1/3 PO dose IV; ↓ in renal/hepatic impair **Caution:** [C, ?] Dose-related risk of nephrotox/hepatotox; live, attenuated vaccines may be less effective **CI:** Renal impair; uncontrolled HTN **Disp:** Caps 25, 100 mg; PO soln 100 mg/mL; Inj 50 mg/mL **SE:** May ↑ BUN & Cr & mimic transplant rejection; HTN; HA; hirsutism **Notes:** Administer in glass container; many drug interactions; Neoral & Sandimmune not interchangeable; monitor BP, Cr, CBC, LFTs, interaction w/ St. John's wort; **Levels:** *Trough:* Just before next dose: *Therapeutic:* Variable 150–300 ng/mL RIA

Cyclosporine, ophthalmic (Restasis)   Uses: *↑ Tear production suppressed due to ocular inflammation* **Action:** Immune modulator, anti-inflammatory **Dose:** 1 gtt bid each eye 12 h apart; OK w/ artificial tears, allow 15 min between **Caution:** [C, –] **CI:** Ocular Infxn, component allergy **Disp:** Single-use vial 0.05% **SE:** Ocular burning/hyperemia **Notes:** Mix vial well

Cyproheptadine (Periactin)   Uses: *Allergic Rxns; itching* **Action:** Phenothiazine antihistamine; serotonin antagonist **Dose:** *Adults.* 4–20 mg PO ÷ q8h; max 0.5 mg/kg/d. *Peds 2–6 y:* 2 mg bid-tid (max 12 mg/24 h). *7–14 y:* 4 mg bid-tid; ↓ in hepatic impair **Caution:** [B, ?] Elderly, CV Dz, Asthma, thyroid Dz, BPH **CI:** Neonates or <2 y; NAG; BOO; acute asthma; GI obst; w/ MAOI **Disp:** Tabs 4 mg; syrup 2 mg/5 mL **SE:** Anticholinergic, drowsiness **Notes:** May stimulate appetite

Cytarabine [ARA-C] (Cytosar-U)   WARNING: Administration by experienced physician in properly equipped facility; potent myelosuppressive agent **Uses:** *Acute leukemias, CML, NHL; IT for leukemic meningitis or prophylaxis* **Action:** Antimetabolite; interferes w/ DNA synth **Dose:** 100–150 mg/m²/d for 5–10 d (low dose); 3 g/m² q12h for 6–12 doses (high dose); 1 mg/kg 1–2/wk (SQ maint); 5–70 mg/m² up to 3/wk IT (per protocols); ↓ in renal/hepatic impair **Caution:** [D, ?] in elderly, w/ marked BM suppression, ↓ dosage by ↓ the number of days of administration **CI:** Component sensitivity **Disp:** Inj 100, 500 mg, 1, 2 g, also 20, 100 mg/mL **SE:** ↓ BM, N/V/D, stomatitis, flu-like syndrome, rash on palms/soles, hepatic/cerebellar dysfunction w/ high doses, noncardiogenic pulm edema, neuropathy, fever **Notes:** Little use in solid tumors; high-dose tox limited by corticosteroid ophthal soln

Cytarabine Liposome (DepoCyt)   WARNING: Can cause chemical arachnoiditis (N/V/HA, fever)↓ severity w/ dexamethasone. Administer by experienced physician in properly equipped facility **Uses:** *Lymphomatous meningitis* **Action:** Antimetabolite; interferes w/ DNA synth **Dose:** 50 mg IT q14d for 5 doses, then 50 mg IT q28d × 4 doses; use dexamethasone prophylaxis **Caution:** [D, ?] May cause neurotox; blockage to CSF flow may ↑ the risk of neurotox; use in peds not established **CI:** Active meningeal Infxn **Disp:** IT Inj 50 mg/5 mL **SE:** Neck pain/rigidity, HA, confusion, somnolence, fever, back pain, N/V, edema, neutropenia, ↓ plt, anemia **Notes:** Cytarabine liposomes are similar in microscopic appearance to WBCs; caution in interpreting CSF studies

Cytomegalovirus Immune Globulin [CMV-IG IV] (CytoGam)
Uses: *Attenuation CMV Dz associated w/ transplantation* **Action:** Exogenous IgG antibodies to CMV **Dose:** 150 mg/kg/dose w/in 72 h of transplant, for 16 wk posttransplant; see insert **Caution:** [C, ?] Anaphylactic Rxns; renal dysfunction **CI:** Allergy to immunoglobulins; IgA deficiency **Disp:** Inj 50 mg/mL **SE:** Flushing, N/V, muscle cramps, wheezing, HA, fever **Notes:** IV only; administer by separate line; do not shake

Dacarbazine (DTIC) WARNING: Causes hematopoietic depression, hepatic necrosis, may be carcinogenic, teratogenic **Uses:** *Melanoma, Hodgkin Dz, sarcoma* **Action:** Alkylating agent; antimetabolite as a purine precursor; ↓ protein synth, RNA, & especially DNA **Dose:** 2–4.5 mg/kg/d for 10 consecutive d or 250 mg/m²/d for 5 d (per protocols); ↓ in renal impair **Caution:** [C, ?] In BM suppression; renal/hepatic impair **CI:** Component sensitivity **Disp:** Inj 100, 200 mg **SE:** ↓ BM, N/V, hepatox, flu-like syndrome, ↓ BP, photosensitivity, alopecia, facial flushing, facial paresthesias, urticaria, phlebitis at Inj site **Notes:** Avoid extrav, ✓ CBC, plt

Daclizumab (Zenapax) WARNING: Administer under skilled supervision in equipped facility **Uses:** *Prevent acute organ rejection* **Action:** IL-2 receptor antagonist **Dose:** 1 mg/kg/dose IV; 1st dose pretransplant, then 1 mg/kg q 14d × 4 doses **Caution:** [C, ?] **CI:** Component sensitivity **Disp:** Inj 5 mg/mL **SE:** Hyperglycemia, edema, HTN, ↓ BP, constipation, HA, dizziness, anxiety, nephrotox, pulm edema, pain, anaphylaxis/hypersensitivity **Notes:** Administer w/in 4 h of preparation

Dactinomycin (Cosmegen) WARNING: Administer under skilled supervision in equipped facility; powder and soln toxic, corrosive, mutagenic, carcinogenic, and teratogenic; avoid exposure and use precautions **Uses:** *Choriocarcinoma, Wilms tumor, Kaposi and Ewing sarcomas, rhabdomyosarcoma, uterine and testicular CA* **Action:** DNA-intercalating agent **Dose:** *Adults.* 0.5 mg/d for 5 d; 2 mg/wk for 3 consecutive wk; 15 mcg/kg or 0.45 mg/m²/d (max 0.5 mg) for 5 d q3–8wk *Peds. Sarcoma* (per protocols); ↓ in renal impair **Caution:** [C, ?] **CI:** Concurrent/recent chickenpox or herpes zoster; infants <6 mo **Disp:** Inj 0.5 mg **SE:** Myelo-/immunosuppression, severe N/V/D, alopecia, acne, hyperpigmentation, radiation recall phenomenon, tissue damage w/ extrav, hepatotox **Notes:** Classified as antibiotic but not used as antimicrobial

Dalteparin (Fragmin) WARNING: ↑ Risk of spinal/epidural hematoma with LP **Uses:** *Unstable angina, non–q-wave MI, prevent & Rx DVT following surgery (hip, Abd), pt w/ restricted mobility, extended therapy for PE DVT in CA pt* **Action:** LMW heparin **Dose:** *Angina/MI:* 120 units/kg (max 10,000 units) SQ q12h w/ ASA. *DVT prophylaxis:* 2500–5000 units SQ 1–2 h pre-op, then daily for 5–10 d. *Systemic anticoagulation:* 200 units/kg/d SQ or 100 units/kg bid SQ. *Cancer:* 200 Int Units/kg (max 18,000 Int Units) SQ q24h × 30 d, mo 2–6 150 Int Units/kg SQ q24h (max 18,000 Int Units) **Caution:** [B, ?] In renal/hepatic impair, active hemorrhage, cerebrovascular Dz, cerebral aneurysm, severe HTN **CI:** HIT; pork product allergy; w/ mifepristone **Disp:** Inj 2500 units (16 mg/0.2 mL), 5000 units (32 mg/0.2 mL), 7500 units (48 mg/0.3 mL), 10,000 units (64 mg/mL), 25,000 units/mL (3.8 mL); prefilled vials 10,000 units/mL (9.5 mL) **SE:** Bleeding, pain at site, ↓ plt **Notes:** Predictable effects eliminates lab monitoring; not for IM/IV use

Dantrolene (Dantrium)   WARNING: Hepatotox reported; D/C after 45 d if no benefit observed
Uses: *Rx spasticity due to upper motor neuron disorders (eg, spinal cord injuries, stroke, CP, MS); malignant hyperthermia* **Action:** Skeletal muscle relaxant **Dose:** *Adults. Spasticity:* 25 mg PO daily; ↑ 25 mg to effect to 100 mg max PO qid PRN. *Peds.* 0.5 mg/kg/dose bid; ↑ by 0.5 mg/kg to effect, to 3 mg/kg/dose max qid PRN. *Adults & Peds. Malignant hyperthermia: Rx:* Cont rapid IV, start 1 mg/kg until Sxs subside or 10 mg/kg is reached. *Postcrisis follow-up:* 4–8 mg/kg/d in 3–4 ÷ doses for 1–3 d to prevent recurrence **Caution:** [C, ?] Impaired cardiac/pulm/hepatic Fxn **CI:** Active hepatic Dz; where spasticity needed to maintain posture or balance **Disp:** Caps 25, 50, 100 mg; powder for Inj 20 mg/vial **SE:** Hepatotox, ↑ LFTs, drowsiness, dizziness, rash, muscle weakness, D/N/V, pleural effusion w/ pericarditis, D, blurred vision, hep, photosensitivity **Notes:** Monitor LFTs; avoid sunlight/EtOH/CNS depressants

Dapsone, oral
Uses: *Rx & prevent PCP; toxoplasmosis prophylaxis; leprosy* **Action:** Unknown; bactericidal **Dose:** *Adults.* PCP prophylaxis 50–100 mg/d PO; Rx PCP 100 mg/d PO w/ TMP 15–20 mg/kg/d for 21 d. *Peds.* PCP prophylaxis alternated dose: (>1 mo) 4 mg/kg/dose once/wk (max 200 mg); prophylaxis of PCP 1–2 mg/kg/24 h PO daily; max 100 mg/d **Caution:** [C, +] G6PD deficiency; severe anemia **CI:** Component sensitivity **Disp:** Tabs 25, 100 mg **SE:** Hemolysis, methemoglobinemia, agranulocytosis, rash, cholestatic jaundice **Notes:** Absorption ↑ by an acidic environment; for leprosy, combine w/ rifampin & other agents

Dapsone, topical (Aczone)
Uses: *Topical for acne vulgaris* **Action:** Unknown; bactericidal **Dose:** Apply pea-size amount and rub into areas bid; wash hands after **Caution:** [C, +] G6PD deficiency; severe anemia **CI:** Component sensitivity **Disp:** 5% gel **SE:** Skin oiliness/peeling, dryness erythema **Notes:** Not for oral, ophthal, or intravag use; check G6PD levels before use; follow CBC if G6PD deficient

Daptomycin (Cubicin)
Uses: *Complicated skin/skin structure Infxns due to gram(+) organisms* S. aureus, bacteremia, MRSA endocarditis **Action:** Cyclic lipopeptide; rapid membrane depolarization & bacterial death. *Spectrum: S. aureus* (including MRSA), *S. pyogenes, S. agalactiae, S. dysgalactiae* subsp *Equisimilis, & E. faecalis* (vancomycin-susceptible strains only) **Dose:** *Skin:* 4 mg/kg IV daily × 7–14 d (over 30 min); *Bacteremia & Endocarditis:* 6 mg/kg q48h; ↓ w/ CrCl <30 mL/min or dialysis: q48h **Caution:** [B, ?] w/ HMG-CoA inhibitors **Disp:** Inj 250, 500 mg/10 mL **SE:** Anemia, constipation, N/V/D, HA, rash, site Rxn, muscle pain/weakness, edema, cellulitis, hypo-/hyperglycemia, ↑ alkaline

phosphatase, cough, back pain, Abd pain, ↓ K⁺, anxiety, chest pain, sore throat, cardiac failure, confusion, *Candida* Infxns **Notes:** ✓ CPK baseline & weekly; consider D/C HMG-CoA reductase inhibitors to ↓ myopathy risk; not for Rx PNA

Darbepoetin Alfa (Aranesp)   **WARNING:** Associated with ↑ CV, thromboembolic events and/or mortality; D/C if Hgb >12 g/dL; may increase tumor progression and death in cancer pts **Uses:** *Anemia associated w/ CRF,* anemia in nonmyeloid malignancy w/ concurrent chemotherapy **Action:** ↑ Erythropoiesis, recombinant erythropoietin variant **Dose:** 0.45 mcg/kg single IV or SQ q wk; titrate, do not exceed target Hgb of 12 g/dL; use lowest doses possible, see insert to convert from Epogen **Caution:** [C, ?] May ↑ risk of CV &/or neurologic SE in renal failure; HTN; w/ Hx Szs **CI:** Uncontrolled HTN, component allergy **Disp:** 25, 40, 60, 100, 200, 300 mcg/mL, 150 mcg/0.075 mL in polysorbate or albumin excipient **SE:** May ↑ cardiac risk, CP, hypo-/hypertension, N/V/D, myalgia, arthralgia, dizziness, edema, fatigue, fever, ↑ risk Infxn **Notes:** Longer half-life than Epogen; weekly CBC until stable

Darifenacin (Enablex)   **Uses:** *OAB* Urinary antispasmodic **Action:** Muscarinic receptor antagonist **Dose:** 7.5 mg/d PO; 15 mg/d max (7.5 mg/d w/ mod hepatic impair or w/ CYP3A4 inhibitors); w/ drugs metabolized by CYP2D (Table 11); swallow whole **Caution:** [C, ?/–] w/ Hepatic impair **CI:** Urinary/gastric retention, uncontrolled NAG, paralytic ileus **Disp:** Tabs ER 7.5 mg, 15 mg **SE:** Xerostomia/eyes, constipation, dyspepsia, Abd pain, retention, abnormal vision, dizziness, asthenia

Darunavir (Prezista)   **Uses:** *Rx HIV w/ resistance to multiple protease inhibitors* **Action:** HIV-1 protease inhibitor **Dose:** 600 mg PO bid, administer w/ ritonavir 100 mg bid; w/ food **Caution:** [B, ?/–] Hx Sulfa allergy, CYP3A4 substrate, changes levels of many meds (↑ amiodarone, ↑ dihydropyridines, ↑ HMG-CoA reductase inhibitors [statins], ↓ SSRIs, ↓ rifampin, ↓ methadone) **CI:** w/ astemizole, terfenadine, dihydroergotamine, ergonovine, ergotamine, methylergonovine, pimozide, midazolam, triazolam **Supplied:** Tabs 300 mg **SE:** ↑ glucose, cholesterol, triglycerides, central redistribution of fat (metabolic syndrome), N, ↓ neutrophils & ↑ amylase

Dasatinib (Sprycel)   **Uses:** CML, Ph + ALL **Action:** multi-TKI **Dose:** 70 mg PO bid; adjust w/ CYP3A4 inhibitors/inducers (Table 11) **Caution:** [D, ?/–] **CI:** None **Disp:** Tabs 20, 50, 70 mg **SE:** ↓ BM, edema, fluid retention, pleural effusions, N/V/D, Abd pain, bleeding, fever, ↑ QT **Notes:** replace K, Mg before Rx

Daunorubicin (Daunomycin, Cerubidine)   **WARNING:** Cardiac Fxn should be monitored due to potential risk for cardiac tox & CHF, renal/hepatic dysfunction **Uses:** *Acute leukemias* **Action:** DNA-intercalating agent; ↓ topoisomerase II; generates oxygen free radicals **Dose:** 45–60 mg/m²/d for 3 consecutive d; 25 mg/m²/wk (per protocols); ↓ in renal/hepatic impair **Caution:** [D, ?] **CI:** Component sensitivity **Disp:** Inj 20, 50 mg **SE:** ↓ BM, mucositis, N/V, orange urine, alopecia, radiation recall phenomenon, hepatotox (hyperbilirubinemia), tissue necrosis w/ extrav, cardiotox (1–2% CHF w/ 550 mg/m² cumulative dose) **Notes:** Prevent cardiotox w/ dexrazoxane (when pt received >300 mg/m² of daunorubicin cum dose); for IV use only; allopurinol prior to ↓ hyperuricemia

Decitabine (Dacogen) Uses: *MDS* **Action:** Inhibits DNA methyltransferase **Dose:** 15 mg/m² cont Inf over 3 h; repeat q8h × 3 d; repeat cycle q6wk, min 4 cycles; delay Tx and ↓ dose if inadequate hematologic recovery at 6 wk (see label protocol); delay Tx w/ Cr >2 mg/dL or bilirubin >2× ULN **Caution:** [D, ?/–]; avoid pregnancy; males should not father a child during or 2 mo after; renal/hepatic impair **Disp:** Powder 50 mg/vial **SE:** Neutropenia, febrile neutropenia, thrombocytopenia, anemia, leukopenia, peripheral edema, petechiae, N/V/D, constipation, stomatitis, dyspepsia, cough, fever, fatigue, ↑ LFTs & bilirubin, hyperglycemia, Infxn, HA **Notes:** ✓ CBC & plt before each cycle and prn; may premedicate w/antiemetic

Deferasirox (Exjade) Uses: *Chronic iron overload due to transfusion in pts >2 y* **Action:** Oral iron chelator **Dose:** Initial: 20 mg/kg PO/d; adjust by 5–10 mg/kg q3–6mo based on monthly ferritin; 30 mg/kg/d max; on empty stomach 30 min before food; hold dose if ferritin <500 mcg/L, dissolve in water, orange, apple juice (<1 g/3.5 oz; >1 g in 7 oz) drink immediately; resuspend residue and swallow; do not chew, swallow whole tabs or take w/ Al-containing antacids **Caution:** [B, ?/–] elderly, renal impair, heme disorders **Disp:** Tabs for oral susp 125, 250, 500 mg **SE:** N/V/D, Abd pain, skin rash, HA, fever, cough, ↑ Cr & LFTs, Infxn, hearing loss, dizziness, cataracts, retinal disorders, ↑ IOP, lens opacities, dizziness **Notes:** ARF, peripheral cytopenias possible; ✓ Cr weekly 1st mo then q mo, ✓ CBC; do not combine w/ other iron-chelator therapies; dose to nearest whole tab; auditory/ophthal testing initially and q12mo; monthly Cr, urine protein, LFTs

Delavirdine (Rescriptor) Uses: *HIV Infxn* **Action:** Nonnucleoside RT inhibitor **Dose:** 400 mg PO tid **Caution:** [C, ?] CDC recommends HIV-infected mothers not breast-feed (transmission risk); w/ renal/hepatic impair **CI:** Use w/ drugs dependent on CYP3A for clearance (Table 11) **Disp:** Tabs 100, 200 mg **SE:** Fat redistribution, immune reconstitution syndrome, HA, fatigue, rash, ↑ transaminases, N/V/D **Notes:** Avoid antacids; ↓ cytochrome P-450 enzymes; numerous drug interactions; monitor LFTs

Demeclocycline (Declomycin) Uses: *SIADH* **Action:** Antibiotic, antagonizes ADH action on renal tubules **Dose:** 300–600 mg PO q12h on empty stomach; ↓ in renal failure; avoid antacids **Caution:** [D, +] Avoid in hepatic/renal impair & children **CI:** Tetracycline allergy **Disp:** Tabs 150, 300 mg **SE:** D, Abd cramps, photosensitivity, DI **Notes:** Avoid sunlight, numerous drug interactions; not for peds <8 y.

Desipramine (Norpramin) **WARNING:** Closely monitor for worsening depression or emergence of suicidality Uses: *Endogenous depression,* chronic pain, peripheral neuropathy **Action:** TCA; ↑ synaptic serotonin or norepinephrine in CNS **Dose:** *Adults.* 100–200 mg/d single or ÷ dose; usually single hs dose (max 300 mg/d) *Peds 6–12 y:* 1–3 mg/kg/d ÷ dose, 5 mg/kg/d max; ↓ dose in elderly **Caution:** [C, ?/–] CV Dz, Sz disorder, hypothyroidism, elderly, liver impair **CI:** MAOIs w/in 14 d; during AMI recovery phase **Disp:** Tabs 10, 25, 50, 75, 100, 150 mg; caps 25, 50 mg **SE:** Anticholinergic (blurred vision, urinary retention, xerostomia); orthostatic ↓ BP; ↑ QT interval, arrhythmias **Notes:** Numerous drug interactions; blue-green urine; avoid sunlight

Desloratadine (Clarinex) Uses: *Seasonal & perennial allergic rhinitis; chronic idiopathic urticaria* Action: Active metabolite of Claritin, H_1-antihistamine, blocks inflammatory mediators **Dose:** *Adults & Peds >12 y:* 5 mg PO daily; 5 mg PO q other day w/ hepatic/renal impair **Caution:** [C, ?/–] RediTabs contain phenylalanine **Disp:** Tabs & RediTabs (rapid dissolving) 5 mg, syrup 0.5 mg/mL **SE:** Allergy, anaphylaxis, somnolence, HA, dizziness, fatigue, pharyngitis, xerostomia, N, dyspepsia, myalgia

Desmopressin (DDAVP, Stimate) **WARNING:** Not for hemophilia B or w/ factor VIII antibody; not for hemophilia A w/ factor VIII levels <5% Uses: *DI (intranasal & parenteral); bleeding due to uremia, hemophilia A, & type I von Willebrand Dz (parenteral), nocturnal enuresis* Action: Synthetic analog of vasopressin (human ADH); ↑ factor VIII **Dose:** *DI: Intranasal: Adults.* 0.1–0.4 mL (10–40 mcg/d in 1–3 ÷ doses). *Peds 3 mo–12 y:* 0.05–0.3 mL/d in 1 or 2 doses. *Parenteral: Adults.* 0.5–1 mL (2–4 mcg/d in 2 ÷ doses); converting from nasal to parenteral, use 1/10 nasal dose. *PO: Adults.* 0.05 mg bid; ↑ to max of 1.2 mg. *Hemophilia A & von Willebrand Dz (type I): Adults & Peds >10 kg:* 0.3 mcg/kg in 50 mL NS, Inf over 15–30 min. *Peds <10 kg:* As above w/ dilution to 10 mL w/ NS. *Nocturnal enuresis: Peds >6 y:* 20 mcg intranasally hs **Caution:** [B, M] Avoid overhydration **CI:** Hemophilia B; factor VIII <50 mL/min, severe classic von Willebrand Dz; pts w/ factor VIII antibodies; hyponatremia **Disp:** Tabs 0.1, 0.2 mg; Inj 4, 15 mcg/mL; nasal soln 0.1, 1.5 mg/mL **SE:** Facial flushing, HA, dizziness, vulval pain, nasal congestion, pain at Inj site, ↓ Na^+, H_2O intoxication **Notes:** In very young & old pts, ↓ fluid intake to avoid H_2O intoxication & ↓ Na^+

Desvenlafaxine (Pristiq) **WARNING:** Monitor for worsening or emergence of suicidality, particularly in ped, adolescent, and young adult pts Uses: *Major depressive disorder* Action: Selective serotonin and norepinephrine reuptake inhibitor **Dose:** 50 mg PO daily, ↓ w/ renal impair **Caution:** [C, ±/M] **CI:** Hypersensitivity, MAOI w/ or w/in 14 d of stopping MAOI **Disp:** Tabs 50, 100 mg **SE:** N, dizziness, insomnia, hyperhidrosis, constipation, somnolence, decreased appetite, anxiety, and specific male sexual Fxn disorders **Notes:** Tabs should be taken whole, allow 7 d after stopping before starting an MAOI

Dexamethasone, nasal (Dexacort Phosphate Turbinaire) Uses: *Chronic nasal inflammation or allergic rhinitis* Action: Anti-inflammatory corticosteroid **Dose:** *Adults & Peds >12 y:* 2 sprays/nostril bid–tid, max 12 sprays/d. *Peds 6–12 y:* 1–2 sprays/nostril bid, max 8 sprays/d **Caution:** [C, ?] **CI:** Untreated Infxn **Disp:** Aerosol, 84 mcg/activation **SE:** Local irritation

Dexamethasone, ophthalmic (AK-Dex Ophthalmic, Decadron Ophthalmic) Uses: *Inflammatory or allergic conjunctivitis* Action: Anti-inflammatory corticosteroid Dose: Instill 1–2 gtt tid-qid Caution: [C, ?/–] CI: Active untreated bacterial, viral, & fungal eye Infxns Disp: Susp & soln 0.1%; oint 0.05% SE: Long-term use associated w/ cataracts

Dexamethasone, systemic, topical (Decadron) See Steroids, Systemic, page 214, & Tables 3 & 4.

Dexpanthenol (Ilopan-Choline PO, Ilopan) Uses: *Minimize paralytic ileus, Rx post-op distention* Action: Cholinergic agent Dose: *Adults. Relief of gas:* 2–3 tabs PO tid. *Prevent post-op ileus:* 250–500 mg IM stat, repeat in 2 h, then q6h PRN. *Ileus:* 500 mg IM stat, repeat in 2 h, then q6h, PRN Caution: [C, ?] CI: Hemophilia, mechanical bowel obst Disp: Inj 250 mg/mL; tabs 50 mg; cream 2% SE: GI cramps

Dexrazoxane (Zinecard, Totect) Uses: *Prevent anthracycline-induced (eg, doxorubicin) cardiomyopathy (Zinecard), extrav of anthracycline chemotherapy (Totect)* Action: Chelates heavy metals; binds intracellular iron & prevents anthracycline-induced free radicals Dose: *Systemic(cardiomyopathy,* Zinecard) 10:1 ratio dexrazoxane:doxorubicin 30 min before each dose, 5:1 ratio w/ CrCl <40 mL/min. *Extrav (Totect):* IV Inf over 1–2 hqd × 3 d, w/in 6 h of extrav. Day 1: 1000 mg/m^2 (max 2000 mg); Day 2: 1000 mg/m^2 (max 2000 mg); Day 3: 500 mg/m^2 (max 1000 mg); w/ CrCl <40 mL/min, ↓ dose by 50% Caution: [D, –] CI: Component sensitivity Disp: Inj powder 250, 500 mg (10 mg/mL) SE: ↓ BM, fever, Infxn, stomatitis, alopecia, N/V/D; ↑ LFTs, Inj site pain

Dextran 40 (Rheomacrodex, Gentran 40) Uses: *Shock, prophylaxis of DVT & thromboembolism, adjunct in peripheral vascular surgery* Action: Expands plasma vol; ↓ blood viscosity Dose: *Shock:* 10 mL/kg Inf rapidly; 20 mL/kg max 1st 24 h; beyond 24 h 10 mL/kg max; D/C after 5 d. *Prophylaxis of DVT & thromboembolism:* 10 mL/kg IV day of surgery, then 500 mL/d IV for 2–3 d, then 500 mL IV q2–3d based on risk for up to 2 wk Caution: [C, ?] Inf Rxns; w/ corticosteroids CI: Major hemostatic defects; cardiac decompensation; renal Dz w/ severe oliguria/anuria Disp: 10% dextran 40 in 0.9% NaCl or 5% dextrose SE: Allergy/anaphylactoid Rxn (observe during 1st min of Inf), arthralgia, cutaneous Rxns, ↓ BP, fever Notes: Monitor Cr & lytes; keep well hydrated

Dextromethorphan (Mediquell, Benylin DM, PediaCare 1, Delsym, others) [OTC] Uses: *Control nonproductive cough* Action: Suppresses medullary cough center Dose: *Adults.* 10–30 mg PO q4h PRN (max 120 mg/24 h). *Peds 2–6 y:* 2.5–7.5 mg q4–8h (max 30 mg/24 h). *7–12 y:* 5–10 mg q4–8h (max 60 mg/24 h) Caution: [C, ?/–] Not for persistent or chronic cough CI: <2 y Disp: Caps 30 mg; lozenges 2.5, 5, 7.5, 15 mg; syrup 15 mg/15 mL, 10 mg/5 mL; liq 10 mg/15 mL, 3.5, 7.5, 15 mg/5 mL; sustained-action liq 30 mg/5 mL SE: GI disturbances Notes: Found in combo OTC products w/ guaifenesin; deaths reported in pts <2 y; abuse potential; efficacy in children debated; do not use w/in 14 d of D/C MAOI

Diazepam (Valium, Diastat) [C-IV]   Uses: *Anxiety, EtOH withdrawal, muscle spasm, status epilepticus, panic disorders, amnesia, pre-op sedation* **Action:** Benzodiazepine **Dose:** *Adults. Status epilepticus:* 5–10 mg q10–20min to 30 mg max in 8-h period. *Anxiety, muscle spasm:* 2–10 mg PO bid-qid or IM/IV q3–4h PRN. *Pre-op:* 5–10 mg PO or IM 20–30 min or IV just prior to procedure. *EtOH withdrawal:* Initial 2–5 mg IV, then 5–10 mg q5–10min, 100 mg in 1 h max. May require up to 1000 mg/24 h for severe withdrawal; titrate to agitation; avoid excessive sedation; may lead to aspiration or resp arrest. *Peds. Status epilepticus:* <5 *y:* 0.05–0.3 mg/kg/dose IV q15–30min up to a max of 5 mg. >5 *y:* to max of 10 mg. *Sedation, muscle relaxation:* 0.04–0.3 mg/kg/dose q2–4h IM or IV to max of 0.6 mg/kg in 8 h, or 0.12–0.8 mg/kg/24 h PO ÷ tid-qid; ↓ w/ hepatic impair **Caution:** [D, ?/–] **CI:** Coma, CNS depression, resp depression, NAG, severe uncontrolled pain, PRG **Disp:** Tabs 2, 5, 10 mg; soln 1, 5 mg/mL; Inj 5 mg/mL; rectal gel 2.5, 5, 10, 20 mg/mL **SE:** Sedation, amnesia, bradycardia, ↓ BP, rash, ↓ resp rate **Notes:** 5 mg/min IV max in adults or 1–2 mg/min in peds (resp arrest possible); IM absorption erratic; avoid abrupt D/C

Diazoxide (Proglycem)   Uses: *Hypoglycemia due to hyperinsulinism (Proglycem); hypertensive crisis (Hyperstat)* **Action:** ↓ Pancreatic insulin release; antihypertensive **Dose:** Repeat in 5–15 min until BP controlled; repeat q4–24h; monitor BP closely. *Hypoglycemia: Adults & Peds.* 3–8 mg/kg/24 h PO ÷ q8–12h. *Neonates.* 8–15 mg/kg/24 h ÷ in 3 equal doses; maint 8–10 mg/kg/24 h PO in 2–3 equal doses **Caution:** [C, ?] ↓ Effect w/ phenytoin; ↑ effect w/ diuretics, warfarin **CI:** Allergy to thiazides or other sulfonamide-containing products; HTN associated w/ aortic coarctation, AV shunt, or pheochromocytoma **Disp:** Caps 50 mg; PO susp 50 mg/mL; IV 15 mg/mL **SE:** Hyperglycemia, ↓ BP, dizziness, Na⁺ & H₂O retention, N/V, weakness **Notes:** Can give false-negative insulin response to glucagons; Rx extrav w/ warm compress

Dibucaine (Nupercainal)   Uses: *Hemorrhoids & minor skin conditions* **Action:** Topical anesthetic **Dose:** Insert PR w/ applicator & after each bowel movement; apply sparingly to skin **Caution:** [C, ?] topical use only **CI:** Component sensitivity **Disp:** 1% oint w/ rectal applicator; 0.5% cream **SE:** Local irritation, rash

Diclofenac (Arthrotec, Cataflam, Flector, Flector patch, Voltaren, Voltaren XR, Voltaren gel)   WARNING: May ↑ risk of cv events & GI bleeding; CI in post-op CABG Uses: *Arthritis & pain, oral and topical, actinic keratosis* **Action:** NSAID **Dose:** 50–75 mg PO bid; w/ food or milk; 1 patch to painful area bid. Topical gel upper extremity 2 g qid (max 8 g/d); lower extremity 4 g qid (max 16 g/d) **Caution:** [C, ?] CHF, HTN, renal/hepatic dysfunction, & Hx PUD, asthma **CI:** NSAID/aspirin allergy; porphyria; following CABG **Disp:** Tabs 50 mg; tabs DR 25, 50, 75, 100 mg; XR tabs 100 mg; *Flector Patch 1.3%* 10 × 14 cm, gel 1% **SE:** *Oral:* Abd cramps, heartburn, GI ulceration, rash, interstitial nephritis; *patch/gel:* pruritus, dermatitis, burning,

N, HA **Notes:** Do not crush tabs; watch for GI bleed; do not apply patch/gel to damaged skin or while bathing; ✓ CBC, LFTs periodically

Diclofenac, ophthalmic (Voltaren ophthalmic) **Uses:** *Inflammation postcataract or pain/photophobia postcorneal refractive surgery* **Action:** NSAID **Dose:** *Post-op cataract:* 1 gtt qid, start 24 h post-op× 2 wk. *Post-op refractive:* 1–2 gtts w/in 1 h pre- and w/in 15 min post-op then qid up to 3 d **Caution:** [C, ?] May ↑ bleed risk in ocular tissues **CI:** NSAID/aspirin allergy **Disp:** ophthal soln 0.1% 2.5, 5 mL bottle **SE:** Burning/stinging/itching, keratitis, ↑ IOP, lacrimation, abnormal vision, conjunctivitis, lid swelling, discharge, iritis.

Dicloxacillin (Dynapen, Dycill) **Uses:** *Rx of pneumonia, skin, & soft-tissue Infxns, & osteomyelitis caused by penicillinase-producing staphylococci* **Action:** Bactericidal; ↓ cell wall synth. *Spectrum: S. aureus & Streptococcus* **Dose:** *Adults.* 150–500 mg qid (2 g/d max) *Peds <40 kg:* 12.5–100 mg/kg/d ÷ qid; take on empty stomach **Caution:** [B, ?] **CI:** Component or PCN sensitivity **Disp:** Caps 125, 250, 500 mg; soln 62.5 mg/5 mL **SE:** N/D, Abd pain **Notes:** Monitor PTT if pt on warfarin

Dicyclomine (Bentyl) **Uses:** *Functional IBS* **Action:** Smooth-muscle relaxant **Dose:** *Adults.* 20 mg PO qid; ↑ to 160 mg/d max or 20 mg IM q6h, 80 Mg/d ÷ qid then ↑ to 160 mg/d, max 2 wk *Peds Infants >6 mo:* 5 mg/dose tid-qid. *Children:* 10 mg/dose tid-qid **Caution:** [B, –] **CI:** Infants <6 mo, NAG, MyG, severe UC, BOO, GI obst, reflux esophagitis **Disp:** Caps 10, 20 mg; tabs 20 mg; syrup 10 mg/5 mL; Inj 10 mg/mL **SE:** Anticholinergic SEs may limit dose **Notes:** Take 30–60 min ac; avoid EtOH, do not administer IV

Didanosine [ddI] (Videx) **WARNING:** Allergy manifested as fever, rash, fatigue, GI/resp Sxs reported; stop drug immediately & do not rechallenge; lactic acidosis & hepatomegaly/steatosis reported **Uses:** *HIV Infxn in zidovudine-intolerant pts* **Action:** NRTI **Dose:** *Adults. >60 kg:* 400 mg/d PO or 200 mg PO bid. *<60 kg:* 250 mg/d PO or 125 mg PO bid; adults should take 2 tabs/administration. *Peds 2 wk–8 mo:* 100 mg/m². *>8 mo:* 120 mg/m² PO bid on empty stomach; ↓ w/ renal impair **Caution:** [B, –] CDC recommends HIV-infected mothers not breast-feed **CI:** Component sensitivity **Disp:** Chew tabs 25, 50, 100, 150, 200 mg; powder packets 100, 167, 250, 375 mg; powder for soln 2, 4 g **SE:** Pancreatitis, peripheral neuropathy, D, HA **Notes:** Do not take w/ meals; thoroughly chew tabs, do not mix w/ fruit juice or acidic beverages; reconstitute powder w/ H₂O; many drug interactions

Diflunisal (Dolobid) **WARNING:** May ↑ risk of cv events & GI bleeding; CI in post-op CABG **Uses:** *Mild–mod pain; osteoarthritis* **Action:** NSAID **Dose:** *Pain:* 500 mg PO bid. *Osteoarthritis:* 500–1500 mg PO in 2–3 ÷ doses; ↓ in renal impair, take w/ food/milk **Caution:** [C (D 3rd tri or near delivery), ?] CHF, HTN, renal/hepatic dysfunction, & Hx PUD **CI:** Allergy to NSAIDs or aspirin, active GI bleed, post-CABG **Disp:** Tabs 250, 500 mg **SE:** May ↑ bleeding time; HA, Abd cramps, heartburn, GI ulceration, rash, interstitial nephritis, fluid retention

Digoxin (Lanoxin, Lanoxicaps, Digitek)   Uses: *CHF, AF & flutter, & PAT* **Action:** Positive inotrope; ↑ AV node refractory period **Dose:** *Adults. PO digitalization:* 0.5–0.75 mg PO, then 0.25 mg PO q6–8h to total 1–1.5 mg. *IV or IM digitalization:* 0.25–0.5 mg IM or IV, then 0.25 mg q4–6h to total 0.125–0.5 mg PO, IM, or IV (average daily dose 0.125–0.25 mg). *Peds preterm infants: Digitalization:* 30 mcg/kg PO or 25 mcg/kg IV; give 1/2 of dose initial, then 1/4 of dose at 8–12-h intervals for 2 doses. *Maint:* 5–7.5 mcg/kg/24 h PO or 4–6 mcg/kg/24 h IV ÷ q12h. *Term infants: Digitalization:* 25–35 mcg/kg PO or 20–30 mcg/kg IV; give 1/2 the initial dose, then 1/4 dose at 8–12 h. *Maint:* 6–10 mcg/kg/24 h PO or 5–8 mcg/kg/24 h ÷ q12h. *1 mo–2 y: Digitalization:* 35–60 mcg/kg PO or 30–50 mcg/kg/24 h IV; give 1/2 the initial dose, then 1/3 dose at 8–12-h intervals for 2 doses. *Maint:* 10–15 mcg/kg/24 h PO or 7.5–15 mcg/kg/24 h IV ÷ q12h. *2–10 y: Digitalization:* 30–40 mcg/kg PO or 25 mcg/kg IV; give 1/2 initial dose, then 1/3 of the dose at 8–12-h intervals for 2 doses. *Maint:* 8–10 mcg/kg/24 h PO or 6–8 mcg/kg/24 h IV ÷ q12h. *7–10 y:* Same as for adults; ↓ renal impair **Caution:** [C, +] w/ ↓ K⁺, Mg²⁺, renal failure **CI:** AV block; idiopathic hypertrophic subaortic stenosis; constrictive pericarditis **Disp:** Caps 0.05, 0.1, 0.2 mg; tabs 0.125, 0.25, 0.5 mg; elixir 0.05 mg/mL; Inj 0.1, 0.25 mg/mL **SE:** Can cause heart block; ↓ K⁺ potentiates sx; N/V, HA, fatigue, visual disturbances (yellow-green halos around lights), cardiac arrhythmias **Notes:** Multiple drug interactions; IM Inj painful, as erratic absorption & should not be used. Levels: *Trough: Just before next dose: Therapeutic:* 0.8–2.0 ng/mL; *Toxic:* >2 ng/mL; *Half-life:* 36 h

Digoxin Immune Fab (Digibind, DigiFab)   Uses: *Life-threatening digoxin intoxication* **Action:** Antigen-binding fragments bind & inactivate digoxin **Dose:** *Adults & Peds.* Based on serum level & pt's wgt; see charts provided w/ drug **Caution:** [C, ?] **CI:** Sheep product allergy **Disp:** Inj 38 mg/vial **SE:** Worsening of cardiac output or CHF, ↓ K⁺, facial swelling, & redness **Notes:** Each vial binds ≈ 0.6 mg of digoxin; renal failure may require redosing in several days

Diltiazem (Cardizem, Cardizem CD, Cardizem LA, Cardizem SR, Cartia XT, Dilacor XR, Diltia XT, Taztia XT, Tiamate, Tiazac)   Uses: *Angina, prevention of reinfarction, HTN, AF or flutter, & PAT* **Action:** CCB **Dose:** *Stable angina PO:* Initial, 30 mg PO qid; ↑ to 180–360 mg/d in 3–4 ÷ doses PRN; XR 120 mg/d (540 mg/d max), LA: 180–360 mg/d. *HTN:* SR: 60–120 mg PO bid; ↑ to 360 mg/d max. *CD or XR:* 120–360 mg/d (max 540 mg/d) or LA 180–360 mg/d. *IV:* 0.25 mg/kg IV bolus over 2 min; may repeat in 15 min at 0.35 mg/kg; begin Inf of 5–15 mg/h. *Acute rate control:* 15–20 mg (0.25 mg/kg) IV over 2 min, repeat in 15 min at 20–25 mg (0.35 mg/kg) over 2 min *(ECC 2005)* **Caution:** [C, +] ↑ effect w/ amiodarone, cimetidine, fentanyl, lithium, cyclosporine, digoxin, β-blockers, theophylline **CI:** SSS, AV block, ↓ BP, AMI, pulm congestion **Disp:** *Cardizem CD:* Caps 120, 180, 240, 300, 360 mg; *Cardizem LA:* 120, 180, 240, 300, 360, 420 mg; *Cardizem SR:* caps 60, 90, 120 mg; *Cardizem:* Tabs 30, 60, 90, 120 mg; *Cartia XT:* Caps 120, 180, 240, 300 mg; *Dilacor XR:* Caps 180, 240 mg;

Diltia XT: Caps 120, 180, 240 mg; *Tiazac:* Caps 120, 180, 240, 300, 360, 420 mg; *Tiamate (XR):* Tabs 120, 180, 240 mg; Inj 5 mg/mL; *Taztia XT:* 120, 180, 240, 300, 360 mg **SE:** Gingival hyperplasia, bradycardia, AV block, ECG abnormalities, peripheral edema, dizziness, HA **Notes:** Cardizem CD, Dilacor XR, & Tiazac not interchangeable

Dimenhydrinate (Dramamine, others)
Uses: *Prevention & Rx of N/V, dizziness, or vertigo of motion sickness* **Action:** Antiemetic, action unknown **Dose:** *Adults.* 50–100 mg PO q4–6h, max 400 mg/d; 50 mg IM/IV PRN. *Peds 2–6 y:* 12.5–25 mg q6–8h max 75 mg/d. *6–12 y:* 25–50 mg q6–8h max 150 mg/d **Caution:** [B, ?] **CI:** Component sensitivity **Disp:** Tabs 50 mg; chew tabs 50 mg; liq 12.5 mg/4 mL, 12.5 mg/5 mL, 15.62 mg/5 mL **SE:** Anticholinergic SE **Notes:** Take 30 min before travel for motion sickness

Dimethyl Sulfoxide [DMSO] (Rimso-50)
Uses: *Interstitial cystitis* **Action:** Unknown **Dose:** Intravesical, 50 mL, retain for 15 min; repeat q2wk until relief **Caution:** [C, ?] **CI:** Component sensitivity **Disp:** 50% & 100% soln **SE:** Cystitis, eosinophilia, GI, & taste disturbance

Dinoprostone (Cervidil Vaginal Insert, Prepidil Vaginal Gel, Prostin E2)
WARNING: Should only be used by trained personnel in an appropriate hospital setting **Uses:** *Induce labor; terminate PRG (12–20 wk); evacuate uterus in missed abortion or fetal death* **Action:** Prostaglandin, changes consistency, dilatation, & effacement of the cervix; induces uterine contraction **Dose:** *Gel:* 0.5 mg; if no cervical/uterine response, repeat 0.5 mg q6h (max 24-h dose 1.5 mg). *Vaginal insert:* 1 insert (10 mg = 0.3 mg dinoprostone/h over 12 h); remove w/ onset of labor or 12 h after insertion. *Vaginal supp:* 20 mg repeated q3–5h; adjust PRN supp: 1 high in vagina, repeat at 3–5-h intervals until abortion (240 mg max) **Caution:** [X, ?] **CI:** Ruptured membranes, allergy to prostaglandins, placenta previa or AUB, when oxytocic drugs CI or if prolonged uterine contractions are inappropriate (Hx C-section, cephalopelvic disproportion, etc) **Disp:** *Endocervical gel:* 0.5 mg in 3-g syringes (w/ 10- & 20-mm shielded catheter). *Vaginal gel:* 0.5 mg/3 g *Vaginal supp:* 20 mg. *Vaginal insert, CR:* 10 mg **SE:** N/V/D, dizziness, flushing, HA, fever, abnormal uterine contractions

Diphenhydramine (Benadryl) [OTC]
Uses: *Rx & prevent allergic Rxns, motion sickness, potentiate narcotics, sedation, cough suppression, & Rx of extrapyramidal Rxns* **Action:** Antihistamine, antiemetic **Dose:** *Adults.* 25–50 mg PO, IV, or IM bid–tid. *Peds >2 y:* 5 mg/kg/24 h PO or IM ÷ q6h (max 300 mg/d); ↑ dosing interval w/ mod–severe renal Insuff **Caution:** [B, –] elderly, NAG, BPH, w/ MAOI **CI:** acute asthma **Disp:** Tabs, caps 25, 50 mg; chew tabs 12.5 mg; elixir 12.5 mg/5 mL; syrup 12.5 mg/5 mL; liq 6.25 mg/5 mL, 12.5 mg/5 mL; Inj 50 mg/mL, cream 2% **SE:** Anticholinergic (xerostomia, urinary retention, sedation)

Diphenoxylate + Atropine (Lomotil, Lonox) [C-V]
Uses: *D* **Action:** Constipating meperidine congener, ↓ GI motility **Dose:** *Adults.* Initial, 5 mg PO tid-qid until controlled, then 2.5–5 mg PO bid; 20 mg/d max *Peds >2 y:*

0.3–0.4 mg/kg/24 h (of diphenoxylate) bid-qid, 10 mg/d max **Caution:** [C, +] elderly, w/ renal impair **CI:** Obstructive jaundice, D due to bacterial Infxn; children <2 y **Disp:** Tabs 2.5 mg diphenoxylate/0.025 mg atropine; liq 2.5 mg diphenoxylate/0.025 mg atropine/5 mL **SE:** Drowsiness, dizziness, xerostomia, blurred vision, urinary retention, constipation

Diphtheria, Tetanus Toxoids, & Acellular pertussis adsorbed, Hep B (Recombinant), & Inactivated Poliovirus Vaccine [IPV] combined (Pediarix) **Uses:** *Vaccine against diphtheria, tetanus, pertussis, HBV, polio (types 1, 2, 3) as a 3-dose primary series in infants & children <7, born to HBsAg(−) mothers* **Actions:** Active immunization **Dose:** *Infants:* Three 0.5-mL doses IM, at 6–8-wk intervals, start at 2 mo; child given 1 dose of hep B vaccine, same; previously vaccinated w/ one or more doses inactivated poliovirus vaccine, use to complete series **Caution:** [C, N/A] **CI:** HBsAg(+) mother, adults, children >7 y, immunosuppressed, allergy to yeast, neomycin, polymyxin B, or any component, encephalopathy, or progressive neurologic disorders; caution in bleeding disorders **Disp:** Single-dose vials 0.5 mL **SE:** Drowsiness, restlessness, fever, fussiness, ↓ appetite, nodule redness, Inj site pain/swelling **Notes:** If IM use only preservative-free Inj

Dipivefrin (Propine) **Uses:** *Open-angle glaucoma* **Action:** α-Adrenergic agonist **Dose:** 1 gtt in eye q12h **Caution:** [B, ?] **CI:** NAG **Disp:** 0.1% soln **SE:** HA, local irritation, blurred vision, photophobia, HTN

Dipyridamole (Persantine) **Uses:** *Prevent post-op thromboembolic disorders, often in combo w/ ASA or warfarin (eg, CABG, vascular graft); w/ warfarin after artificial heart valve; chronic angina; w/ ASA to prevent coronary artery thrombosis; dipyridamole IV used in place of exercise stress test for CAD* **Action:** Anti-plt activity; coronary vasodilator **Dose:** *Adults.* 75–100 mg PO tid-qid; stress test 0.14 mg/kg/min (max 60 mg over 4 min). *Peds >12 y;* 3–6 mg/kg/d divided tid (safety/efficacy not established) **Caution:** [B, ?/−] w/ Other drugs that affect coagulation **CI:** Component sensitivity **Disp:** Tabs 25, 50, 75 mg; Inj 5 mg/mL **SE:** HA, ↓ BP, N, Abd distress, flushing rash, dizziness, dyspnea **Notes:** IV use can worsen angina

Dipyridamole & Aspirin (Aggrenox) **Uses:** *↓ Reinfarction after MI; prevent occlusion after CABG; ↓ risk of stroke* **Action:** ↓ Plt aggregation (both agents) **Dose:** 1 cap PO bid **Caution:** [C, ?] **CI:** Ulcers, bleeding diathesis **Disp:** Dipyridamole (XR) 200 mg/aspirin 25 mg **SE:** ASA component: allergic Rxns, skin Rxns, ulcers/GI bleed, bronchospasm; dipyridamole component: dizziness, HA, rash **Notes:** Swallow caps whole

Disopyramide (Norpace, Norpace CR, NAPAmide, Rythmodan) **WARNING:** Excessive mortality or nonfatal cardiac arrest rate with use in asymptomatic non–life-threatening ventricular arrhythmias with MI 6 d to 2 y prior. Restrict use to life-threatening arrhythmias only **Uses:** *Suppression & prevention of VT* **Action:** Class 1A antiarrhythmic; stabilizes membranes, depresses action potential **Dose:** *Adults.* Immediate <50 kg 200 mg, >50 kg 300 mg, maint 400–800 mg/d ÷ q6h or q12h for CR, max 1600 mg/d. *Peds <1 y:* 10–30 mg/kg/24 h PO (÷ qid). *1–4 y:* 10–20 mg/kg/24 h PO (÷ qid). *4–12 y:* 10–15 mg/kg/24 h PO (÷ qid). *12–18 y:* 6–15 mg/kg/24 h PO (÷ qid); ↓ in renal/hepatic impair **Caution:** [C, +] Elderly, w/ abnormal ECG, lytes, liver/renal impair, NAG **CI:** AV block, cardiogenic shock, ↓ BP, CHF **Disp:** Caps 100, 150 mg; CR caps 100, 150 mg **SE:** Anticholinergic SEs; negative inotrope, may induce CHF **Notes:** Levels: *Trough:* just before next dose; *Therapeutic:* 2–5 mcg/mL; *Toxic* >5 mcg/mL; half-life: 4–10 h

Dobutamine (Dobutrex) Uses: *Short-term in cardiac decompensation secondary to ↓ contractility* **Action:** Positive inotrope **Dose:** *Adults & Peds.* Cont IV Inf of 2.5–15 mcg/kg/min; rarely, 40 mcg/kg/min required; titrate; 2–20 mcg/kg/min; titrate to HR not >10% of baseline *(ECC 2005)* **Caution:** [C, ?] w/ Arrhythmia, MI, severe CAD, ↓ vol **CI:** Sensitivity to sulfites, IHSS **Disp:** Inj 250 mg/20 mL, 12.5/mL **SE:** Chest pain, HTN, dyspnea **Notes:** Monitor PWP & cardiac output if possible; ✓ ECG for ↑ HR, ectopic activity; follow BP

Docetaxel (Taxotere) WARNING: Do not administer if neutrophil count <1500 cells/mm³; severe Rxns possible in hepatic dysfunction Uses: *Breast (anthracycline-resistant), ovarian, lung, & prostate CA* **Action:** Antimitotic agent; promotes microtubular aggregation; semisynthetic taxoid **Dose:** 100 mg/m² over 1 h IV q3wk (per protocols); dexamethasone 8 mg bid prior & continue for 3–4 d; ↓ dose w/ ↑ bilirubin levels **Caution:** [D, –] Sensitivity to meds w/ polysorbate 80, component sensitivity **Disp:** Inj 20 mg/0.5 mL, 80 mg/2 mL **SE:** ↓ BM, neuropathy, N/V, alopecia, fluid retention syndrome; cumulative doses of 300–400 mg/m² w/o steroid preparation & posttreatment & 600–800 mg/m² w/ steroid preparation; allergy possible (rare w/ steroid preparation) **Notes:** ✓ Bilirubin, SGOT and SGPT prior to each cycle; frequent CBC during therapy

Docusate Calcium (Surfak)/Docusate Potassium (Dialose)/ Docusate Sodium (DOSS, Colace) Uses: *Constipation; adjunct to painful anorectal conditions (hemorrhoids)* **Action:** Stool softener **Dose:** *Adults.* 50–500 mg PO ÷ daily–qid. *Peds Infants–3 y:* 10–40 mg/24 h ÷ daily–qid. *3–6 y:* 20–60 mg/24 h ÷ daily–qid. *6–12 y:* 40–120 mg/24 h ÷ daily–qid **Caution:** [C, ?] **CI:** Use w/ mineral oil; intestinal obst, acute Abd pain, N/V **Disp:** *Ca:* Caps 50, 240 mg. *K:* Caps 100, 240 mg. *Na:* Caps 50, 100 mg; syrup 50, 60 mg/15 mL; liq 150 mg/15 mL; soln 50 mg/mL **SE:** Rare Abd cramping, D **Notes:** Take w/ full glass of H_2O; no laxative action; do not use >1 wk

Dofetilide (Tikosyn) WARNING: To minimize the risk of induced arrhythmia, hospitalize for minimum of 3 d to provide calculations of CrCl, cont ECG monitoring, & cardiac resuscitation Uses: *Maintain nl sinus rhythm in AF/A flutter after conversion* **Action:** Type III antiarrhythmic, prolongs action potential **Dose:** Based on CrCl & QTc; CrCl >60 mL/min 500 mcg PO q12h, ✓ QTc 2–3 h after, if QTc >15% over baseline or >500 msec, ↓ to 250 mcg q 12h, ✓ after each dose; if CrCl <60 mL/sec, see insert; D/C if QTc >500 msec after dosing adjustments **Caution:** [C, –] w/ AV block, renal Dz, electrolyte imbalance **CI:** Baseline QTc >440 msec, CrCl <20 mL/min; w/ verapamil, cimetidine, trimethoprim, ketoconazole, quinolones, ACE inhibitors/HCTZ combo **Disp:** Caps 125, 250, 500 mcg **SE:** Ventricular arrhythmias, QT ↑, torsade de pointes, rash, HA, CP, dizziness **Notes:** Avoid w/ other drugs that ↑ QT interval; hold class I/III antiarrhythmics for 3 half-lives prior to dosing; amiodarone level should be <0.3 mg/L before use, do not initiate if HR <60 BPM; restricted to participating prescribers; correct K⁺ and Mg²⁺ before use.

Dolasetron (Anzemet)
Uses: *Prevent chemotherapy and post–op–associated N/V* **Action:** 5-HT₃ receptor antagonist **Dose:** *Adults & Peds. IV:* 1.8 mg/kg IV as single dose 30 min prior to chemotherapy **Adults. PO:** 100 mg PO as a single dose 1 h prior to chemotherapy. *Post-op:* 12.5 mg IV, 100 mg PO 2 h pre-op *Peds 2–16 y:* 1.8 mg/kg PO (max 100 mg) as single dose. *Post-op:* 0.35 mg/kg IV or 1.2 mg/kg PO **Caution:** [B, ?] w/ Cardiac conduction problems **CI:** Component sensitivity **Disp:** Tabs 50, 100 mg; Inj 20 mg/mL **SE:** ↑ QT interval, D, HTN, HA, Abd pain, urinary retention, transient ↑ LFTs

Donepezil (Aricept)
Uses: *Severe Alzheimer dementia* ADHD; behavioral syndromes in dementia; dementia w/ Parkinson Dz; Lewy-body dementia **Action:** ACH inhibitor **Dose:** *Adults.* 5 mg qhs, ↑ to 10 mg PO qhs after 4–6 wk *Peds. ADHD:* 5 mg/d **Caution:** [C, ?] risk for bradycardia w/ preexisting conduction abnormalities, may exaggerate succinylcholine-type muscle relaxation w/ anesthesia, ↑ gastric acid secretion **CI:** Hypersensitivity **Disp:** Tabs 5, 10 mg; orally disintegrating tab 5, 10 mg **SE:** N/V/D, insomnia, Infxn, muscle cramp, fatigue, anorexia **Notes:** N/V/D dose-related & resolves in 1–3 wk

Dopamine (Intropin)
WARNING: Vesicant, give phentolamine w/ extrav **Uses:** *Short-term use in cardiac decompensation secondary to ↓ contractility; ↑ organ perfusion (at low dose)* **Action:** Positive inotropic agent w/ dose response: 1–10 mcg/kg/min δ effects (↑ CO & renal perfusion); 10–20 mcg/kg/min β effects (peripheral vasoconstriction, pressor); >20 mcg/kg/min peripheral & renal vasoconstriction **Dose:** *Adults & Peds.* 5 mcg/kg/min by cont Inf, ↑ by 5 mcg/kg/min to 50 mcg/kg/min max to effect *(ECC 2005)* **Caution:** [C, ?] ↓ Dose w/ MAOI **CI:** Pheochromocytoma, VF, sulfite sensitivity **Disp:** Inj 40, 80, 150 mg/mL, premixed 0.8, 1.6, 3.2 mg/mL **SE:** Tachycardia, vasoconstriction, ↓ BP, HA, N/V, dyspnea **Notes:** >10 mcg/kg/min ↓ renal perfusion; monitor urinary output & ECG for ↑ HR, BP, ectopy; monitor PCWP & cardiac output if possible, phentolamine used for extrav 10 to 15 mL NS w/5 to 10 mg of phentolamine

Doripenem (Doribax)
Uses: *Complicated intra-Abd and UTI including pyelo* **Action:** Carbapenem, ↓ cell wall synth, a β-lactam **Spectrum:** Excellent gram(+) (except MRSA and *Enterococcus* sp.), excellent gram(–) coverage including β-lactamase producers, good anaerobic **Dose:** 500 mg IV q8h, w/ ↓

renal impair **Caution:** [B, ?] **CI:** carbapenem β-lactams hypersensitivity **Disp:** 500 mg single-use vial **SE:** HA, N/D, rash, phlebitis **Notes:** May ↓ valproic acid levels; overuse may ↑ bacterial resistance; monitor for *C. difficile*-associated D

Dornase Alfa (Pulmozyme, DNase) **Uses:** *↓ Frequency of resp Infxns in CF* **Action:** Enzyme cleaves extracellular DNA, ↓ mucous viscosity **Dose:** *Adults.* Inh 2.5 mg/bid dosing w/ FVC >85% w/ recommended nebulizer *Peds* >5 y: Inh 2.5 mg/daily-bid if forced vital capacity >85% **Caution:** [B, ?] **CI:** Chinese hamster product allergy **Disp:** Soln for Inh 1 mg/mL **SE:** Pharyngitis, voice alteration, CP, rash

Dorzolamide (Trusopt) **Uses:** *Open-angle glaucoma, ocular hypertension* **Action:** Carbonic anhydrase inhibitor **Dose:** 1 gtt in eye(s) tid **Caution:** [C, ?] w/ NAG, CrCl <30 mL/min **CI:** Component sensitivity **Disp:** 2% soln **SE:** irritation, bitter taste, punctate keratitis, ocular allergic Rxn

Dorzolamide & Timolol (Cosopt) **Uses:** *Open-angle glaucoma, ocular hypertension* **Action:** Carbonic anhydrase inhibitor w/ β-adrenergic blocker **Dose:** 1 gtt in eye(s) bid **Caution:** [C, ?] CrCl <30 **CI:** Component sensitivity, asthma, severe COPD, sinus bradycardia, AV block **Disp:** Soln dorzolamide 2% & timolol 0.5% **SE:** Irritation, bitter taste, superficial keratitis, ocular allergic Rxn

Doxazosin (Cardura, Cardura XL) **Uses:** *HTN & symptomatic BPH* **Action:** α₁-Adrenergic blocker; relaxes bladder neck smooth muscle **Dose:** *HTN:* Initial 1 mg/d PO; may be ↑ to 16 mg/d PO. *BPH:* Initial 1 mg/d PO, may ↑ to 8 mg/d; XL 2–8 mg q A.M. **Caution:** [B, ?] w/ Liver impair **CI:** Component sensitivity **Disp:** Tabs 1, 2, 4, 8 mg; XL 4, 8 mg **SE:** Dizziness, HA, drowsiness, fatigue, malaise, sexual dysfunction, doses >4 mg ↑ postural ↓ BP risk **Notes:** 1st dose hs; syncope may occur w/in 90 min of initial dose

Doxepin (Adapin) **WARNING:** Closely monitor for worsening depression or emergence of suicidality **Uses:** *Depression, anxiety, chronic pain* **Action:** TCA; ↑ synaptic CNS serotonin or norepinephrine **Dose:** 25–150 mg/d PO, usually hs but can ÷ doses; up to 300 mg/d for depression ↓ in hepatic impair **Caution:** [C, ?/–] w/ EtOH abuse, elderly, w/ MAOI **CI:** NAG, urinary retention, MAOI use w/in 14 d; in recovery phase of MI **Disp:** Caps 10, 25, 50, 75, 100, 150 mg; PO conc 10 mg/mL **SE:** Anticholinergic SEs, ↓ BP, tachycardia, drowsiness, photosensitivity

Doxepin, Topical (Zonalon, Prudoxin) **Uses:** *Short-term Rx pruritus (atopic dermatitis or lichen simplex chronicus)* **Action:** Antipruritic; H₁- & H₂-receptor antagonism **Dose:** Apply thin coating qid, 8 d max **Caution:** [C, ?/–] **CI:** Component sensitivity **Disp:** 5% cream **SE:** ↓ BP, tachycardia, drowsiness, photosensitivity **Notes:** Limit application area to avoid systemic tox

Doxorubicin (Adriamycin, Rubex) **Uses:** *Acute leukemias; Hodgkin Dz & NHLs; soft tissue, osteo- & Ewing sarcoma; Wilms tumor; neuroblastoma; bladder, breast, ovarian, gastric, thyroid, & lung CAs* **Action:** Intercalates DNA; ↓ DNA topoisomerases I & II **Dose:** 60–75 mg/m² q3wk; ↓ w/ hepatic impair;

IV use only ↓ cardiotox w/ weekly (20 mg/m²/wk) or cont Inf (60–90 mg/m² over 96 h); (per protocols) **Caution:** [D, ?] **CI:** Severe CHF, cardiomyopathy, preexisting ↓ BM, previous Rx w/ total cumulative doses of doxorubicin, idarubicin, daunorubicin **Disp:** Inj 20, 50, 75, 150, 200 mg **SE:** ↓ BM, venous streaking & phlebitis, N/V/D, mucositis, radiation recall phenomenon, cardiomyopathy rare (dose-related) **Notes:** Limit of 550 mg/m² cumulative dose (400 mg/m² w/ prior mediastinal irradiation); dexrazoxane may limit cardiac tox; tissue damage w/ extrav; red/orange urine; vesicant w/ extrav, Rx with dexrazoxane

Doxycycline (Adoxa, Periostat, Oracea, Vibramycin, Vibra-Tabs) Uses: *Broad-spectrum antibiotic* acne vulgaris, uncomplicated GC, chlamydia, PID, Lyme Dz, skin Infxns, anthrax, malaria prophylaxis **Action:** Tetracycline; bacteriostatic; ↓ protein synth. *Spectrum:* Limited gram(+) and (–), *Rickettsia* sp, *Chlamydia, M. pneumoniae, B. anthracis* **Dose:** *Adults.* 100 mg PO q12h on 1st d, then 100 mg PO daily–bid or 100 mg IV q12h; acne q day, chlamydia × 7d, Lyme × 21 d, PID × 14 d *Peds >8 y:* 5 mg/kg/24 h PO, 200 mg/d max ÷ daily-bid **Caution:** [D, +] hepatic impair **CI:** Children <8 y, severe hepatic dysfunction **Disp:** Tabs 20, 50, 75, 100, 150 mg; caps 50, 100 mg; Oracea 40 mg caps (30 mg timed release, 10 mg DR); syrup 50 mg/5 mL; susp 25 mg/5 mL; Inj 100, 200 mg/vial **SE:** D, GI disturbance, photosensitivity **Notes:** ↓ effect w/ antacids; tetracycline of choice w/ renal impair; for inhalational anthrax use w/ 1–2 additional antibiotics, not for CNS anthrax

Dronabinol (Marinol) [C-II] Uses: *N/V associated w/ CA chemotherapy; appetite stimulation* **Action:** Antiemetic; ↓ V center in the medulla **Dose:** *Adults & Peds.* Antiemetic: 5–15 mg/m²/dose q4–6h PRN. *Adults.* Appetite stimulant: 2.5 mg PO before lunch & dinner; max 20 mg/d **Caution:** [C, ?] elderly, Hx psychological disorder, Sz disorder, substance abuse **CI:** Hx schizophrenia, sesame oil hypersensitivity **Disp:** Caps 2.5, 5, 10 mg **SE:** Drowsiness, dizziness, anxiety, mood change, hallucinations, depersonalization, orthostatic ↓ BP, tachycardia **Notes:** Principal psychoactive substance present in marijuana

Droperidol (Inapsine) **WARNING:** Cases of QT interval prolongation and torsades de pointes (same fatal) reported Uses: *N/V; anesthetic premedication* **Action:** Tranquilizer, sedation, antiemetic **Dose:** *Adults.* N: initial dose 2.5 mg IV/IM, may repeat 1.25 mg based on response; *Premed:* 2.5–10 mg IV, 30–60 min pre-op. *Peds. Premed:* 0.1–0.15 mg/kg/dose **Caution:** [C, ?]w/ Hepatic/renal impair **CI:** Component sensitivity **Disp:** Inj 2.5 mg/mL **SE:** Drowsiness, ↓ BP, occasional tachycardia & extrapyramidal Rxns, ↑ QT interval, arrhythmias **Notes:** Give IV push slowly over 2–5 min

Drotrecogin Alfa (Xigris) Uses: *↓ Mortality in adults w/ severe sepsis (w/ acute organ dysfunction) at high risk of death (eg, determined by APACHEII score [www.ncemi.org])* **Action:** Recombinant human-activated protein C; antithrombotic and anti-inflammatory, unclear mechanism **Dose:** 24 mcg/kg/h, total of 96 h **Caution:** [C, ?] w/ Anticoagulation, INR >3, plt <30,000, GI bleed w/in 6 wk **CI:** Active bleeding, recent stroke/CNS surgery, head trauma/CNS lesion w/ herniation risk, trauma w/ ↑ bleeding risk, epidural catheter, mifepristone **Disp:** 5-, 20-mg vials **SE:** Bleeding **Notes:** Single-organ dysfunction & renal surgery may not be at high risk of death irrespective of APACHE II score & therefore not indicated. Percutaneous procedures: Stop Inf 2 h before & resume 1 h after; major surgery: stop Inf 2 h before & resume 12 h after in absence of bleeding

Duloxetine (Cymbalta)   **WARNING:** Antidepressants may ↑ risk of suicidality; consider risks/benefits of use. Closely monitor for clinical worsening, suicidality, or behavior changes **Uses:** *Depression, DM peripheral neuropathic pain, generalized anxiety disorder (GAD)* **Action:** Selective serotonin & norepinephrine reuptake inhibitor (SSNRI) **Dose:** *Depression:* 40–60 mg/d PO ÷ bid. *DM neuropathy:* 60 mg/d PO; *GAD:* 30–60 mg/d max 120 mg/d **Caution:** [C, ?/–]; use in 3rd tri; avoid if CrCl <30 mL/min, NAG, w/ fluvoxamine, inhibitors of CYP2D6 (Table 11), TCAs, phenothiazines, type 1C antiarrhythmics (Table 10) **CI:** MAOI use w/in 14 d, w/ thioridazine, NAG, hepatic Insuff **Disp:** Caps delayed-release 20, 30, 60 mg **SE:** N, dizziness, somnolence, fatigue, sweating, xerostomia, constipation, ↓ appetite, sexual dysfunction, urinary hesitancy, ↑ LFTs, HTN **Notes:** Swallow whole; monitor BP; avoid abrupt D/C

Dutasteride (Avodart)   **Uses:** *Symptomatic BPH to improve Sxs, ↓ risk of retention and BPH surgery alone or in combo w/ tamsulosin* **Action:** 5α-Reductase inhibitor; ↓ intracellular dihydrotestosterone (DHT) **Dose:** *Monotherapy:* 0.5 mg PO/d. *Combo:* 0.5 mg PO q day w/ tamsulosin 0.4 mg q day **Caution:** [X, –] Hepatic impair; pregnant women should not handle pills **CI:** Women, peds **Disp:** Caps 0.5 mg **SE:** ↑ testosterone, thyroid-stimulating hormone ↑, ↓ PSA levels, impotence, ↓ libido, gynecomastia, ejaculatory disturbance **Notes:** No blood donation until 6 mo after D/C, new baseline PSA at 6 mo; corrected PSA × 2; under study for PCa chemotherapy prevention

Echothiophate Iodine (Phospholine Ophthalmic)   **Uses:** *Glaucoma* **Action:** Cholinesterase inhibitor **Dose:** 1 gtt eye(s) bid w/ 1 dose hs **Caution:** [C, ?] **CI:** Active uveal inflammation, inflammatory Dz of iris/ciliary body, glaucoma iridocyclitis **Disp:** Powder, reconstitute 1.5 mg/0.03%; 3 mg/0.06%; 6.25 mg/0.125%; 12.5 mg/0.25% **SE:** Local irritation, myopia, blurred vision, ↓ BP, bradycardia

Econazole (Spectazole)   **Uses:** *Tinea, cutaneous Candida, & tinea versicolor Infxns* **Action:** Topical antifungal **Dose:** Apply to areas bid (daily for tinea versicolor) for 2–4 wk **Caution:** [C, ?] **CI:** Component sensitivity **Disp:** Topical cream 1% **SE:** Local irritation, pruritus, erythema **Notes:** Early Sx/clinical improvement; complete course to avoid recurrence

Eculizumab (Soliris)   **WARNING:** ↑ Risk of meningococcal infections (give meningococcal vaccine 2 wk prior to 1st dose and revaccinate per guidelines) **Uses:** *Rx paroxysmal nocturnal hemoglobinuria* **Action:** Complement inhibitor **Dose:** 600 mg IV q 7 d × 4 wk, then 900 mg IV 5th dose 7 d later, then 900 mg IV q14d **Caution:** [C; ?] **CI:** Active *Neisseria meningitidis* Infxn; if not vaccinated against *N. meningitidis* **Disp:** 300-mg vial **SE:** Meningococcal Infxn, HA, nasopharyngitis, N, back pain, Infxns, fatigue, severe hemolysis on D/C **Notes:** IV over 35 min (2-h max Inf time); monitor for 1 h for S/Sx of Inf Rxn

Edrophonium (Tensilon, Reversol) **Uses:** *Diagnosis of *MyG;* acute MyG crisis; curare antagonist, reverse of nondepolarizing neuromuscular blockers* **Action:** Anticholinesterase **Dose:** *Adults. Test for MyG:* 2 mg IV in 1 min; if tolerated, give 8 mg IV; (+) test is brief ↑ in strength. *Peds. Test for MyG:* Total dose 0.2 mg/kg; 0.04 mg/kg test dose; if no Rxn, give remainder in 1 mg increments to 10 mg max; ↓ in renal impair **Caution:** [C, ?] **CI:** GI or GU obst; allergy to sulfite **Disp:** Inj 10 mg/mL **SE:** N/V/D, excessive salivation, stomach cramps, ↑ aminotransferases **Notes:** Can cause severe cholinergic effects; keep atropine available

Efalizumab (Raptiva) **WARNING:** Associated w/ serious Infxns, malignancy, thrombocytopenia **Uses:** Chronic mod–severe plaque psoriasis **Action:** MoAb **Dose:** *Adults.* 0.7 mg/kg SQ conditioning dose, followed by 1 mg/kg/wk; single doses should not exceed 200 mg **Caution:** [C, +/–], chronic Infxn elderly **CI:** Administration of most vaccines **Disp:** 125-mg vial **SE:** 1st-dose Rxn, HA, worsening psoriasis, ↑ LFTs, hemolytic anemia immunosuppressive-related Rxns (see Warning) **Notes:** Minimize 1st-dose Rxn by conditioning dose; ✓ plts monthly, then q3mo & w/ dose ↑; pts may be trained in self-administration

Efavirenz (Sustiva) **Uses:** *HIV Infxns* **Action:** Antiretroviral; nonnucleoside RT inhibitor **Dose:** *Adults.* 600 mg/d PO q hs. *Peds ≥3 y 10–<15 kg:* 200 mg PO q day; *15–<20 kg:* 250 mg PO q day; *20–<25 kg:* 300 mg PO q day; *25–<32.5 kg:* 350 mg PO q day; *32.5–<40 kg:* 400 mg PO q day; *≥40 kg:* 600 mg PO q day; on empty stomach **Caution:** [D, ?] CDC recommends HIV-infected mothers not breast-feed **CI:** w/ Astemizole, bepridil, cisapride, midazolam, pimozide, triazolam, ergot derivatives, voriconazole **Disp:** Caps 50, 100, 200; 600 mg tab **SE:** Somnolence, vivid dreams, depression, CNS Sxs, dizziness, rash, N/V/D **Notes:** ✓ LFTs, cholesterol; not for monotherapy

Efavirenz, Emtricitabine, Tenofovir (Atripla) **WARNING:** Lactic acidosis and severe hepatomegaly with steatosis, including fatal cases, reported w/ nucleoside analogs alone or combo w/ other antiretrovirals **Uses:** *HIV Infxns* **Action:** Triple fixed-dose combo nonnucleoside RT inhibitor/nucleoside analog **Dose:** *Adults.* 1 tab q day on empty stomach; HS dose may ↓ CNS SE **Caution:** [D, ?] CDC recommends HIV-infected mothers not breast-feed, w/ obesity **CI:** <18 y, w/ astemizole, midazolam, triazolam, or ergot derivatives (CYP3A4 competition by efavirenz could cause serious/life-threatening SE) **Disp:** Tab efavirenz 600 mg/emtricitabine 200 mg/tenofovir 300 mg **SE:** Somnolence, vivid dreams, HA, dizziness, rash, N/V/D, ↓ BMD **Notes:** Monitor LFTs, cholesterol; see individual agents for additional info, not for HIV/hep B coinfection

Eletriptan (Relpax) **Uses:** *Acute Rx of migraine* **Action:** Selective serotonin receptor (5-HT$_{1B/1D}$) agonist **Dose:** 20–40 mg PO, may repeat in 2 h;

80 mg/24 h max **Caution:** [C, +] **CI:** Hx ischemic heart Dz, coronary artery spasm, stroke or TIA, peripheral vascular Dz, IBD, uncontrolled HTN, hemiplegic or basilar migraine, w/in 24 h of another 5-HT₁ agonist or ergot, w/in 72 h of CYP3A4 inhibitors **Disp:** Tabs 20, 40 mg **SE:** Dizziness, somnolence, N, asthenia, xerostomia, paresthesias; pain, pressure, or tightness in chest, jaw, or neck; serious cardiac events

Emedastine (Emadine) **Uses:** *Allergic conjunctivitis* **Action:** Antihistamine; selective H₁-antagonist **Dose:** 1 gtt in eye(s) up to qid **Caution:** [B, ?] **CI:** Allergy to ingredients (preservatives benzalkonium, tromethamine) **Disp:** 0.05% soln **SE:** HA, blurred vision, burning/stinging, corneal infiltrates/staining, dry eyes, foreign body sensation, hyperemia, keratitis, tearing, pruritus, rhinitis, sinusitis, asthenia, bad taste, dermatitis, discomfort **Notes:** Do not use contact lenses if eyes are red

Emtricitabine (Emtriva) **WARNING:** Lactic acidosis, & severe hepatomegaly w/ steatosis reported; not for HBV Infxn **Uses:** *HIV-1 Infxn* **Action:** NRTI **Dose:** 200 mg caps or 240 mg soln PO daily; ↓ w/ renal impair **Caution:** [B, –] risk of liver Dz **CI:** Component sensitivity **Disp:** Soln 10 mg/mL, caps 200 mg **SE:** HA, N/D, rash, rare hyperpigmentation of feet & hands, posttreatment exacerbation of hep **Notes:** 1st one-daily NRTI; caps/soln not equivalent; not ok as monotherapy; screen for hep B, do not use w/ HIV and HBV coinfection

Enalapril (Vasotec) **WARNING:** ACE inhibitors used during PRG can cause fetal injury & death **Uses:** *HTN, CHF, LVD,* DN **Action:** ACE inhibitor **Dose:** *Adults.* 2.5–40 mg/d PO; 1.25 mg IV q6h. *Peds.* 0.05–0.08 mg/kg/d PO q12–24h; ↓ w/ renal impair **Caution:** [C (1st tri; D 2nd & 3rd tri), +] D/C immediately w/PRG, w/ NSAIDs, K⁺ supls **CI:** Bilateral RAS, angioedema **Disp:** Tabs 2.5, 5, 10, 20 mg; IV 1.25 mg/mL (1, 2 mL) **SE:** ↓ BP w/ initial dose (especially w/ diuretics), ↑ K⁺, ↑ Cr nonproductive cough, angioedema **Notes:** Monitor Cr; D/C diuretic for 2–3 d prior to start

Enfuvirtide (Fuzeon) **WARNING:** Rarely causes allergy; never rechallenge **Uses:** *w/ Antiretroviral agents for HIV-1 in treatment-experienced pts w/ viral replication despite ongoing therapy* **Action:** Viral fusion inhibitor **Dose:** *Adults.* 90 mg (1 mL) SQ bid in upper arm, anterior thigh, or abdomen; rotate site **Peds.** see insert **Caution:** [B, –] **CI:** Previous allergy to drug **Disp:** 90 mg/mL recons; pt kit w/ supplies × 1 mo **SE:** Inj site Rxns; pneumonia, D, N, fatigue, insomnia, peripheral neuropathy **Notes:** Available via restricted distribution system; use immediately on recons or refrigerate (24 h max)

Enoxaparin (Lovenox) **WARNING:** Recent or anticipated epidural/ spinal anesthesia ↑ risk of spinal/epidural hematoma w/ subsequent paralysis **Uses:** *Prevention & Rx of DVT; Rx PE; unstable angina & non–q–wave MI* **Action:** LMW heparin; inhibit thrombin by complexing w/ antithrombin III **Dose:** *Adults. Prevention:* 30 mg SQ bid or 40 mg SQ q24h. *DVT/PE Rx:* 1 mg/kg SQ q12h or 1.5 mg/kg SQ q24h. *Angina:* 1 mg/kg SQ q12h; *Ancillary to AMI fibrinolysis:*

30 mg IV bolus, then 1 mg/kg SQ bid *(ECC 2005);* CrCl <30 mL/min ↓ to 1 mg/kg SQ q day *Peds. Prevention:* 0.5 mg/kg SQ q12h. *DVT/PE Rx:* 1 mg/kg SQ q12h; ↓ dose w/ CrCl <30 mL/min **Caution:** [B, ?] Not for prophylaxis in prosthetic heart valves **CI:** Active bleeding, HIT Ab **Disp:** Inj 10 mg/0.1 mL (30-, 40-, 60-, 80-, 100-, 120-, 150-mg syringes); 300-mg/mL multidose vial **SE:** Bleeding, hemorrhage, bruising, thrombocytopenia, fever, pain/hematoma at site, ↑ AST/ALT **Notes:** No effect on bleeding time, plt Fxn, PT, or aPTT; monitor plt for HIT, clinical bleeding; may monitor antifactor Xa; not for IM

Entacapone (Comtan) Uses: *Parkinson Dz* **Action:** Selective & reversible carboxymethyl transferase inhibitor **Dose:** 200 mg w/ each levodopa/carbidopa dose; max 1600 mg/d; ↓ levodopa/carbidopa dose 25% w/ levodopa dose >800 mg **Caution:** [C, ?] Hepatic impair **CI:** Use w/ MAOI **Disp:** Tabs 200 mg **SE:** Dyskinesia, hyperkinesia, N, D, dizziness, hallucinations, orthostatic ↓ BP, brown-orange urine **Notes:** ✓ LFTs; do not D/C abruptly

Ephedrine Uses: *Bronchospasm, bronchial asthma, nasal congestion,* ↓ BP, narcolepsy, enuresis, & MyG **Action:** Sympathomimetic; stimulates α- & β-receptors; bronchodilator **Dose:** *Adults. Congestion:* 25–50 mg PO q6h PRN; ↓ *BP:* 25–50 mg IV q5–10min, 150 mg/d max. *Peds.* 0.2–0.3 mg/kg/dose IV q4–6h PRN **Caution:** [C, ?/–] **CI:** Arrhythmias; NAG **Disp:** Nasal soln 0.48%, 0.5%; caps 25 mg; Inj 50 mg/mL; nasal spray 0.25% **SE:** CNS stimulation (nervousness, anxiety, trembling), tachycardia, arrhythmia, HTN, xerostomia, dysuria **Notes:** Protect from light; monitor BP, HR, urinary output; can cause false ↑ amphetamine EMIT; take last dose 4–6 h before hs; abuse potential, OTC sales mostly banned/restricted

Epinephrine (Adrenalin, Sus-Phrine, EpiPen, EpiPen Jr, others) Uses: *Cardiac arrest, anaphylactic Rxn, bronchospasm, open-angle glaucoma* **Action:** β-Adrenergic agonist, some α effects **Dose:** *Adults.* 1 mg IV push, repeat q3–5min; (0.2 mg/kg max) if 1-mg dose fails. Inf: 30 mg (30 mL of 1:1000 soln) in 250 mL NS or D₅W, at 100 mL/h, titrate. ET 2–2.5 mg in 20 mL NS. *Profound bradycardia/hypotension:* 2–10 mcg/min (1 mg of 1:1000 in 500 mL NS, infuse 1–5 mL/min) *(ECC 2005).* *Anaphylaxis:* 0.3–0.5 mL SQ of 1:1000 dilution, repeat PRN q5–15min to max 1 mg/dose & 5 mg/d. *Asthma:* 0.1–0.5 mL SQ of 1:1000 dilution, repeat q 20 min to 4 h, or 1 Inh (metered-dose) repeat in 1–2 min, or susp 0.1–0.3 mL SQ for extended effect. *Peds. ACLS:* 1st dose 0.1 mL/kg IV of 1:10,000 dilution, then 0.1 mL/kg IV of 1:1000 dilution q3–5min to response. *Anaphylaxis:* 0.15–0.3 mg IM depending on wgt <30 kg 0.01 mg/kg. *Asthma:* 0.01 mL/kg SQ of 1:1000 dilution q8–12h **Caution:** [C, ?] ↓ bronchodilation with β-blockers **CI:** Cardiac arrhythmias, NAG **Disp:** Inj 1:1000, 1:2000, 1:10,000, 1:100,000; susp for Inj 1:200; aerosol 220 mcg/spray; 1% Inh soln; EpiPen Autoinjector 1 dose = 0.30 mg; EpiPen Jr 1 dose = 0.15 mg **SE:** CV (tachycardia, HTN, vasoconstriction); CNS stimulation (nervousness, anxiety, trembling), ↓ renal blood flow **Notes:**

Can give via ET tube if no central line (use 2–2.5 × IV dose); EpiPen for pt self-use (www.EpiPen.com)

Epinastine (Elestat) Uses: Itching w/ allergic conjunctivitis **Action:** Anti-histamine **Dose:** 1 gtt bid **Caution:** [C, ?/–] **Disp:** Soln 0.05% **SE:** Burning, folliculosis, hyperemia, pruritus, URI, HA, rhinitis, sinusitis, cough, pharyngitis **Notes:** Remove contacts before, reinsert in 10 min

Epirubicin (Ellence) **WARNING:** Do not give IM or SQ. Extrav causes tissue necrosis; potential cardiotox; severe myelosuppression; ↓ dose w/ hepatic impair **Uses:** *Adjuvant therapy for + axillary nodes after resection of primary breast CA* **Actions:** Anthracycline cytotoxic agent **Dose:** Per protocols; ↓ dose w/ hepatic impair **Caution:** [D, –] **CI:** Baseline neutrophil count <1500 cells/mm³, severe cardiac Insuff, recent MI, severe arrhythmias, severe hepatic dysfunction, previous anthracyclines Rx to max cumulative dose **Disp:** Inj 50 mg/25 mL, 200 mg/100 mL **SE:** Mucositis, N/V/D, alopecia, ↓ BM, cardiotox, secondary AML, tissue necrosis w/ extrav (see Adriamycin for Rx), lethargy **Notes:** ✓ CBC, bilirubin, AST, Cr, cardiac Fxn before/during each cycle

Eplerenone (Inspra) Uses: *HTN* **Action:** Selective aldosterone antagonist **Dose:** *Adults.* 50 mg PO daily-bid, doses >100 mg/d no benefit w/ ↑ K⁺; ↓ to 25 mg PO daily if giving w/ CYP3A4 inhibitors **Caution:** [B, +/–] w/ CYP3A4 inhibitors (Table 11); monitor K⁺ with ACE inhibitor, ARBs, NSAIDs, K⁺-sparing diuretics; grapefruit juice, St. John's wort **CI:** K⁺ >5.5 mEq/L; non–insulin-dependent diabetes mellitus (NIDDM) w/ microalbuminuria; SCr >2 mg/dL (males), >1.8 mg/dL (females); CrCl <30 mL/min; w/ K⁺ supls/K⁺-sparing diuretics, ketoconazole **Disp:** Tabs 25, 50 mg **SE:** ↑ cholesterol/triglycerides, ↑ K⁺, HA, dizziness, gynecomastia, D, orthostatic ↓ BP **Notes:** May take 4 wk for full effect

Epoetin Alfa [Erythropoietin, EPO] (Epogen, Procrit) **WARNING:** ↑ Mortality, serious CV/thromboembolic events, and tumor progression. Renal failure pts experienced ↑ greater risks (death/CV events) on erythropoiesis-stimulating agents (ESAs) to target higher Hgb levels. Maintain Hgb 10–12g/dL. In cancer pt, ESAs ↓ survival/time-to progression in some cancers when dosed Hgb ≥12 g/dL. Use lowest dose needed. Use only for myelosuppressive chemotherapy. D/C following chemotherapy. Pre-op ESA ↑ DVT. Consider DVT prophylaxis **Uses:** *CRF-associated anemia, zidovudine Rx in HIV-infected pts, CA chemotherapy; ↓ transfusions associated w/ surgery* **Action:** Induces erythropoiesis **Dose:** *Adults & Peds.* 50–150 units/kg IV/SQ 3×/wk; adjust dose q4–6wk PRN. *Surgery:* 300 units/kg/d × 10 d before to 4 d after; ↓ dose if Hct ≈ 36% or Hgb, ↑ > ≈ 12 g/dL or Hgb ↑ >1 g/dL in 2-wk period; hold dose if Hgb >12 g/dL **Caution:** [C, +] **CI:** Uncontrolled HTN **Disp:** Inj 2000, 3000, 4000, 10,000, 20,000, 40,000 units/mL **SE:** HTN, HA, fatigue, fever, tachycardia, N/V **Notes:** Refrigerate; monitor baseline & posttreatment Hct/Hgb, BP, ferritin

Epoprostenol (Flolan) Uses: *Pulm HTN* **Action:** Dilates pulm/systemic arterial vascular beds; ↓ plt aggregation **Dose:** Initial 2 ng/kg/min; ↑ by

2 ng/kg/min q15min until dose-limiting SE (CP, dizziness, N/V, HA, ↓ BP, flushing); IV cont Inf 4 ng/kg/min < max tolerated rate; adjust based on response; see package insert **Caution:** [B, ?] ↑ tox w/ diuretics, vasodilators, acetate in dialysis fluids, anticoagulants **CI:** Chronic use in CHF 2nd degree, if pt develops pulm edema w/ dose initiation, severe LVSD **Disp:** Inj 0.5, 1.5 mg **SE:** Flushing, tachycardia, CHF, fever, chills, nervousness, HA, N/V/D, jaw pain, flu-like Sxs **Notes:** Abrupt D/C can cause rebound pulm HTN; monitor bleeding w/ other antiplatelet/anticoagulants; watch ↓ BP w/ other vasodilators/diuretics

Eprosartan (Teveten) **Uses:** *HTN,* DN, CHF **Action:** ARB **Dose:** 400–800 mg/d single dose or bid **Caution:** [C (1st tri); D (2nd & 3rd tri), D/C immediately when pregnancy detected] w/ Lithium, ↑ K+ with K+-sparing diuretics/supls/high-dose trimethoprim **CI:** Bilateral RAS, 1st-degree aldosteronism **Disp:** Tabs 400, 600 mg **SE:** Fatigue, depression, URI, UTI, Abd pain, rhinitis/pharyngitis/cough, hypertriglyceridemia

Eptifibatide (Integrilin) **Uses:** *ACS, PCI* **Action:** Glycoprotein IIb/IIIa inhibitor **Dose:** 180 mcg/kg IV bolus, then 2 mcg/kg/min cont Inf; ↓ in renal impair (SCr >2 mg/dL, <4 mg/dL: 135 mcg/kg bolus & 0.5 mcg/kg/min Inf); ACS: 180 mcg/kg IV bolus then 2 mcg/kg/min. PCI: 135 mcg/kg IV bolus then 0.5 mcg/kg/min; bolus again in 10 min *(ECC 2005)* **Caution:** [B, ?] Monitor bleeding w/ other anticoagulants **CI:** Other glycoprotein IIb/IIIa inhibitors, Hx abnormal bleeding, hemorrhagic stroke (within 30 d), severe HTN, major surgery (w/in 6 wk), plt count <100,000 cells/mm³, renal dialysis **Disp:** Inj 0.75, 2 mg/mL **SE:** Bleeding, ↓ BP, Inj site Rxn, thrombocytopenia **Notes:** Monitor bleeding, coagulants, plts, SCr, activated coagulation time (ACT) with prothrombin consumption index (keep ACT 200–300 s)

Erlotinib (Tarceva) **Uses:** *NSCLC after failing 1 chemotherapy; CA pancreas* **Action:** HER2/EGFR TKI **Dose:** *CA Pancreas* 100 mg, *others* 150 mg/d PO 1 h ac or 2 h pc; ↓ (in 50-mg decrements) w/ severe Rxn or w/ CYP3A4 inhibitors (Table 11); per protocols **Caution:** [D, ?/–]; w/ CYP3A4 (Table 11) inhibitors **Disp:** Tabs 25, 100, 150 mg **SE:** Rash, N/V/D, anorexia, Abd pain, fatigue, cough, dyspnea, edema, stomatitis, conjunctivitis, pruritus, dry skin, Infxn, ↑ LFTs, interstitial lung Dz **Notes:** May ↑ INR w/ warfarin, monitor INR

Ertapenem (Invanz) **Uses:** *Complicated intra-Abd, acute pelvic, & skin Infxns, pyelonephritis, CAP* **Action:** A carbapenem; β-lactam antibiotic, ↓ cell wall synth **Spectrum:** Good gram(+/–) & anaerobic coverage, not *Pseudomonas, Acinetobacter* sp, PCN-resistant pneumococci, MRSA, *Enterococcus,* β-lactamase (+) *H. influenzae, Mycoplasma, Chlamydia* **Dose:** *Adults.* 1 g IM/IV daily; mg/d in CrCl <30 mL/min. *Peds 3 mo–12 y:* 15 mg/kg bid IM/IV, max 1 g/d **Caution:** [B, ?/–] Sz Hx, CNS disorders, β-lactam & multiple allergies, probenecid ↓ renal clearance **CI:** component hypersensitivity or amide anesthetics **Disp:** Inj 1 g/vial **SE:** HA, N/V/D, Inj site Rxns, thrombocytosis, ↑ LFTs **Notes:** Can give IM × 7 d, IV × 14 d; 137 mg Na+ (6 mEq)/g ertapenem

Erythromycin (E-Mycin, E.E.S., Ery-Tab, EryPed, Ilotycin)

Uses: *Bacterial Infxns; bowel preparation*; ↑ GI motility (*prokinetic*); *acne vulgaris* **Action:** Bacteriostatic; interferes w/ protein synth. **Spectrum:** Group A streptococci (*S. pyogenes*), *S. pneumoniae*, *N. meningitidis*, *N. gonorrhoeae* (if PCN-allergic), *Legionella*, *M. pneumoniae* **Dose: Adults.** Base 250–500 mg PO q6–12h or ethylsuccinate 400–800 mg q6–12h; 500 mg–1 g IV q6h. *Prokinetic:* 250 mg PO tid 30 min ac. **Peds.** 30–50 mg/kg/d PO ÷ q6–8h or 20–40 mg/kg/d IV ÷ q6h, max 2 g/d **Caution:** [B, +] ↑ tox of carbamazepine, cyclosporine, digoxin, methylprednisolone, theophylline, felodipine, warfarin, simvastatin/lovastatin; ↓ sildenafil dose w/ use **CI:** Hepatic impair, preexisting liver Dz (estolate), use with pimozide **Disp:** *lactobionate (Ilotycin):* Powder for Inj 500 mg, 1 g. *Base:* Tabs 250, 333, 500 mg; caps 250 mg. *Estolate (Ilosone):* Susp 125, 250 mg/5 mL. *Stearate (Erythrocin):* Tabs 250, 500 mg. *Ethylsuccinate (EES, EryPed):* Chew tabs 200 mg; tabs 400 mg; susp 200, 400 mg/5 mL **SE:** HA, Abd pain, N/V/D; [QT prolongation, torsade de pointes, ventricular arrhythmias/tachycardias (rarely)]; cholestatic jaundice (estolate) **Notes:** 400 mg ethylsuccinate = 250 mg base/estolate; w/ food minimizes GI upset; lactobionate contains benzyl alcohol (caution in neonates)

Erythromycin & Benzoyl Peroxide (Benzamycin)

Uses: *Topical for acne vulgaris* **Action:** Macrolide antibiotic w/ keratolytic **Dose:** Apply bid (A.M. & P.M.). **Caution:** [C, ?] **CI:** Component sensitivity **Disp:** Gel erythromycin 30 mg/benzoyl peroxide 50 mg **SE:** Local irritation, dryness

Erythromycin & Sulfisoxazole (Eryzole, Pediazole)

Uses: *Upper & lower resp tract; bacterial Infxns; H. influenzae otitis media in children*; Infxns in PCN-allergic pts **Action:** Macrolide antibiotic w/ sulfonamide **Dose: Adults.** Based on erythromycin content; 400 mg erythromycin/1200 mg sulfisoxazole PO q6h. **Peds >2 mo:** 40–50 mg/kg/d erythromycin & 150 mg/kg/d sulfisoxazole PO ÷ q6h; max 2 g/d erythromycin or 6 g/d sulfisoxazole × 10 d; ↓ in renal impair **Caution:** [C (D if near term), +] w/ PO anticoagulants, hypoglycemics, phenytoin, cyclosporine **CI:** Infants <2 mo **Disp:** Susp erythromycin ethylsuccinate 200 mg/sulfisoxazole 600 mg/5 mL (100, 150, 200 mL) **SE:** GI upset

Erythromycin, ophthalmic (Ilotycin Ophthalmic)

Uses: *Conjunctival/corneal Infxns* **Action:** Macrolide antibiotic **Dose:** 1/2 inch 2–6×/day **Caution:** [B, +] **CI:** Erythromycin hypersensitivity **Disp:** 0.5% oint **SE:** Local irritation

Erythromycin, topical (A/T/S, Eryderm, Erycette, T-Stat)

Uses: *Acne vulgaris* **Action:** Macrolide antibiotic **Dose:** Wash & dry area, apply 2% product over area bid **Caution:** [B, +] **CI:** Component sensitivity **Disp:** Soln 1.5%, 2%; gel 2%; pads & swabs 2% **SE:** Local irritation

Escitalopram (Lexapro)   WARNING: Closely monitor for worsening depression or emergence of suicidality, particularly in ped pts **Uses:** Depression,

anxiety **Action:** SSRI **Dose:** *Adults.* 10–20 mg PO daily; 10 mg/d in elderly & hepatic impair **Caution:** [C, +/–] Serotonin syndrome (Table 12); use of escitalopram, w/ NSAID, ASA or other drugs affecting coagulation associated w/ ↑ bleeding risk **CI:** w/ or w/in 14 d of MAOI **Disp:** Tabs 5, 10, 20 mg; soln 1 mg/mL **SE:** N/V/D, sweating, insomnia, dizziness, xerostomia, sexual dysfunction **Notes:** Full effects may take 3 wk

Esmolol (Brevibloc) **Uses:** *SVT & noncompensatory sinus tachycardia, AF/flutter* **Action:** β_1-Adrenergic blocker; class II antiarrhythmic **Dose:** *Adults & Peds.* Initial 500 mcg/kg load over 1 min, then 50 mcg/kg/min × 4 min; if inadequate response, repeat load & maint Inf of 100 mcg/kg/min × 4 min; titrate by repeating load, then incremental ↑ in the maint dose of 50 mcg/kg/min for 4 min until desired HR reached or ↓ BP; average dose 100 mcg/kg/min; 0.5 mg/kg over 1 min, then 0.05 mg/kg/min *(ECC 2005)* **Caution:** [C (1st tri; D 2nd or 3rd tri), ?] **CI:** Sinus bradycardia, heart block, uncompensated CHF, cardiogenic shock, ↓ BP **Disp:** Inj 10, 20, 250 mg/mL; premix Inf 10 mg/mL **SE:** ↓ BP; bradycardia, diaphoresis, dizziness, pain on Inj **Notes:** Hemodynamic effects back to baseline w/in 30 min after D/C Inf

Esomeprazole (Nexium) **Uses:** *Short-term (4–8 wk) for erosive esophagitis/GERD; H. pylori Infxn in combo with antibiotics* **Action:** Proton pump inhibitor, ↓ gastric acid **Dose:** *Adults. GERD/erosive gastritis:* 20–40 mg/d PO × 4–8 wk; 20–40 mg IV 10–30 min Inf or >3 min IV push, 10 d max; *Maint:* 20 mg/d PO. *H. pylori Infxn:* 40 mg/d PO, plus clarithromycin 500 mg PO bid & amoxicillin 1000 mg/bid for 10 d; **Caution:** [B, ?/–] **CI:** Component sensitivity **Disp:** Caps 20, 40 mg; IV 20, 40 mg **SE:** HA, D, Abd pain **Notes:** Do not chew; may open caps & sprinkle on applesauce

Estazolam (ProSom) [C-IV] **Uses:** *Short-term management of insomnia* **Action:** Benzodiazepine **Dose:** 1–2 mg PO qhs PRN; ↓ in hepatic impair/elderly/debilitated **Caution:** [X, –] ↑ Effects w/ CNS depressants; cross-sensitivity w/ other benzodiazepines **CI:** PRG, component hypersensitivity, w/ itraconazole or ketoconazole **Disp:** Tabs 1, 2 mg **SE:** Somnolence, weakness, palpitations, anaphylaxis, angioedema, amnesia **Notes:** May cause psychological/physical dependence; avoid abrupt D/C after prolonged use

Esterified Estrogens (Estratab, Menest) **WARNING:** ↑ Risk endometrial cancer. Do not use in the prevention of CV Dz or dementia; ↑ risk of MI, stroke, breast CA, PE, DVT, in postmenopausal **Uses:** *Vasomotor Sxs or vulvar/vaginal atrophy w/ menopause*; female hypogonadism, PCa, prevent osteoporosis **Action:** Estrogen supl **Dose:** *Menopausal vasomotor Sx:* 0.3–1.25 mg, cyclically 3 wk on, 1 wk off; add progestin 10–14 d w/ 28-d cycle w/ uterus intact; *Vulvovaginal atrophy:* same regimen except use 0.3–1.25 mg; *Hypogonadism:* 2.5–7.5 mg/d PO × 20 d, off × 10 d; add progestin 10–14 d w/ 28-d cycle w/uterus intact **Caution:** [X, –] **CI:** Undiagnosed genital bleeding, breast CA, estrogen-dependent tumors, thromboembolic disorders, thrombophlebitis, recent MI, PRG, severe hepatic Dz **Disp:** Tabs 0.3, 0.625, 1.25, 2.5 mg **SE:** N, HA, bloating, breast enlargement/tenderness, edema, venous thromboembolism, hypertriglyceridemia, gallbladder Dz **Notes:** Use lowest dose for shortest time (see WHI data [www.whi.org])

Esterified Estrogens + Methyltestosterone (Estratest, Estratest HS, Syntest DS, HS)
WARNING: ↑ Risk endometrial cancer. Avoid in PRG. Do not use in the prevention of CV Dz or dementia; ↑ risk of MI, stroke, breast CA, PE, DVT in postmenopausal women **Uses:** *Vasomotor Sxs*; postpartum breast engorgement **Action:** Estrogen & androgen supl **Dose:** 1 tab/d × 3 wk, 1 wk off **Caution:** [X, –] **CI:** Genital bleeding of unknown cause, breast CA, estrogen-dependent tumors, thromboembolic disorders, thrombophlebitis, recent MI, PRG **Disp:** Tabs (estrogen/methyltestosterone) 0.625 mg/1.25 mg, 1.25 mg/2.5 mg **SE:** N, HA, bloating, breast enlargement/tenderness, edema, ↑ triglycerides, venous thromboembolism, gallbladder Dz **Notes:** Use lowest dose for shortest time; (see WHI data [www.whi.org])

Estradiol, gel (Divigel)
WARNING: ↑ Risk of endometrial CA. Do not use in the prevention of CV Dz or dementia; ↑ risk MI, stroke, breast CA, PE, and DVT in postmenopausal women (50–79 y). ↑ Dementia risk in postmenopausal women (≥65 y) **Uses:** *Vasomotor Sx in menopause* **Action:** Estrogen **Dose:** 0.25 g q day on right or left upper thigh **Caution:** [X, +/–] may ↑ PT/PTT/plt aggregation w/ thyroid Dz **CI:** Undiagnosed genital bleeding, breast CA, estrogen-dependent tumors, thromboembolic disorders, thrombophlebitis, recent MI, PRG, severe hepatic Dz **Disp:** 0.1% gel 0.25/0.5/ 1 g single-dose foil packets w/ 0.25, 0.5, 1-mg estradiol, respectively **SE:** N, HA, bloating, breast enlargement/tenderness, edema, venous thromboembolism, ↑ BP, hypertriglyceridemia, gallbladder Dz **Notes:** if person other than pt applies, glove should be used, keep dry immediately after, rotate site; contains alcohol, caution around flames until dry, not for Vag use

Estradiol, gel (Elestrin)
WARNING: Do not use in the prevention of CV Dz or dementia; ↑ risk MI, stroke, breast CA, PE, and DVT in postmenopausal women **Uses:** *Postmenopausal vasomotor Sxs* **Action:** Estrogen **Dose:** Apply 0.87–1.7 g to skin q day; add progestin × 10–14 d/28-d cycle w/ intact uterus; use lowest effective estrogen dose **Caution:** [X, ?] **CI:** AUB, breast CA, estrogen-dependent tumors, thromboembolic disorders, recent MI, PRG, severe hepatic Dz **Disp:** Gel 0.06% **SE:** Thromboembolic events, MI, stroke, ↑ BP, breast/ovarian/endometrial CA, site Rxns, vag spotting, breast changes, Abd bloating, cramps, HA, fluid retention **Notes:** Apply to upper arm, wait >25 min before sunscreen; avoid concomitant use for >7 d; BP, breast exams

Estradiol, oral (Estrace, Delestrogen, Femtrace)
WARNING: ↑ Risk of endometrial CA; avoid in PRG **Uses:** *Atrophic vaginitis, menopausal vasomotor Sxs,*↑ low estrogen levels, palliation breast and PCa* **Action:** Estrogen **Dose:** *PO:* 1–2 mg/d, adjust PRN to control Sxs. *Vaginal cream:* 2–4 g/d × 2 wk, then 1 g 1–3×/wk. Vasomotor Sx/Vag Atrophy: 10–20 mg IM q4wk, D/C or taper at

3–6-mo intervals. Hypoestrogenism: 10–20 mg IM q4wk. PCa: 30 mg IM q12wk **Caution:** [X, –] **CI:** Genital bleeding of unknown cause, breast CA, porphyria, estrogen-dependent tumors, thromboembolic disorders, thrombophlebitis; recent MI; hepatic impair **Disp** Ring 0.05, 0.1, 2 mg; gel 0.061%; tabs 0.5, 1, 2 mg; vag cream 0.1 mg/g, depot Inj *(Delestrogen)* 10, 20, 40 mg/mL **SE:** N, HA, bloating, breast enlargement/tenderness, edema, ↑ triglycerides, venous thromboembolism, gallbladder Dz

Estradiol, spray (Evamist)   **WARNING:** ↑ Risk of endometrial CA. Do not use in the prevention of CV Dz or dementia; ↑ risk MI, stroke, breast CA, PE, and DVT in postmenopausal women (50–79 y). ↑ Dementia risk in postmenopausal women (≥65 y) **Uses:** *Vasomotor Sx in menopause* **Action:** Estrogen **Dose:** 1 spray on inner surface of forearm **Caution:** [X, +/–] May ↑ PT/PTT/plt aggregation w/ thyroid Dz **CI:** Undiagnosed genital bleeding, breast CA, estrogen-dependent tumors, thromboembolic disorders, thrombophlebitis, recent MI, PRG, severe hepatic Dz **Disp:** 1.53 mg/spray (56 sprays container) **SE:** N, HA, bloating, breast enlargement/tenderness, edema, venous thromboembolism, ↑ BP, hypertriglyceridemia, gallbladder Dz **Notes:** Contains alcohol, caution around flames until dry; not for Vag use

Estradiol, transdermal (Estraderm, Climara, Vivelle, Vivelle Dot)   **WARNING:** ↑ Risk of endometrial CA. Do not use in the prevention of CV Dz or dementia; ↑ risk MI, stroke, breast CA, PE, and DVT in postmenopausal women (50–79 y). ↑ Dementia risk in postmenopausal women (≥65 y) **Uses:** *Severe menopausal vasomotor Sxs; female hypogonadism* **Action:** Estrogen supl **Dose:** Start 0.0375–0.05 mg/d patch 2× /wk based on product; adjust PRN to control Sxs; w/ intact uterus cycle 3 wk on 1 wk off or use cyclic progestin 10–14 d **Caution:** [X, –] See estradiol **CI:** PRG, AUB, porphyria, breast CA, estrogen-dependent tumors, Hx thrombophlebitis, thrombosis **Disp:** Transdermal patches (mg/24 h) 0.025, 0.0375, 0.05, 0.06, 0.075, 0.1 **SE:** N, bloating, breast enlargement/tenderness, edema, HA, hypertriglyceridemia, gallbladder Dz **Notes:** Do not apply to breasts, place on trunk, rotate sites

Estradiol, vaginal (Estring, Femring, Vagifem)   **WARNING:** ↑ Risk of endometrial CA. Do not use in the prevention of CV Dz or dementia; ↑ risk MI, stroke, breast CA, PE, and DVT in postmenopausal women (50–79 y) **Uses:** *Postmenopausal vaginal atrophy (Estring)* *vasomotor Sxs and vulvar/vaginal atrophy associated with menopause(Femring)* *atrophic vaginitis (Vagifem)* **Action:** Estrogen **Dose:** *Estring:* Insert ring into upper third of vaginal vault; remove and replace after 90 d; reassess 3–6 mo; *Femring* use lowest effective dose, insert vaginally, replace q3mo; *Vagifem* 1 tab vaginally q day × 2 wk, then maint 1 tab 2×/wk, D/C or taper at 3–6 mo **Caution:** [X, –] May ↑ PT/PTT/plt aggregation w/ thyroid Dz, toxic shock reported **CI:** Undiagnosed genital bleeding, breast CA, estrogen-dependent tumors, thromboembolic disorders, thrombophlebitis, recent MI, PRG, severe hepatic Dz **Disp:** *Estring* Ring: 0.0075 mg/24 h; *Femring*

Ring: 0.05 and 0.1 mg/d; *Vagifem* tab (vaginal) 25 mcg **SE:** HA, leukorrhea, back pain, candidiasis, vaginitis, vaginal discomfort/hemorrhage, arthralgia, insomnia, Abd pain

Estradiol Cypionate & Medroxyprogesterone Acetate (Lunelle)
WARNING: Cigarette smoking ↑ risk of serious CV side effects from contraceptives w/ estrogen. This risk ↑ w/ age & w/ heavy smoking (>15 cigarettes/d) & is marked in women >35 y. Women who use Lunelle should not smoke **Uses:** *Contraceptive* **Action:** Estrogen & progestin **Dose:** 0.5 mL IM (deltoid, anterior thigh, buttock) monthly, do not exceed 33 d **Caution:** [X, M] HTN, gallbladder Dz, ↑ lipids, migraines, sudden HA, valvular heart Dz with comps **CI:** PRG, heavy smokers >35 y, DVT, PE, cerebro-/CV Dz, estrogen-dependent neoplasm, undiagnosed AUB, porphyria, hepatic tumors, cholestatic jaundice **Disp:** Estradiol cypionate (5 mg), medroxyprogesterone acetate (25 mg) single-dose vial or syringe (0.5 mL) **SE:** Arterial thromboembolism, HTN, cerebral hemorrhage, MI, amenorrhea, acne, breast tenderness **Notes:** Start w/in 5 d of menstruation

Estradiol/Levonorgestrel, transdermal (Climara Pro)
WARNING: ↑ Risk of endometrial CA. Do not use in the prevention of CV Dz or dementia; ↑ risk MI, stroke, breast CA, PE, and DVT in postmenopausal women (50–79 y). ↑ Dementia risk in postmenopausal women (≥65 y) **Uses:** *Menopausal vasomotor Sx; prevent postmenopausal osteoporosis* **Action:** Estrogen & progesterone **Dose:** 1 Patch 1×/wk **Caution:** [X, –] w/ ↓ Thyroid **CI:** AUB, estrogen-sensitive tumors, Hx thromboembolism, liver impair, PRG, hysterectomy **Disp:** Estradiol 0.045 mg/levonorgestrel 0.015/mg day patch **SE:** Site Rxn, Vag bleed/spotting, breast changes, Abd bloating/cramps, HA, retention fluid, edema, ↑ BP **Notes:** Apply lower Abd; for osteoporosis give CA^{2+}/vit D supl; follow breast exams

Estradiol/Norethindrone Acetate (Femhrt, Activella)
WARNING: ↑ Risk of endometrial CA. Do not use in the prevention of CV Dz or dementia; ↑ risk MI, stroke, breast CA, PE, and DVT in postmenopausal women (50–79 y). ↑ Dementia risk in postmenopausal women (≥65 y) **Uses:** *Menopause vasomotor Sxs; prevent osteoporosis* **Action:** Estrogen/progestin; plant derived **Dose:** 1 tab/d start w/ lowest dose combo **Caution:** [X, –] w/ ↓ CA^{2+}/thyroid **CI:** PRG; Hx breast CA; estrogen-dependent tumor; abnormal genital bleeding; Hx DVT, PE, or related disorders; arterial arterial thromboembolic Dz (CVA, MI) **Disp:** *Femhrt* tabs 2.5/0.5, 5 mcg/1 mg; *Activella* tabs 1.0/0.5, 0.5 mg/0.1 mg **SE:** Thrombosis, dizziness, HA, libido changes, insomnia, emotional stability, breast pain **Notes:** Use in women w/ intact uterus; caution in heavy smokers

Estramustine Phosphate (Emcyt)
Uses: *Advanced PCa* **Action:** estradiol w/ nornitrogen mustard; exact mechanism unknown **Dose:** 14 mg/kg/d in 3–4 ÷ doses; on empty stomach, no dairy products **Caution:** [NA, not used in females] **CI:** Active thrombophlebitis or thromboembolic disorders **Disp:** Caps

140 mg **SE:** N/V, exacerbation of preexisting CHF, edema, hepatic disturbances, thrombophlebitis, MI, PE, gynecomastia in 20–100% **NOTE:** low-dose breast irradiation before may ↓ gynecomastia

Estrogen, Conjugated (Premarin) **WARNING:** ↑ Risk of endometrial CA. Do not use in the prevention of CV Dz or dementia; ↑ risk MI, stroke, breast CA, PE, and DVT in postmenopausal women (50–79 y). ↑ Dementia risk in postmenopausal women (≥65 y) **Uses:** *Mod–severe menopausal vasomotor Sxs; atrophic vaginitis; palliative advanced CAP; prevention & Tx of estrogendeficiency osteoporosis* **Action:** Estrogen hormonal replacement **Dose:** 0.3–1.25 mg/d PO cyclically; prostatic CA 1.25–2.5 mg PO tid; *Vag* cream 0.625 mg/d **Caution:** [X, –] **CI:** Severe hepatic impair, genital bleeding of unknown cause, breast CA, estrogen-dependent tumors, thromboembolic disorders, thrombosis, thrombophlebitis, recent MI **Disp:** Tabs 0.3, 0.45, 0.625, 0.9, 1.25, 2.5 mg; Vag cream 0.625 mg/g **SE:** ↑ Risk of endometrial CA, gallbladder Dz, thromboembolism, HA, & possibly breast CA **Notes:** generic products not equivalent

Estrogen, Conjugated Synthetic (Cenestin, Enjuvia) **WARNING:** ↑ Risk of endometrial CA. Do not use in the prevention of CV Dz or dementia; ↑ risk MI, stroke, breast CA, PE, and DVT in postmenopausal women (50–79 y). ↑ Dementia risk in postmenopausal women (≥65 y) **Uses:** *Vasomotor menopausal Sxs, vulvovaginal atrophy, prevent postmenopausal osteoporosis* **Action:** Multiple estrogen hormonal replacement **Dose:** For all w/ intact uterus progestin × 10–14 d/ 28-d cycle; *Vasomotor* 0.3–1.25 mg (Enjuvia) 0.625–1.25 mg (Cenestin) PO daily; *Vag atrophy* 0.3 mg/d; *Osteoporosis* (Cenestin) 0.625 mg/d **Caution:** [X, –] **CI:** See estrogen, conjugated **Disp:** Tabs Cenestin 0.3, 0.45, 0.625, 0.9 mg; Enjuvia ER 0.3, 0.45, 0.625, 1.25 mg **SE:** ↑ Risk endometrial/breast CA, gallbladder Dz, thromboembolism

Estrogen, Conjugated + Medroxyprogesterone (Prempro, Premphase) **WARNING:** Should not be used for the prevention of CV Dz or dementia; ↑ risk of MI, stroke, breast CA, PE, & DVT; ↑ risk of dementia in postmenopausal women (≥65 y) **Uses:** *Mod–severe menopausal vasomotor Sxs; atrophic vaginitis; prevent postmenopausal osteoporosis* **Action:** Hormonal replacement **Dose:** Prempro 1 tab PO daily; Premphase 1 tab PO daily **Caution:** [X, –] **CI:** Severe hepatic impair, genital bleeding of unknown cause, breast CA, estrogen-dependent tumors, thromboembolic disorders, thrombosis, thrombophlebitis **Disp:** (As estrogen/ medroxyprogesterone) *Prempro:* Tabs 0.625/2.5, 0.625/5 mg; *Premphase:* Tabs 0.625/0 (d 1–14) & 0.625/5 mg (d 15–28) **SE:** Gallbladder Dz, thromboembolism, HA, breast tenderness **Notes:** See WHI (www.whi.org)

Estrogen, Conjugated + Methylprogesterone (Premarin + Methylprogesterone) **WARNING:** Do not use in the prevention of CV Dz or dementia; ↑ risk of endometrial cancer **Uses:** *Menopausal vasomotor Sxs; osteoporosis* **Action:** Estrogen & androgen combo **Dose:** 1 tab/d **Caution:** [X, –] **CI:** Severe hepatic impair, AUB, breast CA, estrogen-dependent tumors, thromboembolic disorders, thrombosis, thrombophlebitis **Disp:** Tabs 0.625 mg estrogen, conjugated, & 2.5 or 5 mg of methylprogesterone **SE:** N, bloating, breast enlargement/tenderness, edema, HA, hypertriglyceridemia, gallbladder Dz

Estrogen, Conjugated + Methyltestosterone (Premarin + Methyltestosterone) **WARNING:** Do not use in the prevention of CV Dz or dementia; ↑ risk of endometrial cancer **Uses:** *Mod–severe menopausal vasomotor Sxs*; postpartum breast engorgement **Action:** Estrogen & androgen combo **Dose:** 1 tab/d × 3 wk, then 1 wk off **Caution:** [X, –] **CI:** Severe hepatic impair, genital bleeding of unknown cause, breast CA, estrogen-dependent tumors, thromboembolic disorders, thrombophlebitis **Disp:** Tabs (estrogen/methyltestosterone) 0.625 mg/5 mg, 1.25 mg/10 mg **SE:** N, bloating, breast enlargement/tenderness, edema, HA, hypertriglyceridemia, gallbladder Dz

Eszopiclone (Lunesta) [C-IV] **Uses:** *Insomnia* **Action:** Nonbenzodiazepine hypnotic **Dose:** 2–3 mg/d hs *Elderly:* 1–2 mg/d hs; w/ hepatic impair use w/ CYP3A4 inhibitor (Table 11): 1 mg/d hs **Caution:** [C, ?/–] **Disp:** Tabs 1, 2, 3 mg **SE:** HA, xerostomia, dizziness, somnolence, hallucinations, Infxn, unpleasant taste, anaphylaxis, angioedema **Notes:** High-fat meals ↓ absorption

Etanercept (Enbrel) **WARNING:** Serious Infxns (bacterial sepsis, TB, reported); D/C w/ severe Infxn. Evaluate for TB risk; test for TB before use **Uses:** *↓ Sxs of RA in pts who fail other DMARD,* Crohn Dz **Action:** TNF receptor blocker **Dose:** *Adults.* RA 50 mg SQ weekly or 25 mg SQ 2×/wk (separated by at least 72–96 h). *Peds 4–17 y:* 0.8 mg/kg/wk (max 50 mg/wk) or 0.4 mg/kg (max 25 mg/dose) 2×/wk 72–96 h apart **Caution:** [B, ?] w/ Predisposition to Infxn (ie, DM); may ↑ risk of malignancy in peds and young adults **CI:** Active Infxn **Disp:** Inj 25 mg/vial, 50 mg/mL syringe **SE:** HA, rhinitis, Inj site Rxn, URI **Notes:** Rotate Inj sites

Ethambutol (Myambutol) **Uses:** *Pulm TB* & other mycobacterial Infxns, MAC **Action:** ↓ RNA synth **Dose:** *Adults & Peds >12 y:* 15–25 mg/kg/d PO single dose; ↓ in renal impair, take w/ food, avoid antacids **Caution:** [C, +] **CI:** unconscious pts, optic neuritis **Disp:** Tabs 100, 400 mg **SE:** HA, hyperuricemia, acute gout, Abd pain; ↑ LFTs, optic neuritis, GI upset

Ethinyl Estradiol (Estinyl, Feminone) **WARNING:** ↑ Risk endometrial cancer. Avoid in PRG. Do not use in the prevention of CV Dz or dementia; ↑ risk of MI, stroke, breast CA, PE, DVT, in postmenopausal women **Uses:** *Menopausal vasomotor Sxs; female hypogonadism* **Action:** Estrogen supl **Dose:** 0.02–1.5 mg/d ÷ daily–tid **Caution:** [X, –] **CI:** Severe hepatic impair; genital bleeding of unknown cause, breast CA, estrogen-dependent tumors, thromboembolic disorders, thrombophlebitis **Disp:** Tabs 0.02, 0.05, 0.5 mg **SE:** N, bloating, breast enlargement/tenderness, edema, HA, hypertriglyceridemia, gallbladder Dz

Ethinyl Estradiol & Norelgestromin (Ortho Evra) **Uses:** *Contraceptive patch* **Action:** Estrogen & progestin **Dose:** Apply patch to abdomen, buttocks, upper torso (not breasts), or upper outer arm at the beginning of the menstrual cycle; new patch is applied weekly for 3 wk; wk 4 is patch-free **Caution:** [X, M] **CI:** PRG, Hx or current DVT/PE, stroke, MI, CV Dz, CAD; severe HTN; severe HA w/ focal neurologic Sx; breast/endometrial CA; estrogen-dependent neoplasms; hepatic dysfunction; jaundice; major surgery w/ prolonged immobilization; heavy smoking if >35 y **Disp:** 20 cm^2 patch (6 mg norelgestromin [active metabolite norgestimate] & 0.75 mg of ethinyl estradiol) **SE:** Breast discomfort, HA, site Rxns, N, menstrual cramps; thrombosis risks similar to OCP **Notes:** Less effective in women >90 kg; instruct pt does not protect against STD/HIV

Ethosuximide (Zarontin) **Uses:** *Absence (petit mal) Szs* **Action:** Anticonvulsant; ↑ Sz threshold **Dose:** *Adults and peds >6 y:* Initial, 500 mg PO ÷ bid; ↑ by 250 mg/d q4–7d PRN (max 1500 mg/d) usual maint 20–30 mg/kg. *Peds 3–6 y:* Initial: 15 mg/kg/d PO ÷ bid. *Maint:* 15–40 mg/kg/d ÷ bid (max 1500 mg/d) **Caution:** [D, +] In renal/hepatic impair; antiepileptics may ↑ risk of suicidal behavior or ideation **CI:** Component sensitivity **Disp:** Caps 250 mg; syrup 250 mg/5 mL **SE:** Blood dyscrasias, GI upset, drowsiness, dizziness, irritability **Notes:** Levels: *Trough:* just before next dose; *Therapeutic: Peak* 40–100 mcg/mL; *Toxic Trough:* >100 mcg/mL; *Half-life:* 25–60 h

Etidronate Disodium (Didronel) **Uses:** *↑ Ca^{2+} of malignancy, Paget Dz, & heterotopic ossification* **Action:** ↓ Nl & abnormal bone resorption **Dose:** *Paget Dz:* 5–10 mg/kg/d PO ÷ doses (for 3–6 mo). ↑ Ca^{2+}: 7.5 mg/kg/d IV Inf over 2 h × 3 d, then 20 mg/kg/d PO on last day of Inf × 1–3 mo **Caution:** [B PO (C parenteral), ?] Bisphosphonates may cause severe musculoskeletal pain **CI:** Overt osteomalacia, SCr >5 mg/dL **Disp:** Tabs 200, 400 mg; Inj 50 mg/mL **SE:** GI intolerance (↓ by ÷ daily doses); hyperphosphatemia, hypomagnesemia, bone pain, abnormal taste, fever, convulsions, nephrotox **Notes:** Take PO on empty stomach 2 h before or 2 h pc

Etodolac **WARNING:** May ↑ risk of cv events & GI bleeding; may worsen ↑ BP **Uses:** *Osteoarthritis & pain,* *RA* **Action:** NSAID **Dose:** 200–400 mg PO bid-qid (max 1200 mg) **Caution:** [C (D 3rd tri), ?] ↑ Bleeding risk w/ aspirin, warfarin; ↑ nephrotox w/ cyclosporine; Hx CHF, HTN, renal/hepatic impair, PUD **CI:** Active GI ulcer **Disp:** Tabs 400, 500 mg; ER tabs 400, 500, 600 mg; caps 200, 300 mg **SE:** N/V/D, gastritis, Abd cramps, dizziness, HA, depression, edema, renal impair **Notes:** Do not crush tabs

Etonogestrel/Ethinyl Estradiol vaginal insert (NuvaRing) **Uses:** *Contraceptive* **Action:** Estrogen & progestin combo **Dose:** Rule out PRG first; insert ring vaginally for 3 wk, remove for 1 wk; insert new ring 7 d after last removed (even if bleeding) at same time of day ring removed. 1st day of menses is day 1, insert before day 5 even if bleeding. Use other contraception for 1st 7 d of starting therapy. See insert if converting from other contraceptive; after delivery or 2nd tri abortion, insert 4 wk postpartum (if not breast-feeding) **Caution:** [X, ?/–] HTN, gallbladder Dz, ↑ lipids, migraines, sudden HA **CI:** PRG, heavy smokers >35 y, DVT, PE, cerebro-/CV Dz, estrogen-dependent neoplasm, undiagnosed abnormal genital bleeding, hepatic tumors, cholestatic jaundice **Disp:** Intravag ring: ethinyl estradiol 0.015 mg/d & etonogestrel 0.12 mg/d **Notes:** If ring removed, rinse w/ cool/lukewarm H_2O (not hot) & reinsert ASAP; if not reinserted w/in 3 h, effectiveness ↓; do not use with diaphragm

Etonogestrel implant (Implanon) **Uses:** *Contraception* **Action:** Transforms endometrium from proliferative to secretory **Dose:** 1 Implant subdermally q3y **Caution:** [X, +] Exclude pregnancy before implant **CI:** PRG, hormonally responsive tumors, breast CA, AUB, hepatic tumor, active liver Dz, hx thromboembolic Dz **Disp:** 68-mg implant **SE:** Spotting, irregular periods, amenorrhea, dysmenorrhea, HA, tender breasts, N, wgt gain, acne, ectopic pregnancy, PE, ovarian cysts, stroke, ↑ BP **Notes:** 99% Effective; remove implant and replace; restricted distribution; physician must register and train; does not protect against STDs

Etoposide [VP-16] (VePesid, Toposar) **Uses:** *Testicular, NSCLC, Hodgkin Dz, & NHLs, peds ALL, & allogeneic/autologous BMT in high doses* **Action:** Topoisomerase II inhibitor **Dose:** 50 mg/m²/d IV for 3–5 d; 50 mg/m²/d PO for 21 d (PO availability = 50% of IV); 2–6 g/m² or 25–70 mg/kg in BMT (per protocols); ↓ in renal/hepatic impair **Caution:** [D, –] IT administration **Disp:** Caps 50 mg; Inj 20 mg/mL **SE:** N/V (Emesis in 10–30%), ↓ BM, alopecia, ↓ BP w/ rapid IV, anorexia, anemia, leukopenia, ↑ risk secondary leukemias

Etravirine (Intelence) **Uses:** *HIV* **Action:** Non-NRTI **Dose:** 200 mg PO bid following a meal **Caution:** [B, ±] Many interactions: substrate/inducer (CYP3A4), substrate/inhibitor (CYP2C9, CYP2C19); do not use w/ tipranavir/ritonavir, fosamprenavir/ritonavir, atazanavir/ritonavir, protease inhibitors w/o ritonavir, and non-NRTIs **CI:** None **Disp:** Tabs 100 mg **SE:** N/V/D, rash, severe/potentially life-threatening skin Rxns, fat redistribution

Exemestane (Aromasin) **Uses:** *Advanced breast CA in postmenopausal women w/ progression after tamoxifen* **Action:** Irreversible, steroidal aromatase inhibitor; ↓ estrogens **Dose:** 25 mg PO daily after a meal **Caution:** [D, ?/–] **CI:** PRG, component sensitivity **Disp:** Tabs 25 mg **SE:** Hot flashes, N, fatigue,↑ alkaline phosphate

Exenatide (Byetta) **Uses:** Type 2 DM combined w/ metformin &/or sulfonylurea **Action:** An incretin mimetic: ↑ insulin release, ↓ glucagon secretion, ↓ gastric emptying, promotes satiety **Dose:** 5 mcg SQ bid w/in 60 min before A.M. & P.M. meals; ↑ to 10 mcg SQ bid after 1 mo PRN; do not give pc **Caution:** [C, ?/–] may ↓ absorption of other drugs (take antibiotics/contraceptives 1 h before) **CI:** CrCl <30 mL/min **Disp:** Soln 5, 10 mcg/dose in prefilled pen **SE:** Hypoglycemia, N/V/D, dizziness, HA, dyspepsia, ↓ appetite, jittery; acute pancreatitis **Notes:** Consider ↓ sulfonylurea to ↓ risk of hypoglycemia; discard pen 30 d after 1st use

Ezetimibe (Zetia) **Uses:** *Hypercholesterolemia alone or w/ a HMG-CoA reductase inhibitor* **Action:** ↓ cholesterol & phytosterols absorption **Dose:** *Adults & Peds >10 y:* 10 mg/d PO **Caution:** [C, +/–] Bile acid sequestrants ↓ bioavailability

CI: Hepatic impair **Disp:** Tabs 10 mg **SE:** HA, D, Abd pain, ↑ transaminases w/ HMG-CoA reductase inhibitor **Notes:** See ezetimibe/simvastatin

Ezetimibe/Simvastatin (Vytorin) **Uses:** *Hypercholesterolemia* **Action:** ↓ Absorption of cholesterol & phytosterols w/ HMG-CoA-reductase inhibitor **Dose:** 10/10–10/80 mg/d PO; w/ cyclosporine or danazol: 10/10 mg/d max; w/ amiodarone or verapamil: 10/20 mg/d max; ↓ w/ severe renal Insuff; give 2 h before or 4 h after bile acid sequestrants **Caution:** [X, –]; w/ CYP3A4 inhibitors (Table 11), gemfibrozil, niacin >1 g/d, danazol, amiodarone, verapamil **CI:** PRG/lactation; liver Dz, ↑ LFTs **Disp:** Tabs (ezetimibe/simvastatin) 10/10, 10/20, 10/40, 10/80 mg **SE:** HA, GI upset, myalgia, myopathy (muscle pain, weakness, or tenderness w/ creatine kinase 10 × ULN), rhabdomyolysis, hep, Infxn **Notes:** Monitor LFTs, lipids; ezetimibe/simvastatin combo lowered LDL more than simvastatin alone in ENHANCE study, but there was no difference in carotid-intima media thickness

Famciclovir (Famvir) **Uses:** *Acute herpes zoster (shingles) & genital herpes* **Action:** ↓ Viral DNA synth **Dose:** *Zoster:* 500 mg PO q8h × 7 d. *Simplex:* 125–250 mg PO bid; ↓ w/ renal impair **Caution:** [B, –] **CI:** Component sensitivity **Disp:** Tabs 125, 250, 500 mg **SE:** Fatigue, dizziness, HA, pruritus, N/D **Notes:** Best w/in 72 h of initial lesion

Famotidine (Pepcid, Pepcid AC) [OTC] **Uses:** *Short-term Tx of duodenal ulcer & benign gastric ulcer; maint for duodenal ulcer, hypersecretory conditions, GERD, & heartburn* **Action:** H₂-antagonist; ↓ gastric acid **Dose:** *Adults. Ulcer:* 20 mg IV q12h or 20–40 mg PO qhs × 4–8 wk. *Hypersecretion:* 20–160 mg PO q6h. *GERD:* 20 mg PO bid × 6 wk; maint: 20 mg PO hs. *Heartburn:* 10 mg PO PRN q12h. *Peds.* 0.5–1 mg/kg/d; ↓ in severe renal Insuff **Caution:** [B, M] **CI:** Component sensitivity **Disp:** Tabs 10, 20, 40 mg; chew tabs 10 mg; susp 40 mg/5 mL; gelatin caps 10 mg; Inj 10 mg/2 mL **SE:** Dizziness, HA, constipation, D, thrombocytopenia **Notes:** Chew tabs contain phenylalanine

Felodipine (Plendil) **Uses:** *HTN & CHF* **Action:** CCB **Dose:** 2.5–10 mg PO daily; swallow whole; ↓ in hepatic impair **Caution:** [C, ?] ↑ effect with azole antifungals, erythromycin, grapefruit juice **CI:** Component sensitivity **Disp:** ER tabs 2.5, 5, 10 mg **SE:** Peripheral edema, flushing, tachycardia, HA, gingival hyperplasia **Notes:** Follow BP in elderly & w/ hepatic impair

Fenofibrate (TriCor, Antara, Lofibra, Lipofen, Triglide) **Uses:** *Hypertriglyceridemia, hypercholesteremia* **Action:** ↓ Triglyceride synth **Dose:** 43–160 mg/d; ↓ w/ renal impair; take w/ meals **Caution:** [C, ?] Hepatic/ severe renal Insuff, primary biliary cirrhosis, unexplained ↑ LFTs, gallbladder Dz **Disp:** Caps 50, 100, 150 mg; caps (micronized): *(Lofibra)* 67, 134, 200 mg, *(Antara)* 43, 130 mg; tabs 54, 160 mg **SE:** GI disturbances, cholecystitis, arthralgia, myalgia, dizziness, ↑ LFTs **Notes:** Monitor LFTs

Fenoldopam (Corlopam) **Uses:** *Hypertensive emergency* **Action:** Rapid vasodilator **Dose:** Initial 0.03–0.1 mcg/kg/min IV Inf, titrate q15min by

1.6 mcg/kg/min to max 0.05–0.1 mcg/kg/min Caution: [B, ?] ↓ BP w/ β-blockers CI: Allergy to sulfites Disp: Inj 10 mg/mL SE: ↓ BP, edema, facial flushing, N/V/D, atrial flutter/fibrillation, ↑ IOP Notes: Avoid concurrent β-blockers

Fenoprofen (Nalfon) WARNING: May ↑ risk of cv events and GI bleeding Uses: *Arthritis & pain* Action: NSAID Dose: 200–600 mg q4–8h, to 3200 mg/d max; w/ food Caution: [B (D 3rd tri), +/–] CHF, HTN, renal/hepatic impair, Hx PUD CI: NSAID sensitivity Disp: Caps 200, 300, 600 mg SE: GI disturbance, dizziness, HA, rash, edema, renal impair, hep Notes: Swallow whole

Fentanyl (Sublimaze) [C-II] Uses: *Short-acting analgesic* in anesthesia & PCA Action: Narcotic analgesic Dose: *Adults.* 25–100 mcg/dose IV/IM titrated; *Anesthesia:* 5–15 mcg/kg; *Pain:* 200 mcg over 15 min, titrate to effect *Peds.* 1–2 mcg/kg IV/IM q1–4h titrate; ↓ in renal impair Caution: [B, +] CI: Paralytic ileus ↑ ICP, resp depression, severe renal/hepatic impair Disp: Inj 0.05 mg/mL SE: Sedation, ↓ BP, bradycardia, constipation, N, resp depression, miosis Notes: 0.1 mg fentanyl = 10 mg morphine IM

Fentanyl iontophoretic transdermal system (Ionsys) WARNING: Use only w/ hospitalized pts, D/C on discharge; fentanyl may result in potentially life-threatening resp depression and death Uses: *Short-term in-hospital analgesia* Action: Opioid narcotic, iontophoretic transdermal Dose: 40 mcg/activation by pt; dose given over 10 min; max over 24 h 3.2 mg (80 doses) Caution: [C, –] CI: See fentanyl Disp: Battery-operated self-contained transdermal system, 40 mcg/activation, 80 doses SE: See fentanyl, site Rxn Notes: Choose nl skin site chest or upper outer arm; titrate to comfort, pts must have access to supplemental analgesia; instruct in device use; dispose properly at discharge

Fentanyl, transdermal (Duragesic) [C-II] WARNING: Potential for abuse and fatal overdose Uses: *Persistent mod–severe chronic pain in pts already tolerant to opioids* Action: Narcotic Dose: Apply patch to upper torso q72h; dose based on narcotic requirements in previous 24 h; start 25 mcg/h patch q72h; ↓ in renal impair Caution: [B, +] w/ Cyp3A4 inhibitors (Table 11) may ↑ fentanyl effect, w/ Hx substance abuse CI: Not opioid tolerant, short-term pain management, post-op pain in outpatient surgery, mild pain, PRN use ↑ ICP, resp depression, severe renal/hepatic impair, peds <2 y Disp: Patches 12.5, 25, 50, 75, 100 mcg/h SE: Resp depression (fatal), sedation, ↓ BP, bradycardia, constipation, N, miosis Notes: 0.1 mg fentanyl = 10 mg morphine IM; do not cut patch; peak level 24–72 h

Fentanyl, transmucosal system (Actiq, Fentora) [C-II] WARNING: Potential for abuse and fatal overdose; use only in CA pts with chronic pain who are opioid tolerant; buccal formulation ↑ bioavailability over transmucosal; do not substitute on a mcg-per-mcg basis; use w/ strong CYP3A4 inhibitors may ↑ fentanyl levels Uses: *Breakthrough CA pain* Action: Narcotic analgesic, transmucosal absorption Dose: Start 100 mcg buccal (Fentora) × 1, may repeat in 30 min, 4 tabs/dose max; titrate; start 200 mcg PO (Actiq) × 1, may repeat × 1 after 30 min; titrate **Caution:** [B, +] **CI:** ↑ ICP, resp depression, severe renal/hepatic impair, management of post-op or awake pain **Disp:** *(Actiq)* Lozenges on stick 200, 400, 600, 800, 1200, 1600 mcg; *(Fentora)* buccal tabs 100, 200, 300, 400, 600, 800 mcg **SE:** Sedation, ↓ BP, bradycardia, constipation, N, resp depression, miosis **Notes:** 0.1 mg fentanyl = 10 mg IM morphine; for use in pts already tolerant to opioid therapy

Ferrous Gluconate (Fergon [OTC], others)   WARNING: Accidental overdose of iron-containing products is a leading cause of fatal poisoning in children <6. Keep out of reach of children **Uses:** *Iron-deficiency anemia* & Fe supl **Action:** Dietary supl **Dose:** *Adults.* 100–200 mg of elemental Fe/d ÷ doses. *Peds.* 4–6 mg/kg/d ÷ doses; on empty stomach (OK w/ meals if GI upset occurs); avoid antacids **Caution:** [A, ?] **CI:** Hemochromatosis, hemolytic anemia **Disp:** Tabs Fergon 240 (27 mg Fe), 246 (28 mg Fe), 300 (34 mg Fe), 325 mg (36 mg Fe) **SE:** GI upset, constipation, dark stools, discoloration of urine, may stain teeth **Notes:** 12% Elemental Fe; false (+) stool guaiac; keep away from children; severe tox in overdose

Ferrous Gluconate Complex (Ferrlecit)   **Uses:** *Irondeficiency anemia or supl to erythropoietin therapy* **Action:** Fe supl **Dose:** Test dose: 2 mL (25 mg Fe) IV over 1 h, if OK, 125 mg (10 mL) IV over 1 h. Usual cumulative dose 1 g Fe over 8 sessions (until favorable Hct) **Caution:** [B, ?] **CI:** non–Fe-deficiency anemia; CHF; Fe overload **Disp:** Inj 12.5 mg/mL Fe **SE:** ↓ BP, serious allergic Rxns, GI disturbance, Inj site Rxn **Notes:** Dose expressed as mg Fe; may infuse during dialysis

Ferrous Sulfate (OTC)   **Uses:** *Fe-deficiency anemia & Fe supl* **Action:** Dietary supl **Dose:** *Adults.* 100–200 mg elemental Fe/d in ÷ doses. *Peds.* 1–6 mg/kg/d ÷ daily–tid; on empty stomach (OK w/ meals if GI upset occurs); avoid antacids **Caution:** [A, ?] ↑ Absorption w/ vit C; ↓ absorption w/ tetracycline, fluoroquinolones, antacids, H$_2$ blockers, proton pump inhibitors **CI:** Hemochromatosis, hemolytic anemia **Disp:** Tabs 187 (60 mg Fe), 200 (65 mg Fe), 324 (65 mg Fe), 325 mg (65 mg Fe); SR caplets & tabs 160 (50 mg Fe), 200 mg (65 mg Fe); gtt 75 mg/0.6 mL (15 mg Fe/0.6 mL); elixir 220 mg/5 mL (44 mg Fe/5 mL); syrup 90 mg/5 mL (18 mg Fe/5 mL) **SE:** GI upset, constipation, dark stools, discolored urine

Fexofenadine (Allegra, Allegra-D)   **Uses:** *Allergic rhinitis chronic idiopathic urticaria* **Action:** Selective antihistamine, antagonizes H$_1$-receptors; *Allegra D* contains pseudoephedrine **Dose:** *Adults & Peds >12 y:* 60 mg PO bid or 180 mg/d; 12-h ER form bid, 24-h ER form q day. *Peds 6–11 y:* 30 mg PO bid; ↓ in renal impair **Caution:** [C, ?] w/ Nevirapine **CI:** Component sensitivity **Disp:** Tabs 30, 60, 180 mg; susp 6 mg/mL; *Allegra-D 12-h* ER tab (60 mg fexofenadine/120 mg pseudoephedrine), *Allegra-d 24-h* ER (180 mg fexofenadine/240 mg pseudoephedrine) **SE:** Drowsiness (rare), HA

Filgrastim [G-CSF] (Neupogen) Uses: *↓ Incidence of Infxn in febrile neutropenic pts; Rx chronic neutropenia* Action: Recombinant G-CSF Dose: *Adults & Peds.* 5 mcg/kg/d SQ or IV single daily dose; D/C when ANC >10,000 Caution: [C, ?] w/ Drugs that potentiate release of neutrophils (eg, lithium) CI: Allergy to E. coli-derived proteins or G-CSF Disp: Inj 300, 600 mcg/mL SE: Fever, alopecia, N/V/D, splenomegaly, bone pain, HA, rash Notes: ✓ CBC & plt; monitor for cardiac events; no benefit w/ ANC >10,000/mm³

Finasteride (Proscar, Propecia) Uses: *BPH & androgenetic alopecia* Action: ↓ 5α-Reductase Dose: *BPH:* 5 mg/d PO. *Alopecia:* 1 mg/d PO; food ↓ absorption Caution: [X, –] Hepatic impair CI: Pregnant women should avoid handling pills, teratogen to male fetus Disp: Tabs 1 mg (*Propecia*), 5 mg (*Proscar*) SE: ↓ Libido, vol ejaculate, ED, gynecomastia Notes: ↓ PSA by ~ 50%; reestablish PSA baseline 6 mo (double PSA for "true" reading); 3–6 mo for effect on urinary Sxs; continue to maintain new hair, not for use in women

Flavoxate (Urispas) Uses: *Relief of Sx of dysuria, urgency, nocturia, suprapubic pain, urinary frequency, incontinence* Action: Antispasmodic Dose: 100–200 mg PO tid-qid Caution: [B, ?] CI: GI obst, GI hemorrhage, ileus, achalasia, BPH Disp: Tabs 100 mg SE: Drowsiness, blurred vision, xerostomia

Flecainide (Tambocor) WARNING: ↑ Mortality in pts with ventricular arrhythmias and recent MI; pulm effects reported; ventricular proarrhythmic effects in atrial fibrillation/flutter, not ok for chronic atrial fibrillation Uses: *Prevent AF/flutter & PSVT, *prevent/suppress life-threatening ventricular arrhythmias* Action: Class 1C antiarrhythmic Dose: *Adults.* 100 mg PO q12h; ↑ by 50 mg q12h q4d to max 400 mg/d. *Peds.* 3–6 mg/kg/d in 3 ÷ doses; ↓ w/ renal impair. Caution: [C, +] Monitor w/hepatic impair, ↑ conc with amiodarone, digoxin, quinidine, ritonavir/amprenavir, β-blockers, verapamil; may worsen arrhythmias CI: 2nd-/3rd-degree AV block, right bundle-branch block w/ bifascicular or trifascicular block, cardiogenic shock, CAD, ritonavir/amprenavir, alkalinizing agents Disp: Tabs 50, 100, 150 mg SE: Dizziness, visual disturbances, dyspnea, palpitations, edema, chest pain, tachycardia, CHF, HA, fatigue, rash, N Notes: Initiate Rx in hospital; dose q8h if pt is intolerant/uncontrolled at q12h; Levels: *Trough:* Just before next dose; *Therapeutic:* 0.2–1 mcg/mL; *Toxic:* >1 mcg/mL; *Half-life:* 11–14 h

Floxuridine (FUDR) WARNING: Administration by experienced physician only; pts should be hospitalized for 1st course due to risk for severe Rxn Uses: *GI adenoma, liver, renal cancers*; colon & pancreatic CAs Action: Converted to 5-FU; inhibits thymidylate synthase; ↓ DNA synthase (S-phase specific) Dose: 0.1–0.6 mg/kg/d for 1–6 wk (per protocols) usually intraarterial for liver mets Caution: [D, –] Interaction w/ vaccines CI: BM suppression, poor nutritional status, serious Infxn, PRG, component sensitivity Disp: Inj 500 mg SE: ↓ BM, anorexia, Abd cramps, N/V/D, mucositis, alopecia, skin rash, & hyperpigmentation; rare neurotox (blurred vision, depression, nystagmus, vertigo, & lethargy);

intraarterial catheter-related problems (ischemia, thrombosis, bleeding, & Infxn) **Notes:** Need effective birth control; palliative Rx for inoperable/incurable pts

Fluconazole (Diflucan)

Uses: *Candidiasis (esophageal, oropharyngeal, urinary tract, vaginal, prophylaxis); cryptococcal meningitis, prophylaxis w/ BMT* **Action:** Antifungal; ↓ cytochrome P-450 sterol demethylation. **Spectrum:** All *Candida* sp except *C. krusei* **Dose:** *Adults.* 100–400 mg/d PO or IV. *Vaginitis:* 150, mg PO daily. *Crypto:* doses up to 800 mg/d reported; 400 mg d 1, then 200 mg × 10–12 wk after CSF (−). *Peds.* 3–6 mg/kg/d PO or IV; 12 mg/kg/d/systemic Infxn; ↓ in renal impair **Caution:** [C, −] **CI:** None **Disp:** Tabs 50, 100, 150, 200 mg; susp 10, 40 mg/mL; Inj 2 mg/mL **SE:** HA, rash, GI upset, ↓ K+, ↑ LFTs **Notes:** PO (preferred) = IV levels

Fludarabine Phosphate (Flamp, Fludara)

WARNING: Administer only under supervision of qualified physician experienced in chemotherapy. Can ↓ BM and cause severe CNS effects (blindness, coma, and death). Severe/fatal autoimmune hemolytic anemia reported; monitor for hemolysis. Use w/ pentostatin not ok (fatal pulm tox) **Uses:** *Autoimmune hemolytic anemia, CLL, cold agglutinin hemolysis,* low-grade lymphoma, mycosis fungoides **Action:** ↓ Ribonucleotide reductase; blocks DNA polymerase-induced DNA repair **Dose:** 18–30 mg/m^2/d for 5 d, as a 30-min Inf (per protocols); ↓ w/ renal impair **Caution:** [D, −] Give cytarabine before fludarabine (↓ its metabolism) **CI:** w/ pentostatin, severe Infxns, CrCl <30 mL/min, hemolytic anemia **Disp:** Inj 50 mg **SE:** ↓ BM, N/V/D, ↑ LFTs, edema, CHF, fever, chills, fatigue, dyspnea, nonproductive cough, pneumonitis, severe CNS tox rare in leukemia, autoimmune hemolytic anemia

Fludrocortisone Acetate (Florinef)

Uses: *Adrenocortical Insuff, Addison dz, salt-wasting syndrome* **Action:** Mineralocorticoid **Dose:** *Adults.* 0.1–0.2 mg/d PO. *Peds.* 0.05–0.1 mg/d PO **Caution:** [C, ?] **CI:** Systemic fungal Infxns; known allergy **Disp:** Tabs 0.1 mg **SE:** HTN, edema, CHF, HA, dizziness, convulsions, acne, rash, bruising, hyperglycemia, hypothalamic–pituitary–adrenal suppression, cataracts **Notes:** For adrenal Insuff, use w/ glucocorticoid; dose changes based on plasma renin activity

Flumazenil (Romazicon)

Uses: *Reverse sedative effects of benzodiazepines & general anesthesia* **Action:** Benzodiazepine receptor antagonist **Dose:** *Adults.* 0.2 mg IV over 15 s; repeat PRN, to 1 mg max (5 mg max in benzodiazepine OD). *Peds.* 0.01 mg/kg (0.2 mg/dose max) IV over 15 s; repeat 0.005 mg/kg at 1-min intervals to max 1 mg total; ↓ in hepatic impair **Caution:** [C, ?] **CI:** TCA OD; if pts given benzodiazepines to control life-threatening conditions (ICP/status epilepticus) **Disp:** Inj 0.1 mg/mL **SE:** N/V, palpitations, HA, anxiety, nervousness, hot flashes, tremor, blurred vision, dyspnea, hyperventilation, withdrawal syndrome **Notes:** Does not reverse narcotic Sx or amnesia, use associated w/ Szs

Flunisolide (AeroBid, Aerospan, Nasarel)

Uses: *Asthma in pts requiring chronic steroid therapy; relieve seasonal/perennial allergic rhinitis*

Action: Topical steroid **Dose:** *Adults. Metered-dose Inh:* 2 Inh bid (max 8/d). *Nasal:* 2 sprays/nostril bid (max 8/d). *Peds >6 y: Metered-dose Inh:* 2 Inh bid (max 4/d). *Nasal:* 1–2 sprays/nostril bid (max 4/d) **Caution:** [C, ?] w/ Adrenal Insuff **CI:** Status asthmaticus, viral, TB, fungal, bacterial Infxn; **Disp:** AeroBid 0.25 mg/Inh; Nasarel 29 mcg/spray; Aerospan 80 mcg/Inh (CFC-Free) **SE:** Tachycardia, bitter taste, local effects, oral candidiasis **Notes:** Not for acute asthma

Fluorouracil [5-FU] (Adrucil)   **WARNING:** Administration by experienced chemotherapy physician only; pts should be hospitalized for 1st course due to risk for severe Rxn **Uses:** *Colorectal, gastric, pancreatic, breast, basal cell,* head, neck, bladder, CAs **Action:** Inhibits thymidylate synthetase (↓ DNA synth, S-phase specific) **Dose:** 370–1000 mg/m^2/d × 1–5 d IV push to 24-h cont Inf; protracted venous Inf of 200–300 mg/m^2/d (per protocol); 800 mg/d max **Caution:** [D, ?] ↑ tox w/ allopurinol; do not give *Moraxella catarrhalis* vaccine (MRX) before 5-FU **CI:** Poor nutritional status, depressed BM Fxn, thrombocytopenia, major surgery w/in past mo, G6PD enzyme deficiency, PRG, serious Infxn, bilirubin >5 mg/dL **Disp:** Inj 50 mg/mL **SE:** Stomatitis, esophagopharyngitis, N/V/D, anorexia, ↓ BM, rash/dry skin/photosensitivity, tingling in hands/feet w/ pain (palmar–plantar erythrodysesthesia), phlebitis/discoloration at Inj sites **Notes:** ↑ Thiamine intake; contraception ok

Fluorouracil, Topical [5-FU] (Efudex)   **Uses:** *Basal cell carcinoma; actinic/solar keratosis* **Action:** Inhibits thymidylate synthetase (↓ DNA synth, S-phase specific) **Dose:** 5% cream bid × 2–6 wk **Caution:** [D, ?] Irritant chemotherapy **CI:** Component sensitivity **Disp:** Cream 0.5, 1, 5%; soln 1, 2, 5% **SE:** Rash, dry skin, photosensitivity **Notes:** Healing may not be evident for 1–2 mo; wash hands thoroughly; avoid occlusive dressings; do not overuse

Fluoxetine (Prozac, Sarafem)   **WARNING:** Closely monitor for worsening depression or emergence of suicidality, particularly in ped pts **Uses:** *Depression, OCD, panic disorder, bulimia* (Prozac); *PMDD* (Sarafem) **Action:** SSRI **Dose:** 20 mg/d PO (max 80 mg ÷ dose); weekly 90 mg/wk after 1–2 wk of standard dose. *Bulimia:* 60 mg q A.M.. *Panic disorder:* 20 mg/d. *OCD:* 20–80 mg/d. *PMDD:* 20 mg/d or 20 mg intermittently, start 14 d prior to menses, repeat with each cycle; ↓ in hepatic failure **Caution:** [C, ?/–] Serotonin syndrome w/ MAOI, SSRI, serotonin agonists, linezolid; QT prolongation w/ phenothiazines **CI:** MAOI/thioridazine (wait 5 wk after D/C before MAOI) **Disp:** *Prozac:* Caps 10, 20, 40 mg; scored tabs 10, 20 mg; SR caps 90 mg; soln 20 mg/5 mL. *Sarafem:* Caps 10, 20 mg **SE:** N, nervousness, wgt loss, HA, insomnia

Fluoxymesterone (Halotestin, Androxy)[CIII]   **Uses:** Androgen-responsive metastatic *breast CA, hypogonadism* **Action:** ↓ Secretion of LH & FSH (feedback inhibition) **Dose:** *Breast CA:* 10–40 mg/d ÷ × 1–3 mo. *Hypogonadism:* 5–20 mg/d **Caution:** [X, ?/–] ↑ Effect w/ anticoagulants, cyclosporine, insulin, lithium, narcotics **CI:** Serious cardiac, liver, or kidney Dz; PRG **Disp:** Tabs 10 mg **SE:** Priapism, edema, virilization, amenorrhea & menstrual irregularities, hirsutism, alopecia, acne, N, cholestasis; suppression of factors II, V, VII, & X, & poly-cythemia; ↑ libido, HA, anxiety **Notes:** Radiographic exam of hand/wrist q6mo in prepubertal children; ↓ total T_4 levels

Flurazepam (Dalmane) [C-IV] **Uses:** *Insomnia* **Action:** Benzodi-azepine **Dose:** *Adults & Peds >15 y:* 15–30 mg PO qhs PRN; ↓ in elderly **Caution:** [X, ?/–] Elderly, low albumin, hepatic impair **CI:** NAG; PRG **Disp:** Caps 15, 30 mg **SE:** "Hangover" due to accumulation of metabolites, apnea, anaphylaxis, angioedema, amnesia **Notes:** May cause dependency

Flurbiprofen (Ansaid, Ocufen) **WARNING:** May ↑ risk of cv events and GI bleeding **Uses:** *Arthritis, ocular surgery* **Action:** NSAID **Dose:** 50–300 mg/d ÷ bid-qid, max 300 mg/d w/ food, ocular 1 gtt q 30 min × 4, beginning 2 h pre-op **Caution:** [B (D in 3rd tri), +] PRG (3rd tri); aspirin allergy **Disp:** Tabs 50, 100 mg **SE:** Dizziness, GI upset, peptic ulcer Dz, ocular irritation

Flutamide (Eulexin) **WARNING:** Liver failure & death reported. Mea-sure LFTs before, monthly, & periodically after; D/C immediately if ALT 2 × upper limits of nl or jaundice develops **Uses:** Advanced *PCa* (w/ LHRH agonists, eg, leuprolide or goserelin); w/ radiation & GnRH for localized CAP **Action:** Non-steroidal antiandrogen **Dose:** 250 mg PO tid (750 mg total) **Caution:** [D, ?] CI: Severe hepatic impair **Disp:** Caps 125 mg **SE:** Hot flashes, loss of libido, impo-tence, N/V/D, gynecomastia, hepatic failure **Notes:** ✓ LFTs, avoid EtOH

Fluticasone Furoate, nasal (Veramyst) **Uses:** *Seasonal allergic rhinitis* **Action:** Topical steroid **Dose:** *Adults & Peds > 12 y:* 2 sprays/nostril/d, then 1 spray /d maint. *Peds 2–11 y:* 1–2 sprays/nostril/d **Caution:** [C, M] Avoid w/ ritonavir, other steroids, recent nasal surgery/trauma **CI:** None **Disp:** Nasal spray 27.5 mcg/actuation **SE:** HA, epistaxis, nasopharyngitis, pyrexia, pharyngola-ryngeal pain, cough, nasal ulcers, back pain

Fluticasone Propionate, nasal (Flonase) **Uses:** *Seasonal aller-gic rhinitis* **Action:** Topical steroid **Dose:** *Adults & Peds >12 y:* 2 sprays/nostril/d *Peds 4–11 y:* 1–2 sprays/nostril/d **Caution:** [C, M] **CI:** Primary Rx of status asth-maticus **Disp:** Nasal spray 50 mcg/actuation **SE:** HA, dysphonia, oral candidiasis

Fluticasone Propionate, inhalation (Flovent HFA, Flovent Diskus) **Uses:** *Chronic asthma* **Action:** Topical steroid **Dose:** *Adults & Peds >12 y:* 2–4 puffs bid. *Peds 4–11 y:* 50 or 44 mcg bid **Caution:** [C, M] **CI:** Status asthmaticus **Disp:** *Diskus* dry powder: 50, 100, 250 mcg/actuation; *HFA*; MDI 44/110/220 mcg/Inh **SE:** HA, dysphonia, oral candidiasis **Notes:** Risk of thrush, rinse mouth after; counsel on use of devices

Fluticasone Propionate & Salmeterol Xinafoate (Advair Diskus, Advair HFA, 45/21, 115/21, 230/21 inhaled aerosol) **WARNING:** Increased risk of worsening wheezing or asthma-related death with long acting β₂-adrenergic agonists **Uses:** *Maint therapy for asthma* **Action:** Cor-ticosteroid w/ LA bronchodilator β₂ agonist **Dose:** *Adults & Peds >12 y:* 1 Inh bid q12h; titrate to lowest effective dose (4 Inh or 920/84 mcg/d max) **Caution:** [C, M] **CI:** Acute asthma attack; conversion from PO steroids; w/ phenothiazines **Disp:** Diskus = metered-dose Inh powder (fluticasone/salmeterol) 100/50, 250/50, 500/50; HFA = aerosol 45/21, 115/21, 230/21 mg **SE:** Upper resp Infxn, pharyngitis, HA **Notes:** Combo of *Flovent* & *Serevent*; do not wash mouthpiece, do not exhale into device; *Advair HFA* for pts not controlled on other meds (eg, low-medium dose Inh steroids) or whose Dz severity warrants 2 maint therapies

Fluvastatin (Lescol) **Uses:** *Atherosclerosis, primary hypercholesterolemia, heterozygous familial hypercholesterolemia hypertriglyceridemia* **Action:** HMG-CoA reductase inhibitor **Dose:** 20–40 mg bid PO or XL 80 mg/d ↓ w/ hepatic impair **Caution:** [X, –] **CI:** Active liver Dz, ↑ LFTs, PRG, breast-feeding **Disp:** Caps 20, 40 mg; XL 80 mg **SE:** HA, dyspepsia, N/D, Abd pain **Notes:** Dose no longer limited to HS ✓ LFTs

Fluvoxamine (Luvox) **WARNING:** Closely monitor for worsening depression or emergence of suicidality, particularly in ped pts **Uses:** *OCD* **Action:** SSRI **Dose:** Initial 50-mg single qhs dose, ↑ to 300 mg in ÷ doses; ↓ in elderly/hepatic impair, titrate slowly; ÷ doses >100 mg **Caution:** [C, ?/–] **Interactions** (MAOIs, phenothiazines, SSRIs, serotonin agonists, others) **CI:** MAOI w/in 14 d **Disp:** Tabs 25, 50, 100 mg **SE:** HA, N/D, somnolence, insomnia

Folic Acid **Uses:** *Megaloblastic anemia; folate deficiency* **Action:** Dietary supl **Dose:** *Adults.* Supl 0.4 mg/d PO. *PRG:* 0.8 mg/d PO. *Folate deficiency:* 1 mg PO daily–tid. *Peds.* Supl 0.04–0.4 mg/24 h PO, IM, IV, or SQ. *Folate deficiency:* 0.5–1 mg/24 h PO, IM, IV, or SQ **Caution:** [A, +] **CI:** Pernicious, aplastic, normocytic anemias **Disp:** Tabs 0.4, 0.8, 1 mg; Inj 5 mg/mL **SE:** Well tolerated **Notes:** OK for all women of child-bearing age; ↓ fetal neural tube defects by 50%; no effect on normocytic anemias

Fondaparinux (Arixtra) **WARNING:** When epidural/spinal anesthesia or spinal puncture is used, pts anticoagulated or scheduled to be anticoagulated with LMW heparins, heparinoids, or fondaparinux are at risk for epidural or spinal hematoma, which can result in long-term or permanent paralysis **Uses:** *DVT prophylaxis* w/ hip fracture, hip or knee replacement, Abd surgery; w/ DVT or PE in combo w/ warfarin **Action:** Synth inhibitor of activated factor X; a pentasaccharide **Dose:** 2.5 mg SQ daily, up to 5–9 d; start >6 h post-op; ↓ w/ renal impair **Caution:** [B, ?] ↑ Bleeding risk w/ anticoagulants, antiplatelets, drotrecogin alfa, NSAIDs **CI:** Wgt <50 kg, CrCl <30 mL/min, active bleeding, SBE ↓ plt w/ antiplatelet Ab **Disp:** Prefilled syringes w/ 27-gauge needle: 2.5/0.5, 5/0.4, 7.5 /0.6, 10/0.8, mg/mL **SE:** Thrombocytopenia, anemia, fever, N **Notes:** D/C if plts <100,000 mm³; only give SQ; may monitor antifactor Xa levels

Formoterol Fumarate (Foradil, Perforomist) **WARNING:** May ↑ risk of asthma related death **Uses:** *Long-term Rx of bronchoconstriction in COPD, EIB (only *Foradil*)* **Action:** LA β₂-agonist **Dose:** *Adults. Performist:* 20-mcg Inh q12h; *Foradil:* 12-mcg Inh q12h, 24 mcg/d max; *EIB:* 12 mcg 15 min before exercise *Peds >5y:* (*Foradil*) See Adults **Caution:** [C, M] Not for acute Sx, w/ CV Dz, w/ adrenergic meds, xanthine derivatives meds that ↑ QT; β-blockers may ↓ effect, D/C w/ ECG change **CI:** none **Disp:** *Foradil* caps 12 mcg for Aerolizer Inhaler (12 & 60 doses) **SE:** N/D, nasopharyngitis, dry mouth, angina, HTN, ↓ BP, tachycardia, arrhythmias, nervousness, HA, tremor, muscle cramps, palpitations, dizziness **Notes:** excess use may ↑ CV risks; not for oral use

Fosamprenavir (Lexiva)   **WARNING:** Do not use with severe liver dysfunction, reduce dose with mild–mod liver impair (fosamprenavir 700 mg bid w/o ritonavir) **Uses:** HIV Infxn **Action:** Protease inhibitor **Dose:** 1400 mg bid w/o ritonavir; w/ritonavir, fosamprenavir 1400 mg + ritonavir 200 mg daily or fosamprenavir 700 mg + ritonavir 100 mg bid; w/ efavirenz & ritonavir: fosamprenavir 1400 mg + ritonavir 300 mg daily **Caution:** [C, ?/–] **CI:** w/ Drugs that use CYP A4 for clearance (Table 11) such as w/ rifampin, lovastatin, simvastatin, delavirdine, ergot alkaloids, midazolam, triazolam, or pimozide; sulfa allergy **Disp:** Tabs 700 mg **SE:** N/V/D, HA, fatigue, rash **Notes:** Numerous drug interactions because of hepatic metabolism

Fosaprepitant (Emend, Inj)   **Uses:** *Prevent chemotherapy-associated N/V* **Action:** Substance P/neurokinin 1 receptor antagonist **Dose:** *Chemotherapy:* 115 mg IV 30 min before chemotherapy on d 1 (followed by aprepitant [Emend, Oral] 80 mg PO days 2 and 3) in combo w/ other antiemetics **Caution:** [B, ?/–] Potential for drug interactions, substrate and mod CYP3A4 inhibitor (dosedependent) **CI:** w/ Pimozide, terfenadine, astemizole, or cisapride **Disp:** Inj 115 mg **SE:** N/D, weakness, hiccups, dizziness, HA, dehydration, hot flushing, dyspepsia, Abd pain, neutropenia, ↑ LFTs, Inj site discomfort **Notes:** ↓ Effect of OCP and warfarin

Foscarnet (Foscavir)   **Uses:** *CMV retinitis*; acyclovir-resistant *herpes Infxns* **Action:** ↓ Viral DNA polymerase & RT **Dose:** *CMV retinitis: Induction:* 60 mg/kg IV q8h or 100 mg/kg q12h × 14–21 d. *Maint:* 90–120 mg/kg/d IV (Mon–Fri). *Acyclovir-resistant HSV: Induction:* 40 mg/kg IV q8–12h × 14–21 d; use central line; ↓ with renal impair **Caution:** [C, –] ↑ Sz potential w/ fluoroquinolones; avoid nephrotoxic Rx (cyclosporine, aminoglycosides, amphotericin B, protease inhibitors) **CI:** CrCl <0.4 mL/min/kg **Disp:** Inj 24 mg/mL **SE:** Nephrotox, electrolyte abnormalities **Notes:** Sodium loading (500 mL 0.9% NaCl) before & after helps minimize nephrotox; monitor-ionized Ca^{2+}

Fosfomycin (Monurol)   **Uses:** *Uncomplicated UTI* **Action:** ↓ cell wall synth *Spectrum:* gram(+)*Enterococcus,* staphylococci, pneumococci; gram(−) (*E. coli, Salmonella, Shigella, H. influenzae, Neisseria,* indole-negative *Proteus, Providencia*); *B. fragilis* & anaerobic gram(−) cocci are resistant **Dose:** 3 g PO in 90–120 mL of H_2O single dose; ↓ in renal impair **Caution:** [B, ?] ↓ Absorption w/ antacids/Ca salts **CI:** Component sensitivity **Disp:** Granule packets 3 g **SE:** HA, GI upset **Notes:** May take 2–3 d for Sxs to improve

Fosinopril (Monopril) Uses: *HTN, CHF,* DN Action: ACE inhibitor Dose: 10 mg/d PO initial; max 40 mg/d PO; ↓ in elderly; ↓ in renal impair Caution: [D, +] ↑ K+ w/ K+ supls, ARBs, K+-sparing diuretics; ↑ renal after effects w/ NSAIDs, diuretics, hypovolemia CI: Hereditary/idiopathic angioedema or angioedema w/ ACE inhibitor, bilateral RAS Disp: Tabs 10, 20, 40 mg SE: Cough, dizziness, angioedema, ↑ K+

Fosphenytoin (Cerebyx) Uses: *Status epilepticus* Action: ↓ Sz spread in motor cortex Dose: As phenytoin equivalents (PE). *Load:* 15–20 mg PE/kg. *Maint:* 4–6 mg PE/kg/d; ↓ dosage, monitor levels in hepatic impair Caution: [D, +] May ↑ phenobarbital CI: Sinus bradycardia, SA block, 2nd-/3rd-degree AV block, Adams–Stokes syndrome, rash during Rx Disp: Inj 75 mg/mL SE: ↓ BP, dizziness, ataxia, pruritus, nystagmus Notes: 15 min to convert fosphenytoin to phenytoin; administer <150 mg PE/min to prevent ↓ BP; administer with BP monitoring

Frovatriptan (Frova) Uses: *Rx acute migraine* Action: Vascular serotonin receptor agonist Dose: 2.5 mg PO repeat in 2 h PRN, 7.5 mg/d max PO dose; max 7.5 mg/d Caution: [C, ?/–] CI: Angina, ischemic heart Dz, coronary artery vasospasm, hemiplegic or basilar migraine, uncontrolled HTN, ergot use, MAOI use w/in 14 d Supplied: Tabs 2.5 mg SE: N, V, dizziness, hot flashes, paresthesias, dyspepsia, dry mouth, hot/cold sensation, chest pain, skeletal pain, flushing, weakness, numbness, coronary vasospasm, HTN

Fulvestrant (Faslodex) Uses: *HR(+) metastatic breast CA in postmenopausal women w/ progression following antiestrogen therapy* Action: Estrogen receptor antagonist Dose: 250 mg IM monthly, as single 5-mL Inj or 2 concurrent 2.5-mL IM Inj in buttocks Caution: [X, ?/–] ↓ Effects w/ CYP3A4 inhibitors (Table 11); w/ hepatic impair; PRG Disp: Prefilled syringes 50 mg/mL (single 5 mL, dual 2.5 mL) SE: N/V/D, constipation, Abd pain, HA, back pain, hot flushes, pharyngitis, Inj site Rxns Notes: Only use IM

Furosemide (Lasix) Uses: *CHF, HTN, edema,* ascites Action: Loop diuretic; ↓ Na & Cl reabsorption in ascending loop of Henle & distal tubule Dose: *Adults* 20–80 mg PO or IV bid. *Peds.* 1 mg/kg/dose IV q6–12h; 2 mg/kg/dose PO q12–24h (max 6 mg/kg/dose); ↑ doses w/renal impair Caution: [C, +] ↓ K+, ↑ risk digoxin tox & ototox w/ aminoglycosides, cisplatin (especially in renal dysfunction) CI: Sulfonylurea allergy; anuria; hepatic coma; electrolyte depletion Disp: Tabs 20, 40, 80 mg; soln 10 mg/mL, 40 mg/5 mL; Inj 10 mg/mL SE: ↓ BP, hyperglycemia, ↓ K + Notes: ✓ Lytes, renal Fxn; high doses IV may cause ototox

Gabapentin (Neurontin) Uses: Adjunct in *partial Szs; postherpetic neuralgia (PHN)*; chronic pain syndromes Action: Anticonvulsant; GABA analog Dose: *Adults & Peds >12 y: Anticonvulsant:* 300 mg PO tid, ↑ max 3600 mg/d. *PHN:* 300 mg day 1, 300 mg bid day 2, 300 mg tid day 3, titrate (1800–3600 mg/d); *Peds 3–12 y:* Start 0–15 mg/kg/d ÷ tid, ↑ over 3 d: *3–4 y:* 40 mg/kg/d given ÷ tid *age ≥5 y:* 25–35 mg/kg/d ÷ tid, 50 mg/kg/d max; ↓ w/ renal impair Caution: [C, ?]

Use in peds 3–12 y w/ epilepsy may ↑ CNS-related adverse events **CI:** Component sensitivity **Disp:** Caps 100, 300, 400, soln 250 mg/5 mL; scored tab 600, 800 mg **SE:** Somnolence, dizziness, ataxia, fatigue **Notes:** Not necessary to monitor levels; taper ↑ or ↓ over 1 wk

Galantamine (Razadyne) Uses: *Mild-mod Alzheimer Dz* Action: ? Acetylcholinesterase inhibitor **Dose:** 4 mg PO bid, ↑ to 8 mg bid after 4 wk; may ↑ to 12 mg bid in 4 wk **Caution:** [B, ?] Caution w/ heart block, ↑ effect w/ succinylcholine, bethanechol, amiodarone, diltiazem, verapamil, NSAIDs, digoxin; ↓ effect w/ anticholinergics; ↑ risk of death w/ mild impair **Disp:** Tabs 4, 8, 12 mg; soln 4 mg/mL **SE:** GI disturbances, ↓ wgt, sleep disturbances, dizziness, HA **Notes:** Caution w/ urinary outflow obst, Parkinson Dz, severe asthma/COPD, severe heart Dz or ↓ BP

Gallium Nitrate (Ganite) **WARNING:** ↑ Risk of severe renal Insuff w/ concurrent use of nephrotoxic drugs (eg, aminoglycosides, amphotericin B). D/C if use of potentially nephrotoxic drug is indicated; hydrate several d after administration. D/C if Cr >2.5 mg/dL **Uses:** *↑ Ca²⁺ of malignancy* **Action:** ↓ Bone resorption of Ca²⁺ **Dose:** ↑ Ca²⁺: 100–200 mg/m²/d × 5 d. *CA:* 350 mg/m² cont Inf × 5 d to 700 mg/m² rapid IV Inf q2wk in antineoplastic settings (per protocols) **Caution:** [C, ?] Do not give w/ live or rotavirus vaccine **CI:** SCr >2.5 mg/dL **Disp:** Inj 25 mg/mL **SE:** Renal Insuff, ↓ Ca²⁺, hypophosphatemia, ↓ bicarb, <1% acute optic neuritis **Notes:** Bladder CA, also in combo w/ vinblastine & ifosfamide

Ganciclovir (Cytovene, Vitrasert) Uses: *Rx & prevent CMV retinitis, prevent CMV Dz* in transplant recipients **Action:** ↓ viral DNA synth **Dose:** *Adults & Peds. IV:* 5 mg/kg IV q12h for 14–21 d, then maint 5 mg/kg/d IV × 7 d/wk or 6 mg/kg/d IV × 5 d/wk. *Ocular implant:* One implant q5–8mo. *Adults. PO:* Following induction, 1000 mg PO tid. *Prevention:* 1000 mg PO tid; with food; ↓ in renal impair **Caution:** [C, –] ↑ Effect w/ immunosuppressives, imipenem/cilastatin, zidovudine, didanosine, other nephrotox Rx **CI:** ANC <500, plt <25,000, intravitreal implant **Disp:** Caps 250, 500 mg; Inj 500 mg, ocular implant 4.5 mg **SE:** Granulocytopenia & thrombocytopenia, fever, rash, GI upset **Notes:** Not a cure for CMV; handle Inj w/ cytotoxic cautions; no systemic benefit w/ implant

Gefitinib (Iressa) Uses: *Rx locally advanced or metastatic NSCLC after platinum-based & docetaxel chemotherapy fails* **Action:** selective TKI of EGFR **Dose:** 250 mg/d PO **Caution:** [D, –] **Disp:** Tabs 250 mg **SE:** D, rash, acne, dry skin, N/V, interstitial lung Dz, ↑ transaminases **Notes:** ✓ LFTs, only give to pts who have already received drug; no new pts because it has not been shown to increase survival

Gemcitabine (Gemzar) Uses: *Pancreatic CA, brain mets, NSCLC,* gastric CA **Action:** Antimetabolite; ↓ ribonucleotide reductase; produces false nucleotide base-inhibiting DNA synth **Dose:** 1000–1250 mg/m² over 30 min–1 h IV Inf/wk × 3–4 wk or 6–8 wk; modify dose based on hematologic Fxn (per protocol)

Caution: [D, ?/–] **CI:** PRG **Disp:** Inj 200 mg, 1 g **SE:** ↓ BM, N/V/D, drug fever, skin rash **Notes:** Reconstituted soln 38 mg/mL; hepatic/renal Fxn

Gemfibrozil (Lopid) **Uses:** *Hypertriglyceridemia, coronary heart Dz* **Action:** Fibric acid **Dose:** 1200 mg/d PO ÷ bid 30 min ac A.M. & P.M. **Caution:** [C, ?] ↑ Warfarin effect, sulfonylureas; ↑ risk of myopathy w/ HMG-CoA reductase inhibitors; ↓ effects w/ cyclosporine **CI:** Renal/hepatic impair (SCr >2.0 mg/dL), gallbladder Dz, primary biliary cirrhosis **Disp:** Tabs 600 mg **SE:** Cholelithiasis, GI upset **Notes:** Avoid w/HMG-CoA reductase inhibitors; ✓ LFTs & serum lipids

Gemifloxacin (Factive) **Uses:** *CAP, acute exacerbation of chronic bronchitis* **Action:** ↓ DNA gyrase & topoisomerase IV; *Spectrum:* S. pneumoniae (including multidrug-resistant strains), H. influenzae, H. parainfluenzae, M. catarrhalis, M. pneumoniae, C. pneumoniae, K. pneumoniae **Dose:** 320 mg PO daily × 5–7 d; CrCl <40 mL/min: 160 mg PO/d **Caution:** [C, ?/–]; Peds <18 y; Hx of ↑ QTc interval, electrolyte disorders, w/ class IA/III antiarrhythmics, erythromycin, TCAs, antipsychotics, ↑ INR and bleeding risk w/ warfarin **CI:** Fluoroquinolone allergy **Disp:** Tab 320 mg **SE:** Rash, N/V/D, C. difficile enterocolitis, ↑ risk of Achilles tendon rupture, tendonitis, Abd pain, dizziness, xerostomia, arthralgia, allergy/anaphylactic Rxns, peripheral neuropathy, tendon rupture **Notes:** Take 3 h before or 2 h after Al/Mg antacids, Fe, Z, or other metal cations; ↑ rash risk w/ ↑ duration of therapy

Gemtuzumab Ozogamicin (Mylotarg) **WARNING:** Can cause severe allergic Rxns & other Inf-related Rxns including severe pulm events; hepatotox, including severe hepatic venoocclusive Dz (VOD) reported **Uses:** *Relapsed CD33+ AML in pts >60 who are poor candidates for chemotherapy* **Action:** MoAb linked to calicheamicin; selective for myeloid cells **Dose:** 9 mg/m² IV over 2 h × 2 doses; separate doses by 2 wk or per protocol **Caution:** [D, –] **CI:** Component sensitivity, lactating mothers **Disp:** 5 mg/20 mL vial **SE:** ↓ BM, allergy, anaphylaxis, chills, fever, N/V, HA, pulm events, hepatotox **Notes:** Single-agent use only, not in combo; premedicate w/ diphenhydramine & acetaminophen; ✓ CBC, LFTs, lytes

Gentamicin (Garamycin, G-mycitin, others) **Uses:** *Septicemia, serious bacterial Infxn of CNS, urinary tract, resp tract, GI tract, including peritonitis, skin, bone, soft tissue, including burns; severe Infxn P. aeruginosa w/ carbenicillin; group D streptococci endocarditis w/ PCN-type drug; serious staphylococcal Infxns, but not the antibiotic of 1st choice; mixed Infxn w/ staphylococci and gram-negatives* **Action:** Aminoglycoside, bactericidal; ↓ protein synth *Spectrum:* gram(–) (not Neisseria, Legionella, Acinetobacter); weaker gram(+) but synergy w/ PCNs **Dose:** **Adults.** *Standard:* 1–2 mg/kg IV q8–12h or daily dosing 4–7 mg/kg q24h IV. *Gram(+) Synergy:* 1 mg/kg q8h **Peds Infants <7 d <1200 g:** 2.5 mg/kg/dose q18–24h. **Infants >1200 g:** 2.5 mg/kg/dose q12–18h. **Infants >7 d:** 2.5 mg/kg/dose IV q8–12h. **Children:** 2.5 mg/kg/d IV q8h; ↓ w/ renal Insuff; if obese, dose based on IBW **Caution:** [C, +/–] Avoid other nephrotoxics **CI:** Aminoglycoside sensitivity **Disp:** Premixed Infs 40, 60, 70, 80, 90, 100, 120 mg; ADD-Vantage Inj vials 10 mg/mL; Inj 40 mg/mL; IT preservative-free 2 mg/mL **SE:** Nephro-/oto-/neurotox **Notes:** Follow CrCl, SCr & serum conc for dose adjustments; use IBW for dose (use adjusted if obese >30% IBW);OK to use intraperitoneal for peritoneal dialysis-related Infxns *Levels: Peak:* 30 min after Inf; *Trough* <0.5 h before next dose; *Therapeutic: Peak* 5–8 mcg/mL, *Trough* <2 mcg/mL, if >2 associated w/ renal tox

Gentamicin & Prednisolone, Ophthalmic (Pred-G Ophthalmic)

Uses: *Steroid-responsive ocular & conjunctival Infxns* sensitive to gentamicin **Action:** Bactericidal; ↓ protein synth w/ anti-inflammatory. *Spectrum: Staphylococcus, E. coli, H. influenzae, Klebsiella, Neisseria, Pseudomonas, Proteus, & Serratia* sp **Dose:** *Oint:* 1/2 inch in conjunctival sac daily-tid. *Susp:* 1 gtt bid-qid, up to 1 gtt/h for severe Infxns **CI:** Aminoglycoside sensitivity **Caution:** [C, ?] **Disp:** *Oint, ophthal:* Prednisolone acetate 0.6% & gentamicin sulfate 0.3% (3.5 g). *Susp, ophthal:* Prednisolone acetate 1% & gentamicin sulfate 0.3% (2, 5, 10 mL) **SE:** Local irritation

Gentamicin, ophthalmic (Garamycin, Genoptic, Gentacidin, Gentak, others)

Uses: *Conjunctival Infxns* **Action:** Bactericidal; ↓ protein synth **Dose:** *Oint:* Apply 1/2 inch bid–tid. *Soln:* 1–2 gtt q2–4h, up to 2 gtt/h for severe Infxn **Caution:** [C, ?] **CI:** Aminoglycoside sensitivity **Disp:** Soln & oint 0.1% and 0.3% **SE:** Local irritation **Notes:** Do not use other eye drops w/in 5–10 min; do not touch dropper to eye

Gentamicin, topical (Garamycin, G-mycitin)

Uses: *Skin Infxns* caused by susceptible organisms **Action:** Bactericidal; ↓ protein synth **Dose:** *Adults & Peds >1 y:* Apply tid-qid **Caution:** [C, ?] **CI:** Aminoglycoside sensitivity **Disp:** Cream & oint 0.1% **SE:** Irritation

Glimepiride (Amaryl)

Uses: *Type 2 DM* **Action:** Sulfonylurea; ↑ pancreatic insulin release; ↑ peripheral insulin sensitivity; ↓ hepatic glucose output/production **Dose:** 1–4 mg/d, max 8 mg **Caution:** [C, –] DKA **Disp:** Tabs 1, 2, 4 mg **SE:** HA, N, hypoglycemia **Notes:** Give w/ 1st meal of day

Glimepiride/pioglitazone (Duetact)

Uses: *Adjunct to exercise type 2 DM not controlled by single agent* **Action:** Sulfonylurea (↓ glucose) w/ agent that ↑ insulin sensitivity & ↓ gluconeogenesis **Dose:** initial 30 mg/2 mg PO q A.M.; 45 mg pioglitazone/8 mg glimepiride/d max; w/food **Caution:** [C, ?/–] w/ Liver impair, elderly **CI:** Component hypersensitivity, DKA **Disp:** Tabs 30/2, 30 mg/4 & 4 mg **SE:** Hct, ↑ ALT, ↓ glucose, URI, ↑ wgt, edema, HA, N/D, may ↑ CV mortality **Notes:** Monitor CBC, ALT, Cr, wgt

Glipizide (Glucotrol, Glucotrol XL)

Uses: *Type 2 DM* **Action:** Sulfonylurea; ↑ pancreatic insulin release; ↑ peripheral insulin sensitivity; ↓ hepatic glucose output/production; ↓ intestinal glucose absorption **Dose:** 5 mg initial, ↑ by 2.5–5 mg/d, max 40 mg/d; XL max 20 mg; 30 min ac; hold if NPO **Caution:** [C, ?/–] Severe liver Dz **CI:** DKA, type 1 DM, sulfonamide sensitivity **Disp:** Tabs 5, 10 mg;

XL tabs 2.5, 5, 10 mg **SE:** HA, anorexia, N/V/D, constipation, fullness, rash, urticaria, photosensitivity **Notes:** Counsel about DM management; wait several d before adjusting dose; monitor glucose

Glucagon **Uses:** Severe *hypoglycemic* Rxns in DM with sufficient liver glycogen stores; β-blocker OD **Action:** Accelerates liver gluconeogenesis **Dose:** **Adults.** 0.5–1 mg SQ, IM, or IV; repeat in 20 min PRN. *β-blocker OD:* 3–10 mg IV; repeat in 10 min PRN; may give cont Inf 1–5 mg/h *(ECC 2005)*. *Peds* **Neonates:** 0.3 mg/kg/dose SQ, IM, or IV q4h PRN. *Children:* 0.025–0.1 mg/kg/dose SQ, IM, or IV; repeat in 20 min PRN **Caution:** [B, M] **CI:** Pheochromocytoma **Disp:** Inj 1 mg **SE:** N/V, ↓ BP **Notes:** Administration of dextrose IV necessary; ineffective in starvation, adrenal Insuff, or chronic hypoglycemia

Glyburide (DiaBeta, Micronase, Glynase) **Uses:** *Type 2 DM* **Action:** Sulfonylurea; ↑ pancreatic insulin release; ↑ peripheral insulin sensitivity; ↓ hepatic glucose output/production; ↓ intestinal glucose absorption **Dose:** 1.25–10 mg daily-bid, max 20 mg/d. *Micronized:* 0.75–6 mg daily-bid, max 12 mg/d **Caution:** [C, ?] Renal impair **CI:** DKA, type 1 DM **Disp:** Tabs 1.25, 2.5, 5 mg; micronized tabs 1.5, 3, 6 mg **SE:** HA, hypoglycemia **Notes:** Not OK for CrCl <50 mL/min; hold dose if NPO

Glyburide/Metformin (Glucovance) **Uses:** *Type 2 DM* **Action:** *Sulfonylurea:* ↑ Pancreatic insulin release. *Metformin:* Peripheral insulin sensitivity; ↓ hepatic glucose output/production; ↓ intestinal glucose absorption **Dose:** 1st line (naïve pts), 1.25/250 mg PO daily-bid; 2nd line, 2.5/500 mg or 5/500 mg (max 20/2000 mg); take w/ meals, slowly ↑ dose; hold before & 48 h after ionic contrast media **Caution:** [C, –] **CI:** SCr >1.4 in females or >1.5 in males; hypoxemic conditions (sepsis, recent MI); alcoholism; metabolic acidosis; liver Dz; **Disp:** Tabs 1.25/250 mg, 2.5/500 mg, 5/500 mg **SE:** HA, hypoglycemia, lactic acidosis, anorexia, N/V, rash **Notes:** Avoid EtOH; hold dose if NPO; monitor folate levels (megaloblastic anemia)

Glycerin Suppository **Uses:** *Constipation* **Action:** Hyperosmolar laxative **Dose:** *Adults.* 1 Adult supp PR PRN. *Peds.* 1 Infant supp PR daily-bid PRN **Caution:** [C, ?] **Disp:** Supp (adult, infant); liq 4 mL/applicator-full **SE:** D

Gonadorelin (Factrel) **Uses:** *Primary hypothalamic amenorrhea* **Action:** ↑ Pituitary release of LH & FSH **Dose:** 5 mcg IV over 1 min q 90 min × 21 d using pump kit **Caution:** [B, M] ↑ Levels w/ androgens, estrogens, progestins, glucocorticoids, spironolactone, levodopa; ↓ levels w/ OCP, digoxin, dopamine antagonists **CI:** Condition exacerbated by PRG or reproductive hormones, ovarian cysts, causes of anovulation other than hypothalamic, hormonally dependent tumor **Disp:** Inj 100 mcg **SE:** Multiple pregnancy risk; Inj site pain **Notes:** Monitor LH, FSH

Goserelin (Zoladex) **Uses:** Advanced *CA Prostate* & w/ radiation for localized high-risk Dz, *endometriosis, breast CA* **Action:** LHRH agonist, transient ↑ then ↓ in LH, w/ ↓ testosterone **Dose:** 3.6 mg SQ (implant) q28d or 10.8 mg

SQ q3mo; usually upper Abd wall **Caution:** [X, –] **CI:** PRG, breast-feeding, 10.8-mg implant not for women **Disp:** SQ implant 3.6 (1 mo), 10.8 mg (3 mo) **SE:** Hot flashes, ↓ libido, gynecomastia, & transient exacerbation of CA-related bone pain ("flare Rxn" 7–10 d after 1st dose) **Notes:** Inject SQ into fat in Abd wall; do not aspirate; females must use contraception

Granisetron (Kytril)

Uses: *Rx and Prevention of N/V (chemo/radiation/postoperation)* **Action:** Serotonin (5-HT₃) receptor antagonist **Dose:** *Adults & Peds. Chemotherapy:* 10 mcg/kg/dose IV 30 min prior to chemotherapy *Adults.* Inj 0.1, 1 mg/mL *Chemotherapy:* 2 mg PO q day 1 h before chemotherapy, then 12 h later. *Post-op N/V:* 1 mg IV over 30 s before end of case **Caution:** [B, +/–] St. John's wort ↓ levels **CI:** Liver Dz, children <2 y **Disp:** Tabs 1 mg; Inj 0.1, 1 mg/mL; soln 2 mg/10 mL **SE:** HA, asthenia, somnolence, D, constipation, Abd pain, dizziness, insomnia, ↑ LFTs

Guaifenesin (Robitussin, others)

Uses: *Relief of dry, nonproductive cough* **Action:** Expectorant **Dose:** *Adults.* 200–400 mg (10–20 mL) PO q4h SR 600–1200 mg PO bid, (max 2.4 g/d). *Peds 2–5 y:* 50–100 mg (2.5–5 mL) PO q4h (max 600 mg/d). *6–11 y:* 100–200 mg (5–10 mL) PO q4h (max 1.2 g/d) **Caution:** [C, ?] **Disp:** Tabs 100, 200; SR tabs 600, 1200 mg; caps 200 mg; SR caps 300 mg; liq 100 mg/5 mL **SE:** GI upset **Notes** Give w/ large amount of H₂O; some dosage forms contain EtOH

Guaifenesin & Codeine (Robitussin AC, Brontex, others) [C-V]

Uses: *Relief of dry cough* **Action:** Antitussive w/ expectorant **Dose:** *Adults.* 5–10 mL or 1 tab PO q6–8h (max 60 mL/24 h). *Peds 2–6 y:* 1–1.5 mg/kg codeine/d ÷ dose q4–6h (max 30 mg/24 h). *6–12 y:* 5 mL q4h (max 30 mL/24 h) **Caution:** [C, +] **Disp:** Brontex tab 10 mg codeine/300 mg guaifenesin; liq 2.5 mg codeine/75 mg guaifenesin/5 mL; others 10 mg codeine/100 mg guaifenesin/5 mL **SE:** Somnolence, constipation

Guaifenesin & Dextromethorphan (many OTC brands)

Uses: *Cough* due to upper resp tract irritation **Action:** Antitussive w/ expectorant **Dose:** *Adults & Peds >12 y:* 10 mL PO q6–8h (max 40 mL/24 h). *Peds 2–6 y:* Dextromethorphan 1–2 mg/kg/24 h ÷ 3–4 × d (max 10 mL/d). *6–12 y:* 5 mL q6–8h (max 20 mL/d) **Caution:** [C, +] **CI:** Administration w/ MAOI **Disp:** Many OTC formulations **SE:** Somnolence **Notes:** Give with plenty of fluids; some forms contain EtOH

Haemophilus B Conjugate Vaccine (ActHIB, HibTITER, PedvaxHIB, Prohibit, others)

Uses: Routine *immunization* of children against *H. influenzae* type B Dzs **Action:** Active immunization against *Haemophilus* B **Dose:** *Peds.* 0.5 mL (25 mg) IM in deltoid or vastus lateralis **Caution:** [C, +] **CI:** Febrile illness, immunosuppression, allergy to thimerosal **Disp:** Inj 7.5, 10, 15, 25 mcg/0.5 mL **SE:** Observe for anaphylaxis; edema, ↑ risk of *Haemophilus* B Infxn the wk after vaccination **Notes:** Booster not required; report SAE to Vaccine Adverse Events Reporting System (VAERS: 1-800-822-7967); dosing varies w/ product

Haloperidol (Haldol) **WARNING:** Risk for torsade de pointes and QT prolongation, death w/ IV administration at higher doses **Uses:** *Psychotic disorders, agitation, Tourette disorders, hyperactivity in children* **Action:** Butyrophenone; antipsychotic, neuroleptic **Dose:** *Adults. Mod Sxs:* 0.5–2 mg PO bid–tid. *Severe Sxs/agitation:* 3–5 mg PO bid–tid or 1–5 mg IM q4h PRN (max 100 mg/d). *Peds 3–6 y:* 0.01–0.03 mg/kg/24 h PO daily. *6–12 y:* Initial, 0.5–1.5 mg/24 h PO; ↑ by 0.5 mg/24 h to maint of 2–4 mg/24 h (0.05–0.1 mg/kg/24 h) or 1–3 mg/dose IM q4–8h to 0.1 mg/kg/24 h max; Tourette Dz may require up to 15 mg/24 h PO; ↓ in elderly **Caution:** [C, ?] ↑ Effects w/ SSRIs, CNS depressants, TCA, indomethacin, metoclopramide; avoid levodopa (↓ antiparkinsonian effects) **CI:** NAG, severe CNS depression, coma, Parkinson Dz, BM suppression, severe cardiac/hepatic Dz **Disp:** Tabs 0.5, 1, 2, 5, 10, 20 mg; conc liq 2 mg/mL; Inj 5 mg/mL; decanoate Inj 50, 100 mg/mL **SE:** Extrapyramidal Sxs (EPS), ↓ BP, anxiety, dystonias **Notes:** Do not give decanoate IV; dilute PO conc liq w/ H$_2$O/juice; monitor for EPS; ECG monitoring w/ off-label IV use

Heparin **Uses:** *Rx & prevention of DVT & PE,* unstable angina, AF w/ emboli, & acute arterial occlusion **Action:** Acts w/ antithrombin III to inactivate thrombin & ↓ thromboplastin formation **Dose:** *Adults. Prophylaxis:* 3000–5000 units SQ q8–12h. *DVT/PE Rx:* Load 50–80 units/kg IV (max 10,000 units), then 10–20 units/kg IV qh (adjust based on PTT); bolus 60 units/kg (max 4000 units); then 12 units/kg/h (max 1000 units/h) round to nearest 50 units; keep PTT 1.5–2.0 (control 48 h or until angiography) *(ECC 2005)* *Peds Infants:* Load 50 units/kg IV bolus, then 20 units/kg/h IV by cont Inf. *Children:* Load 50 units/kg IV, then 15–25 units/kg cont Inf or 100 units/kg/dose q4h IV intermittent bolus (adjust based on PTT) **Caution:** [B, +] ↑ Risk of hemorrhage w/ anticoagulants, aspirin, antiplatelets, cephalosporins w/ MTT side chain **CI:** Uncontrolled bleeding, severe thrombocytopenia, suspected ICH **Disp:** Inj 10, 100, 1000, 2000, 2500, 5000, 7500, 10,000, 20,000, 40,000 units/mL **SE:** Bruising, bleeding, thrombocytopenia **Notes:** Follow PTT, thrombin time, or activated clotting time; little PT effect; therapeutic PTT 1.5–2 × control for most conditions; monitor for HIT w/ plt counts

Hep A Vaccine (Havrix, Vaqta) **Uses:** *Prevent hep A* in high-risk individuals (eg, travelers, certain professions, or high-risk behaviors) **Action:** Active immunity **Dose:** (Expressed as ELISA units [EL.U.]) *Havrix: Adults.* 1440 EL.U. single IM dose. *Peds >2 y:* 720 EL.U. single IM dose. *Vaqta: Adults.* 50 units single IM dose. *Peds.* 25 units single IM dose **Caution:** [C, +] **CI:** Component allergy **Disp:** Inj 720 EL.U./0.5 mL, 1440 EL.U./1 mL; 50 units/mL **SE:** Fever, fatigue, HA, Inj site pain **Notes:** Booster OK 6–12 mo after primary; report SAE to Vaccine Adverse Events Reporting System (VAERS: 1-800-822-7967)

Hep A (Inactivated) & Hep B (Recombinant) Vaccine (Twinrix) **Uses:** *Active immunization against hep A/B in pts >18 y* **Action:** Active immunity **Dose:** 1 mL IM at 0, 1, & 6 mo; accelerated regimen 1 mL IM day 0, 7 and 21–20 then booster at 12 mo **Caution:** [C, +/–] **CI:** Component sensitivity **Disp:**

Single-dose vials, syringes **SE:** Fever, fatigue, pain at site, HA **Notes:** Booster OK 6–12 mo after vaccination; report SAE to Vaccine Adverse Events Reporting System (VAERS: 1-800-822-7967)

Hep B Immune Globulin (HyperHep, HepaGam B, H-BIG)

Uses: *Exposure to HBsAg(+) material (eg, blood, accidental needlestick, mucous membrane contact, PO), prevent hep B in HBsAg(+) liver Tx pt* **Action:** Passive immunization **Dose:** *Adults & Peds.* 0.06 mL/kg IM 5 mL max; w/in 24 h of exposure; w/in 14 d of sexual contact; repeat 1 mo if nonresponder or refused initial after exposure; liver Tx per protocols **Caution:** [C, ?] **CI:** Allergies to γ-globulin or anti-immunoglobulin Ab; allergies to thimerosal; IgA deficiency **Disp:** Inj **SE:** Inj site pain, dizziness **Notes:** IM in gluteal or deltoid; w/ continued exposure, give hep B vaccine; not for active hep B; ineffective for chronic hep B

Hep B Vaccine (Engerix-B, Recombivax HB)

Uses: *Prevent hep B* **Action:** Active immunization; recombinant DNA **Dose:** *Adults.* 3 IM doses 1 mL each; 1st 2 doses 1 mo apart, the 3rd 6 mo after the 1st. *Peds.* 0.5 mL IM adult schedule **Caution:** [C, +] ↓ Effect w/ immunosuppressives **CI:** Yeast allergy **Disp:** *Engerix-B:* Inj 20 mcg/mL; peds Inj 10 mcg/0.5 mL. *Recombivax HB:* Inj 10 & 40 mcg/mL; peds Inj 5 mcg/0.5 mL **SE:** Fever, Inj site pain **Notes:** Deltoid IM Inj adults/older peds; younger peds, use anterolateral thigh

Hetastarch (Hespan)

Uses: *Plasma vol expansion* adjunct in shock & leukapheresis **Action:** Synthetic colloid; acts similar to albumin **Dose:** *Vol expansion:* 500–1000 mL (1500 mL/d max) IV (20 mL/kg/h max rate). *Leukapheresis:* 250–700 mL; ↓ in renal failure **Caution:** [C, +] **CI:** Severe bleeding disorders, CHF, oliguric/anuric renal failure **Disp:** Inj 6 g/100 mL **SE:** Bleeding (↑ PT, PTT, bleed time) **Notes:** Not blood or plasma substitute

Human Papillomavirus (Types 6, 11, 16, 18) Recombinant Vaccine (Gardasil)

Uses: *Prevent cervical CA, precancerous genital lesions, and genital warts due to human papillomavirus (HPV) types 6, 11, 16, 18 in females 9–26 y* **Action:** Recombinant vaccine, passive humoral immunity **Dose:** 0.5 mL IM initial, then at 2 and 6 mo **Caution:** [B, ?/–] **Disp:** Single-dose vial & prefilled syringe: 0.5 mL **SE:** Site Rxn (pain, erythema, swelling, pruritus), fever, syncope **Notes:** First approved cancer prevention vaccine; report adverse events to Vaccine Adverse Events Reporting System (VAERS: 1-800-822-7967); IM in upper thigh or deltoid; continue cervical CA screening

Hydralazine (Apresoline, others)

Uses: *Mod–severe HTN; CHF* (w/ Isordil) **Action:** Peripheral vasodilator **Dose:** *Adults.* Initial 10 mg PO 3–4×/d, ↑ to 25 mg 3–4×/d, 300 mg/d max. *Peds.* 0.75–3 mg/kg/24 h PO ÷ q6–12h; ↓ in renal impair; ✓ CBC & ANA before **Caution:** [C, +] ↓ Hepatic Fxn & CAD; ↑ tox w/ MAOI, indomethacin, β-blockers **CI:** Dissecting aortic aneurysm, mitral valve/rheumatic heart Dz **Disp:** Tabs 10, 25, 50, 100 mg; Inj 20 mg/mL **SE:** SLE-like syndrome w/ chronic high doses; SVT following IM route, peripheral neuropathy **Notes:** Compensatory sinus tachycardia eliminated w/ β-blocker

Hydrochlorothiazide (HydroDIURIL, Esidrix, others) Uses: *Edema, HTN*; prevent stones in hypercalcuria Action: Thiazide diuretic; ↓ distal tubule Na+ reabsorption Dose: *Adults.* 25–100 mg/d PO single or ÷ doses; 200 mg/d max. *Peds <6 mo:* 2–3 mg/kg/d in 2 ÷ doses. *>6 mo:* 2 mg/kg/d in 2 ÷ doses Caution: [D, +] CI: Anuria, sulfonamide allergy, renal Insuff Disp: Tabs 25, 50, mg; caps 12.5 mg; PO soln 50 mg/5 mL SE: ↓ K+, hyperglycemia, hyperuricemia, ↓ Na+; sun sensitivity

Hydrochlorothiazide & Amiloride (Moduretic) Uses: *HTN* Action: Combined thiazide & K+-sparing diuretic Dose: 1–2 tabs/d PO Caution: [D, ?] CI: Renal failure, sulfonamide allergy Disp: Tabs (amiloride/HCTZ) 5 mg/50 mg SE: ↓ BP, photosensitivity, ↑ K+/↓ K+, hyperglycemia, ↓ Na+, hyperlipidemia, hyperuricemia

Hydrochlorothiazide & Spironolactone (Aldactazide) Uses: *Edema, HTN* Action: Thiazide & K+-sparing diuretic Dose: 25–200 mg each component/d, ÷ doses Caution: [D, +] CI: Sulfonamide allergy Disp: Tabs (HCTZ/spironolactone) 25 mg/25 mg, 50 mg/50 mg SE: Photosensitivity, ↓ BP, ↑ or ↓ K+, ↓ Na+, hyperglycemia, hyperlipidemia, hyperuricemia

Hydrochlorothiazide & Triamterene (Dyazide, Maxzide) Uses: *Edema & HTN* Action: Combo thiazide & K+-sparing diuretic Dose: *Dyazide:* 1–2 caps PO daily-bid. *Maxzide:* 1 tab/d PO Caution: [D, +/–] CI: Sulfonamide allergy Disp: (Triamterene/HCTZ) 37.5 mg/25 mg, 75 mg/50 mg SE: Photosensitivity, ↓ BP, ↑ or ↓ K+, ↓ Na+, hyperglycemia, hyperlipidemia, hyperuricemia Notes: HCTZ component in Maxzide more bioavailable than in Dyazide

Hydrocodone & Acetaminophen (Lorcet, Vicodin, Hycet, others) [C-III] Uses: *Mod–severe pain*; Action: Narcotic analgesic w/ nonnarcotic analgesic Dose: *Adults.* 1–2 caps or tabs PO q4–6h PRN; soln 15 mL q4–6h *Peds.* Soln (Hycet) 0.27 mL/kg q4–6h Caution: [C, M] CI: CNS depression, severe resp depression Disp: Many formulations; specify hydrocodone/APAP dose; caps 5/500; tabs 2.5/500, 5/325, 5/400, 5/500, 7.5/325, 7.5/400, 7.5/500, 7.5/650, 7.5/750, 10/325, 10/400, 10/500, 10/650, 10/660, 10/750; soln *Hycet* (fruit punch) 7.5 mg hydrocodone/325 mg acetaminophen/15 mL SE: GI upset, sedation, fatigue Notes: Do not exceed >4 g APAP/d

Hydrocodone & Aspirin (Lortab ASA, others) [C-III] Uses: *Mod–severe pain* Action: Narcotic analgesic with NSAID Dose: 1–2 PO q4–6h PRN, w/ food/milk Caution: [C, M] ↓ Renal Fxn, gastritis/PUD, CI: Component sensitivity; children w/chickenpox (Reye syndrome) Disp: 5 mg hydrocodone/ 500 mg ASA/tab SE: GI upset, sedation, fatigue Notes: Monitor for GI bleed

Hydrocodone & Guaifenesin (Hycotuss Expectorant, others) [C-III] Uses: *Nonproductive cough* associated with resp Infxn Action: Expectorant w/ cough suppressant Dose: *Adults & Peds >12 y:* 5 mL q4h pc & hs. *Peds <2 y:* 0.3 mg/kg/d ÷ qid. *2–12 y:* 2.5 mL q4h pc & hs Caution: [C, M] CI: Component sensitivity Disp: Hydrocodone 5 mg/guaifenesin 100 mg/5 mL SE: GI upset, sedation, fatigue

**Hydrocodone & Homatropine (Hycodan, Hydromet, others)
[C-III]**   Uses: *Relief of cough* **Action:** Combo antitussive **Dose:** (Based on hydrocodone) *Adults.* 5–10 mg q4–6h. *Peds.* 0.6 mg/kg/d ÷ tid-qid **Caution:** [C, M] **CI:** NAG, ↑ ICP, depressed ventilation **Disp:** Syrup 5 mg hydrocodone/5 mL; tabs 5 mg hydrocodone **SE:** Sedation, fatigue, GI upset **Notes:** Do not give < q4h; see individual drugs

Hydrocodone & Ibuprofen (Vicoprofen) [C-III]   Uses: *Mod–severe pain (<10 d)* **Action:** Narcotic + NSAID **Dose:** 1–2 tabs q4–6h PRN **Caution:** [C, M] Renal Insuff; ↓ effect w/ ACE inhibitors & diuretics; ↑ effect w/ CNS depressants, EtOH, MAOI, aspirin, TCA, anticoagulants **CI:** Component sensitivity **Disp:** Tabs 7.5 mg hydrocodone/200 mg ibuprofen **SE:** Sedation, fatigue, GI upset

Hydrocodone & Pseudoephedrine (Detussin, Histussin-D, others) [C-III]   Uses: *Cough & nasal congestion* **Action:** Narcotic cough suppressant with decongestant **Dose:** 5 mL qid, PRN **Caution:** [C, M] **CI:** MAOIs **Disp:** hydrocodone/pseudoephedrine 5 mg/60 mg, 3 mg/15 mg 5 mL; tab 5 mg/60 mg **SE:** ↑ BP, GI upset, sedation, fatigue

Hydrocodone, Chlorpheniramine, Phenylephrine, Acetaminophen, & Caffeine (Hycomine Compound) [C-III]   Uses: *Cough & Sxs of URI* **Action:** Narcotic cough suppressant w/ decongestants & analgesic **Dose:** 1 tab PO q4h PRN **Caution:** [C, M] **CI:** NAG **Disp:** Hydrocodone 5 mg/chlorpheniramine 2 mg/phenylephrine 10 mg/APAP 250 mg/caffeine 30 mg/tab **SE:** ↑ BP, GI upset, sedation, fatigue

Hydrocortisone, rectal (Anusol-HC Suppository, Cortifoam Rectal, Proctocort, others)   Uses: *Painful anorectal conditions,* radiation proctitis, ulcerative colitis **Action:** Anti-inflammatory steroid **Dose:** *Adults.* Ulcerative colitis: 10–100 mg PR daily-bid for 2–3 wk **Caution:** [B, ?/–] **CI:** Component sensitivity **Disp:** *Hydrocortisone acetate:* Rectal aerosol 90 mg/applicator; supp 25 mg. *Hydrocortisone base:* Rectal 0.5%, 1%, 2.5%; rectal susp 100 mg/60 mL **SE:** Minimal systemic effect

Hydrocortisone, topical & systemic (Cortef, Solu-Cortef)
See Steroids page 214 and Tables 3 & 4 **Caution:** [B, –] **CI:** Viral, fungal, or tubercular skin lesions; serious Infxns (except septic shock or TB meningitis) **SE:** *Systemic:* ↑ Appetite, insomnia, hyperglycemia, bruising **Notes:** May cause hypothalamic–pituitary–adrenal axis suppression

Hydromorphone (Dilaudid) [C-II]   WARNING: A potent Schedule II opioid agonist; highest potential for abuse and risk of resp depression. HP formula is highly concentrated; do not confuse w/ standard formulations, OD and death could result. Alcohol, other opioids, CNS depressants ↑ resp depressant effects Uses: *Mod/severe pain* **Action:** Narcotic analgesic **Dose:** 1–4 mg PO, IM, IV, or PR q4–6h PRN; 3 mg PR q6–8h PRN; ↓ w/ hepatic failure **Caution:** [B (D if prolonged use or high doses near term), ?] ↑ Resp depression and CNS effects

CNS depressants, phenothiazines, TCA **CI:** CNS lesion w/ ↑ ICP, COPD, cor pulmonale, emphysema, kyphoscoliosis, status asthmaticus; HP-Inj form in OB analgesia **Disp:** Tabs 2, 4 mg, 8 mg scored; liq 5 mg/5 mL or 1 mg/mL; Inj 1, 2, 4, *HP* is 10 mg/mL; supp 3 **SE:** Sedation, dizziness, GI upset **Notes:** Morphine 10 mg IM = hydromorphone 1.5 mg IM

Hydroxocobalamin (Cyanokit)   **Uses:** *Cyanide poisoning* **Action:** Binds cyanide to form nontoxic cyanocobalamin excreted in urine **Dose:** 5 mg IV over 15 min, repeat PRN 5 g IV over 15 min–2 h, total dose 10 g **Caution:** [C, ?] **CI:** None known **Disp:** Kit 2 2.5 g vials w/ Inf set **SE:** ↑ BP (can be severe) anaphylaxis, chest tightness, edema, urticaria, rash, chromaturia, N, HA, Inj site Rxns

Hydroxyurea (Hydrea, Droxia)   **Uses:** *CML, head & neck, ovarian & colon CA, melanoma, ALL, sickle cell anemia, polycythemia vera, HIV* **Action:** ↓ Ribonucleotide reductase **Dose:** (per protocol) 50–75 mg/kg for WBC >100,000 cells/mL; 20–30 mg/kg in refractory CML. *HIV:* 1000–1500 mg/d in single or ÷ doses; ↓ in renal Insuff **Caution:** [D, –] ↑ Effects w/ zidovudine, zalcitabine, didanosine, stavudine, fluorouracil **CI:** Severe anemia, BM suppression, WBC <2500 or plt <100,000, PRG **Disp:** Caps 200, 300, 400, 500 mg, tabs 1000 mg **SE:** ↓ BM (mostly leukopenia), N/V, rashes, facial erythema, radiation recall Rxns, renal impair **Notes:** Empty caps into H$_2$O

Hydroxyzine (Atarax, Vistaril)   **Uses:** *Anxiety, sedation, itching* **Action:** Antihistamine, antianxiety **Dose:** *Adults. Anxiety/sedation:* 50–100 mg PO or IM qid or PRN (max 600 mg/d). *Itching:* 25–50 mg PO or IM tid-qid. *Peds.* 0.5–1.0 mg/kg/24 h PO or IM q6h; ↓ w/hepatic impair **Caution:** [C, +/–] ↑ Effects w/ CNS depressants, anticholinergics, EtOH **CI:** Component sensitivity **Disp:** Tabs 10, 25, 50 mg; caps 25, 50 mg; syrup 10 mg/5 mL; susp 25 mg/5 mL; Inj 25, 50 mg/mL **SE:** Drowsiness, anticholinergic effects **Notes:** Used to potentiate narcotic effects; not for IV/SQ (thrombosis & digital gangrene possible)

Hyoscyamine (Anaspaz, Cystospaz, Levsin, others)   **Uses:** *Spasm w/ GI & bladder disorders* **Action:** Anticholinergic **Dose:** *Adults.* 0.125–0.25 mg (1–2 tabs) SL/PO tid-qid, ac & hs; 1 SR caps q12h **Caution:** [C, +] ↑ Effects w/ amantadine, antihistamines, antimuscarinics, haloperidol, phenothiazines, TCA, MAOI **CI:** BOO, GI obst, NAG, MyG, paralytic ileus, ulcerative colitis, MI **Disp:** (Cystospaz-M, Levsinex) time-release caps 0.375 mg; elixir (EtOH); soln 0.125 mg/5 mL; Inj 0.5 mg/mL; tab 0.125 mg; tab (Cystospaz) 0.15 mg; XR tab (Levbid) 0.375 mg; SL (Levsin SL) 0.125 mg **SE:** Dry skin, xerostomia, constipation, anticholinergic SE, heat prostration w/ hot weather **Notes:** Administer tabs ac

Hyoscyamine, Atropine, Scopolamine, & Phenobarbital (Donnatal, others)   **Uses:** *Irritable bowel, spastic colitis, peptic ulcer, spastic bladder* **Action:** Anticholinergic, antispasmodic **Dose:** 0.125–0.25 mg (1–2 tabs) tid-qid, 1 caps q12h (SR), 5–10 mL elixir tid-qid or q8h **Caution:** [D, M] **CI:** NAG **Disp:** Many combos/manufacturers. Caps (*Donnatal*, others): Hyoscyamine

0.1037 mg/atropine 0.0194 mg/scopolamine 0.0065 mg/phenobarbital 16.2 mg.
Tabs (*Donnatal*, others): Hyoscyamine 0.1037 mg/atropine 0.0194 mg/scopolamine
0.0065 mg/phenobarbital 16.2 mg. LA (*Donnatal*): Hyoscyamine 0.311
mg/atropine 0.0582 mg/scopolamine 0.0195 mg/phenobarbital 48.6 mg. Elixirs (*Don-natal*, others): Hyoscyamine 0.1037 mg/atropine 0.0194 mg/scopolamine 0.0065
mg/phenobarbital 16.2 mg/5 mL **SE:** Sedation, xerostomia, constipation

Ibandronate (Boniva) **Uses:** *Rx & prevent osteoporosis in post-menopausal women* **Action:** Bisphosphonate, ↓ osteoclast-mediated bone-resorption **Dose:** 2.5 mg PO daily or 150 mg once/month on same day (do not lie
down for 60 min after); 3 mg IV over 15–30 s q3mo **Caution:** [C, ?/–] Avoid w/
CrCl <30 mL/min **CI:** Uncorrected ↓ Ca²⁺; inability to stand/sit upright for 60 min
(PO) **Disp:** Tabs 2.5, 150 mg, Inj IV 3 mg/3 mL **SE:** Jaw osteonecrosis (avoid
extensive dental procedures) N/D, HA, dizziness, asthenia, HTN, Infxn, dysphagia,
esophagitis, esophageal/gastric ulcer, musculoskeletal pain **Notes:** Take 1st thing
in A.M. w/ H₂O (6–8 oz) >60 min before 1st food/beverage & any meds w/ multiva-lent cations; give adequate Ca²⁺ & vit D supls; possible association between bis-phosphonates & severe muscle/bone/joint pain

Ibuprofen (Motrin, Motrin IB, Rufen, Advil, others) [OTC]
WARNING: May ↑ risk of cv events & GI bleeding **Uses:** *Arthritis, pain, fever*
Action: NSAID **Dose:** *Adults.* 200–800 mg PO bid-qid (max 2.4 g/d); *Peds.* 30–40
mg/kg/d in 3–4 ÷ doses (max 40 mg/kg/d); w/ food **Caution:** [B, +] May interfere w/
aspirin's antiplatelet effect if given <8 h before aspirin **CI:** 3rd tri PRG, severe
hepatic impair, allergy, use w/ other NSAIDs, upper GI bleeding, ulcers **Disp:** Tabs
100, 200, 400, 600, 800 mg; chew tabs 50, 100 mg; caps 200 mg; susp 100 mg/2.5 mL,
100 mg/5 mL, 40 mg/mL (Motrin IB & Advil OTC 200 mg are the OTC forms)
SE: Dizziness, peptic ulcer, platelet inhibition, worsening of renal Insuff

Ibutilide (Corvert) **Uses:** *Rapid conversion of AF/flutter* **Action:** Class
III antiarrhythmic **Dose:** *Adults* >60 kg 0.01 mg/kg (max 1 mg) IV Inf over 10 min;
may repeat × 1; <60 kg use 0.01 mg/kg (*ECC 2005;* DC cardiovert preferred)
Caution: [C, –] **CI:** w/ Class I/III antiarrhythmics (Table 10); QTc >440 msec
Disp: Inj 0.1 mg/mL **SE:** Arrhythmias, HA **Notes:** Give w/ ECG monitoring;
✓ K⁺, Mg²⁺

Idarubicin (Idamycin) WARNING: Administer only under supervision
of an MD experienced in leukemia and in an institution with resources to maintain
a patient compromised by drug tox **Uses:** *Acute leukemias* (AML, ALL), *CML*
in blast crisis, breast CA* **Action:** DNA-intercalating agent; ↓ DNA topoiso-merases I & II **Dose:** (Per protocol) 10–12 mg/m²/d for 3–4 d; ↓ in renal/hepatic
impair **Caution:** [D, –] **CI:** Bilirubin >5 mg/dL, PRG **Disp:** Inj 1 mg/mL (5, 10,
20 mg vials) **SE:** ↓ BM, cardiotox, N/V, mucositis, alopecia, & IV site Rxns, rarely
↓ renal/hepatic Fxn **Notes:** Avoid extrav, potent vesicant; IV only

Ifosfamide (Ifex, Holoxan) **Uses:** Lung, breast, pancreatic & gastric
CA, Hodgkin lymphoma/NHL, soft-tissue sarcoma **Action:** Alkylating agent

Dose: (Per protocol) 1.2 g/m²/d for 5 d bolus or cont Inf; 2.4 g/m²/d for 3 d; w/ mesna uroprotection; ↓ in renal/hepatic impair **Caution:** [D, M] ↑ Effect w/ phenobarbital, carbamazepine, phenytoin; St. John's wort may ↓ levels [B–M Bxn, PRG **Disp:** Inj 1, 3 g **SE:** Hemorrhagic cystitis, nephrotox, N/V, mild–mod leukopenia, lethargy & confusion, alopecia, ↑ hepatic enzyme **Notes:** Administer w/ mesna to prevent hemorrhagic cystitis

Iloprost (Ventavis)   WARNING: Associated with syncope; may require dosage adjustment Uses: *NYHA class III/IV pulm arterial HTN* Action:
Prostaglandin analog **Dose:** Initial 2.5 mcg; if tolerated, ↑ to 5 mcg Inh 6–9×/d at least 2 h apart while awake **Caution:** [C, ?/–] Antiplatelet effects, ↑ bleeding risk w/ anticoagulants; additive hypotensive effects **CI:** SBP <85 mm Hg **Disp:** Inh soln 10 mcg/mL **SE:** Syncope, ↓ BP, vasodilation, cough, HA, trismus **Notes:** Requires *Pro-Dose AAD* or *I-neb ADD* system nebulizer; counsel on syncope risk; do not mix w/ other drugs

Imatinib (Gleevec)   Uses: *Rx CML Ph +, CML blast crisis, ALL Ph +,
myelodysplastic/myeloproliferative Dz, aggressive systemic mastocytosis, chronic eosinophilic leukemia, GIST, dermatofibrosarcoma protuberans* **Action:** ↓ BCL-ABL; TKI **Dose:** *Adults.* Typical dose 400–600 mg PO daily; w/ meal **Peds.** CML Ph + newly diagnosed 340 mg/m²/d, 600 mg/d max; recurrent 260 mg/m²/d PO ÷ daily-bid, to 340 mg/m²/d max **Caution:** [D, ?/–] w/ CYP3A4 meds (Table 11), warfarin **CI:** Component sensitivity **Disp:** Tab 100, 400 mg **SE:** GI upset, fluid retention, muscle cramps, musculoskeletal pain, arthralgia, rash, HA, neutropenia, thrombocytopenia **Notes:** Follow CBCs & LFTs baseline & monthly; w/ large glass of H₂O & food to ↓ GI irritation

Imipenem–Cilastatin (Primaxin)   Uses: *Serious Infxns* due to sus-
ceptible bacteria **Action:** Bactericidal; ↓ cell wall synth. **Spectrum:** Gram(+) (*S. aureus,* group A & B streptococci), gram(–) (not *Legionella*), anaerobes **Dose:** *Adults.* 250–1000 mg (imipenem) IV q6–8h, 500–750 mg IM. **Peds.** 60–100 mg/kg/24 h IV ÷ q6h; ↓ if CrCl <70 mL/min **Caution:** [C, +/–] Probenecid ↑ tox **CI:** Ped pts w/ CNS Infxn (↑ Sz risk) & <30 kg w/ renal impair **Disp:** Inj (imipenem/cilastatin) 250/250 mg, 500/500 mg **SE:** Szs if drug accumulates, GI upset, thrombocytopenia

Imipramine (Tofranil)   WARNING: Close observation for suicidal
thinking or unusual changes in behavior **Uses:** *Depression, enuresis,* panic attack, chronic pain **Action:** TCA; ↑ CNS synaptic serotonin or norepinephrine **Dose:** *Adults. Hospitalized:* Initial 100 mg/24 h PO in ÷ doses; ↑ over several wk 300 mg/d max. *Outpatient:* Maint 50–150 mg PO qhs; 300 mg/24 h max. **Peds.** *Antidepressant:* 1.5–5 mg/kg/24 h ÷ daily-qid. *Enuresis: >6 y:* 10–25 mg PO qhs; ↑ by 10–25 mg at 1–2-wk intervals (max 50 mg for 6–12 y, 75 mg for >12 y); Rx for 2–3 mo, then taper **Caution:** [D, ?/–] CI: Use with MAOIs, NAG, acute recovery from MI, PRG, CHF, angina, CV Dz, arrhythmias **Disp:** Tabs 10, 25, 50 mg; caps 75, 100, 125, 150 mg **SE:** CV Sxs, dizziness, xerostomia, discolored urine **Notes:** Less sedation than amitriptyline

Imiquimod Cream, 5% (Aldara) **Uses:** *Anogenital warts, HPV, condylomata acuminata* **Action:** Unknown; ? cytokine induction **Dose:** Apply 3×/wk, leave on 6–10 h & wash off w/ soap & water, continue 16 wk max **Caution:** [B, ?] **CI:** Component sensitivity **Disp:** Single-dose packets 5% (250-mg cream) **SE:** Local skin Rxns **Notes:** Not a cure; may weaken condoms/Vag diaphragms, wash hands before & after use

Immune Globulin, IV (Gamimune N, Sandoglobulin, Gammar IV) **Uses:** *IgG Ab deficiency Dz states (eg, congenital agammaglobulinemia, CVH, & BMT), HIV, hep A prophylaxis, ITP* **Action:** IgG supl **Dose:** *Adults & Peds. Immunodeficiency:* 100–200 mg/kg/mo IV at 0.01–0.04 mL/kg/min to 400 mg/kg/dose max. *ITP:* 400 mg/kg/dose IV daily × 5 d. *BMT:* 500 mg/kg/wk; ↓ in renal Insuff **Caution:** [C, ?] Separate administration of live vaccines by 3 mo **CI:** IgA deficiency w/ Abs to IgA, severe thrombocytopenia or coagulation disorders **Disp:** Inj **SE:** Associated mostly w/ Inf rate; GI upset

Immune Globulin, subcutaneous (Vivaglobin) **Uses:** *Primary immunodeficiency* **Action:** IgG supl **Dose:** 100–200 mg/kg body wgt SQ weekly **Caution:** [C, ?] **CI:** Hx anaphylaxis to immune globulin; some IgA deficiency **Disp:** 10-, 20-mL vials w/ 160 mg/IgG/mL **SE:** Inj site Rxns, HA, GI complaint, fever, N, D, rash, sore throat **Notes:** May instruct in home administration; keep refrigerated; discard unused drug; dose >15 mL divide between sites

Inamrinone [Amrinone] (Inocor) **Uses:** *Acute CHF, ischemic cardiomyopathy* **Action:** Inotrope w/ vasodilator **Dose:** IV bolus 0.75 mg/kg over 2–3 min; maint 5–10 mcg/kg/min, 10 mg/kg/d max; ↓ if CrCl <10 mL/min **Caution:** [C, ?] **CI:** Bisulfite allergy **Disp:** Inj 5 mg/mL **SE:** Monitor fluid, electrolyte, & renal changes **Notes:** Incompatible w/ dextrose solns, ↓ LFTs, observe for arrhythmias

Indapamide (Lozol) **Uses:** *HTN, edema, CHF* **Action:** Thiazide diuretic; ↑ Na, Cl, & H_2O excretion in distal tubule **Dose:** 1.25–5 mg/d PO **Caution:** [D, ?] ↑ Effect w/ loop diuretics, ACE inhibitors, cyclosporine, digoxin, Li ↓Eff **CI:** Anuria, thiazide/sulfonamide allergy, renal Insuff, PRG **Disp:** Tabs 1.25, 2.5 mg **SE:** ↓ BP, dizziness, photosensitivity **Notes:** No additional effects w/ doses >5 mg; take early to avoid nocturia; use sunscreen; OK w/ food/milk

Indinavir (Crixivan) **Uses:** *HIV Infxn* **Action:** Protease inhibitor; ↓ maturation of noninfectious virions to mature infectious virus **Dose:** Typical 800 mg PO q8h in combo w/ other antiretrovirals (dose varies); on empty stomach; ↓ w/ hepatic impair **Caution:** [C, ?] Numerous drug interactions, especially CYP3A4 inhibitor (Table 11) **CI:** w/ Triazolam, midazolam, pimozide, ergot alkaloids, simvastatin, lovastatin, sildenafil, St. John's wort, amiodarone **Disp:** Caps 100, 200, 333, 400 mg **SE:** Nephrolithiasis, dyslipidemia, lipodystrophy, N/V, ↑ bilirubin **Notes:** Drink six 8-oz glasses of H_2O/d

Indomethacin (Indocin) **WARNING:** May ↑ risk of cv events & GI bleeding **Uses:** *Arthritis; close ductus arteriosus; ankylosing spondylitis* **Action:** ↓ Prostaglandins **Dose:** *Adults.* 25–50 mg PO bid-tid, max 200 mg/d *Infants:*

0.2–0.25 mg/kg/dose IV; may repeat in 12–24 h up to 3 doses; w/ food **Caution:** [B, +] **CI:** ASA/NSAID sensitivity, peptic ulcer/active GI bleed, precipitation of asthma/urticaria/rhinitis by NSAIDs/aspirin, premature neonates w/ NEC↓ renal Fxn, active bleeding, thrombocytopenia, 3rd tri PRG **Disp:** Inj 1 mg/vial; caps 25, 50 mg; SR caps 75 mg; susp 25 mg/5 mL **SE:** GI bleeding or upset, dizziness, edema **Notes:** Monitor renal Fxn

Infliximab (Remicade)

WARNING: TB, invasive fungal Infxns, & other opportunistic Infxns reported, some fatal; perform TB skin testing prior to use; possible association with rare lymphoma **Uses:** *Mod–severe Crohn Dz; fistulizing Crohn Dz; ulcerative colitis; RA (w/ MTX) psoriasis, ankylosing spondylitis* **Action:** IgG1K neutralizes TNF-α **Dose:** *Adults. Crohn Dz:* Induction: 5 mg/kg IV Inf, w/ doses 2 & 6 wk after. *Maint:* 5 mg/kg IV Inf q8wk. *RA:* 3 mg/kg IV Inf at 0, 2, 6 wk, then q8wk. *Peds >6 y:* 5 mg/kg IV q8wk **Caution:** [B, ?/–] Active Infxn, hepatic impair, Hx or risk of TB, hep B **CI:** Murine allergy, mod–severe CHF, w/ live vaccines (eg, smallpox) **Disp:** 100 mg Inj **SE:** Allergic Rxns; HA, fatigue, GI upset, Inf Rxns; hepatotox; reactivation hep B, pneumonia, BM suppression, systemic vasculitis, pericardial effusion **Notes:** Monitor LFTs, PPD at baseline, monitor hep B carrier, skin exam for malignancy w/ psoriasis; can premedicate w/ antihistamines, APAP, and/or steroids to ↓ Inf Rxns

Influenza Vaccine (Fluarix, FluLaval, Fluzone, Fluvirin)

Uses: *Prevent influenza* in adults >50 y, children 6–23 mo, pregnant women (2nd/3rd tri during flu season), nursing home residents, chronic Dzs, health-care workers, household contacts of high-risk pts, children <9 y receiving vaccine for the first time **Action:** Active immunization **Dose:** *Adults and Peds >9 y:* 0.5 mL dose IM annually. *Peds 6 mo–3 y:* 0.25 mL IM annually; 0.25 mL IM ×2 doses >4 wk apart 1st vaccination; give 2 doses in 2nd vaccination year if only 1 dose given in 1st year. *3–8 y:* 0.5 mL IM annually, start 0.5 mL IM × 2 doses >4 wk apart in 1st vaccination year **Caution:** [C, +] **CI:** Egg, gentamicin, or thimerosal allergy, Infxn at site, acute resp or febrile illness, Hx Guillain–Barré, immunocompromised, children 5–17 y on aspirin **Disp:** Based on manufacturer, 0.25- & 0.5-mL prefilled syringes **SE:** Inj site soreness, fever, myalgia, malaise, Guillain–Barré syndrome (controversial) **Notes:** Fluarix not labeled for peds; optimal in US Oct–Nov, protection begins 1–2 wk after, lasts up to 6 mo; each year, vaccines based on predictions of flu active in flu season (December–spring in US); whole or split virus for adults; peds <13 y split virus or purified surface antigen to ↓ febrile Rxns; see www.cdc.gov/flu for more info

Influenza Virus Vaccine Live, intranasal (FluMist)

Uses: *Prevent influenza* **Action:** Live-attenuated vaccine **Dose:** *Adults 18–49 y:* 0.1 mL each nostril × 1 annually **Peds 5–8 y:* 0.1 mL each nostril × 1 annually; initial 0.1 mL each nostril × 2 doses >6 wk apart in 1st vaccination year *>9 y:* See adult dose **Caution:** [C, ?/–] **CI:** Egg allergy, PRG, Hx Guillain–Barré syndrome, known/suspected immune deficiency, asthma or reactive airway Dz, acute febrile illness, peds 5–17 y on ASA **Disp:** Prefilled, single-use, intranasal sprayer; shipped frozen, store 35–46°F; new refrigerated shipping form for 2008 **SE:** Runny nose, nasal congestion, HA, cough **Notes:** Do not give w/ other vaccines; avoid contact w/immunocompromised individuals for 21 d

Insulin, injectable (see Table 5 page 255)

Uses: *Type 1 or type 2 DM refractory to diet or PO hypoglycemic agents; acute life-threatening ↑ K+* **Action:** Insulin supl **Dose:** Based on serum glucose; usually SQ; can give IV (only regular)/IM; type 1 typical start dose 0.5–1 units/kg/d; type 2 0.3–0.4 units/kg/d; renal failure ↓ insulin needs **Caution:** [B, +] **CI:** Hypoglycemia **Disp:** Table 5 **SE:** Highly purified insulins ↑ free insulin; monitor for several wk when changing doses/agents

Interferon Alfa (Roferon-A, Intron-A)

WARNING: Can cause or aggravate fatal or life-threatening neuropsychological, autoimmune, ischemic, and infectious disorders. Monitor closely **Uses:** *Hairy cell leukemia, Kaposi sarcoma, melanoma, CML, chronic hep B & C, follicular NHL, condyloma acuminata* **Action:** Antiproliferative; modulates host immune response; ↓ viral replication in infected cells **Dose:** Per protocols. *Adults. Hairy cell leukemia:* Alfa-2a (Roferon-A): 3 million units/d for 16–24 wk SQ/IM then 3 million units 3×/wk × 6–24 mo; Alfa-2b (Intron A): 2 million units/m² IM/SQ 3×/wk for 2–6 mo. *Chronic hep B:* Alfa-2b (Intron A): 3 million units/m² SQ 3×/wk × 1 wk, then 6 million units/m² 3×/wk (max 10 million units 3×/wk, total duration 16–24 wk). *Follicular NHL* (Intron A): 5 million units SQ 3×/wk for 18 mo. *Melanoma* (Intron A): 20 million units/m² IV × 5 d/wk × 4 wk, then 10 million units/m² SQ 3×/wk × 48 wk. *Kaposi sarcoma* (Intron A): 30 million units/m² IM/SQ 3×/wk × 10–12 wk, then 36 million units IM/SQ 3×/wk. *Chronic hep C* (Intron A): 3 million units 3×/wk × 16 wk (continue 18–24 mo if response). *Roferon A:* 3 million units 3×/wk for 12 mo SQ/IM. *Condyloma* (Intron A): 1 million units/lesion (max 5 lesions) 3×/wk for 3 wk. *Peds. CML:* Alfa-2a (Roferon-A): 2.5–5 million units/m² IM daily. **CI:** Benzyl alcohol sensitivity, decompensated liver Dz, autoimmune Dz, immunosuppressed, neonates, infants **Disp:** Inj forms (see also polyethylene glycol [PEG]-interferon) **SE:** Flu-like Sxs, fatigue, anorexia, neurotox at high doses; up to 40% neutralizing Ab w/ therapy

Interferon Alfa-2b & Ribavirin Combo (Rebetron)

WARNING: Can cause or aggravate fatal or life-threatening neuropsychological, autoimmune, ischemic, and infectious disorders. Monitor pts closely. CI in pregnant females & their male partners **Uses:** *Chronic hep C w/ compensated liver Dz who relapse after α-interferon therapy* **Action:** Combo antiviral agents (see individual agents) **Dose:** 3 million units Intron A SQ 3× w/ 1000–1200 mg of Rebetron PO ÷ bid dose for 24 wk. *Pts <75 kg:* 1000 mg of Rebetron/d **Caution:** [X, ?] **CI:** PRG, males w/ PRG female partner, autoimmune hep, CrCl <50 mL/min **Disp:** *Pts <75 kg:* Combo packs: 6 vials Intron A (3 Munits/0.5 mL) w/ 6 syringes & EtOH swabs, 70 Rebetol caps; one 18-MU multidose vial of Intron A Inj (22.8 million units/3.8 mL;

3 million units/0.5 mL) & 6 syringes & swabs, 70 Rebetol caps; one 18-million units Intron A Inj multidose pen (22.5 million units/1.5 mL; 3 million units/0.2 mL) w/ 6 needles & swabs, 70 Rebetol caps. *Pts >75 kg:* Identical except 84 Rebetol caps/pack **SE:** See warning, flu-like syndrome, HA, anemia **Notes:** Monthly PRG test; instruct in self-administration of SQ Intron A

Interferon Alfacon-1 (Infergen)   WARNING: Can cause or aggra-
vate fatal or life-threatening neuropsychological, autoimmune, ischemic, & infectious disorders. Monitor closely **Uses:** *Chronic hep C* **Action:** Biologic response modifier **Dose:** 9 mcg SQ 3×/wk × 24 wk **Caution:** [C, M] **CI:** *E. coli* product allergy **Disp:** Inj 9, 15 mcg **SE:** Flu-like syndrome, depression, blood dyscrasias, colitis, pancreatitis, hepatic decompensation, ↑ SCr, eye disorders, ↓ thyroid **Notes:** Allow >48 h between Inj; monitor CBC, plt, SCr, TFTs

Interferon Beta-1a (Rebif)   WARNING: Can cause or aggravate fatal
or life-threatening neuropsychological, autoimmune, ischemic, & infectious disorders. Monitor closely **Uses:** *MS, relapsing* **Action:** Biologic response modifier **Dose:** 44 mcg SQ 3×/wk; start 8.8 mcg SQ 3×/wk × 2 wk, then 22 mcg SQ 3×/wk × 2 wk **Caution:** [C, ?] w/ Hepatic impair, depression, Sz disorder, thyroid Dz **CI:** Human albumin allergy **Disp:** 0.5 mL prefilled syringes w/ 29-gauge needle Titrate Pak 8.8 and 22 mcg; 22 or 44 mcg **SE:** Inj site Rxn, HA, flu-like Sx, malaise, fatigue, rigors, myalgia, depression w/ suicidal ideation, hepatotox, ↓ BM **Notes:** Dose >48 h apart; ✓ CBC 1, 3, 6 mo; ✓ TFTs q6mo w/ hx thyroid Dz

Interferon Beta-1b (Betaseron)   Uses: *MS, relapsing/remitting/
secondary progressive* **Action:** Biologic response modifier **Dose:** 0.625 mg (2 MU) q other day SQ, ↑ by 0.0625 mg q2wk to target dose 0.25 mg q other day **Caution:** [C, ?] **CI:** Human albumin sensitivity **Disp:** Powder for Inj 0.3 mg (32 MU interferon [IFN]) **SE:** Flu-like syndrome, depression, blood dyscrasias, Inj site necrosis, anaphylaxis **Notes:** Teach pt self-injection, rotate sites; ✓ LFTs, CBC 1, 3, 6 mo, TFT q6mo

Interferon Gamma-1b (Actimmune)   Uses: *↓ Incidence of serious
Infxns in chronic granulomatous Dz (CGD), osteoporosis* **Action:** Biologic response modifier **Dose:** *Adults. CGD:* 50 mcg/m² SQ (1.5 MU/m²) BSA >0.5 m²; if BSA <0.5 m², give 1.5 mcg/kg/dose; given 3× wk **Caution:** [C, ?] **CI:** Allergy to E. *coli*-derived products **Disp:** Inj 100 mcg (2 MU) **SE:** Flu-like syndrome, depression, blood dyscrasias, dizziness, altered mental status, gait disturbance, hepatic tox **Notes:** may ↑ deaths in interstitial pulm fibrosis

Ipecac Syrup [OTC]   Uses: *Drug OD, certain cases of poisoning*
NOTE: Usage is falling out of favor & is no longer recommended by some groups **Action:** Irritation of the GI mucosa; stimulation of the chemoreceptor trigger zone **Dose:** *Adults.* 15–30 mL PO, followed by 200–300 mL of H₂O; if no emesis in 20 min, repeat once. *Peds 6–12 y:* 5–10 mL PO, followed by 10–20 mL/kg of H₂O; if no emesis in 20 min, repeat once. *1–12 y:* 15 mL PO followed by 10–20 mL/kg of H₂O; if no emesis in 20 min, repeat once **Caution:** [C, ?] **CI:** Ingestion of petroleum distillates, strong acid, base, or other caustic agents; comatose/unconscious

Disp: Syrup 15, 30 mL (OTC) **SE:** Lethargy, D, cardiotox, protracted V **Notes:** Caution in CNS depressant OD; activated charcoal considered more effective (www.clintox.org/PosStatements/Ipecac.html)

Ipratropium (Atrovent HFA, Atrovent nasal) **Uses:** *Bronchospasm w/ COPD, rhinitis, rhinorrhea* **Action:** Synthetic anticholinergic similar to atropine; antagonizes acetylcholine receptors, inhibits mucous gland secretions **Dose:** *Adults & Peds >12 y:* 2–4 puffs qid, max 12 Inh/d *Nasal:* 2 sprays/nostril bid-tid; *Nebulization:* 500 mcg 3–4 times/d **Caution:** [B, +/–] w/ Inhaled insulin **CI:** Allergy to soya lecithin-related foods **Disp:** HFA Metered-dose inhaler 18 mcg/dose; Inh soln 0.02%; nasal spray 0.03, 0.06% **SE:** Nervousness, dizziness, HA, cough, bitter taste, nasal dryness, URI, epistaxis **Notes:** Not for acute bronchospasm

Irbesartan (Avapro) **Uses:** *HTN, DN,* *? CHF* **Action:** Angiotensin II receptor antagonist **Dose:** 150 mg/d PO, may ↑ to 300 mg/d **Caution:** [C (1st tri; D 2nd/3rd), ?/–] **Disp:** 75, 150, 300 mg tabs **SE:** Fatigue, ↓ BP ↑ K

Irinotecan (Camptosar) **WARNING:** D & myelosuppression **Uses:** *Colorectal* & lung CA **Action:** Topoisomerase I inhibitor; ↓ DNA synth **Dose:** Per protocol; 125–350 mg/m² q wk–q3wk (↓ hepatic dysfunction, as tolerated per tox) **Caution:** [D, –] Allergy to component **Disp:** Inj 20 mg/mL **SE:** ↓ BM, N/V/D, Abd cramping, alopecia; D is dose limiting; Rx acute D w/ atropine; Rx subacute D w/ loperamide **Notes:** D correlated to levels of metabolite SN-38

Iron Dextran (Dexferrum, INFeD) **WARNING:** Anaphylactic Rxns with use; use only if oral iron not possible; administer where resuscitation techniques available **Uses:** *Fe deficiency when cannot supplement PO* **Action:** Fe supl **Dose:** *Adults.* *Iron*deficiency anemia: Estimate Fe deficiency, give 25–100 mg IM/IV/d until total dose; total dose (mL) = [0.0442 × (desired Hgb – observed Hgb) × lean body wgt] + (0.26 × lean body wgt); *Iron replacement, blood loss:* total dose (mg) = blood loss (mL) × Hct (as decimal fraction) max 100 mg/d; *Peds >4 mo:* As above; max: 0.5 mL (wgt <5 kg), 1 mL (5–10 kg), 2 mL (>10 kg) per dose IM or direct IV **Caution:** [C, M] **CI:** Anemia w/o Fe deficiency **Disp:** Inj 50 mg (Fe)/mL **SE:** Anaphylaxis, flushing, dizziness, Inj site & Inf Rxns, metallic taste **Notes:** Give IM w/ "Z-track" technique; IV preferred; give test dose >1 h before

Iron Sucrose (Venofer) **Uses:** *Fe deficiency anemia w/ chronic HD in those receiving erythropoietin* **Actions:** Fe replacement **Dose:** 5 mL (100 mg) IV on dialysis, 1 mL (20 mg)/min max **Caution:** [C, M] **CI:** Anemia w/o Fe deficiency **Disp:** 20 mg elemental Fe/mL, 5-mL vials. **SE:** Anaphylaxis, ↓ BP, cramps, N/V/D, HA **Notes:** Most pts require cumulative doses of 1000 mg; give slowly

Isoniazid (INH) **Uses:** *Rx & prophylaxis of TB* **Action:** Bactericidal; interferes w/ mycolic acid synth, disrupts cell wall **Dose:** *Adults. Active TB:* 5 mg/kg/24 h PO or IM (usually 300 mg/d) or DOT: 15 mg/kg (max 900 mg) 3×/wk. *Prophylaxis:* 300 mg/d PO for 6–12 mo or 900 mg 2×/wk. *Peds. Active TB:* 10–15 mg/kg/d daily-bid PO or IM 300 mg/d max. *Prophylaxis:* 10 mg/kg/24 h PO; ↓ in hepatic/renal dysfunction **Caution:** [C, +] Liver Dz, dialysis; avoid EtOH

CI: Acute liver Dz, Hx INH hep **Disp:** Tabs 100, 300 mg; syrup 50 mg/5 mL; Inj 100 mg/mL **SE:** Hep, peripheral neuropathy, GI upset, anorexia, dizziness, skin Rxn **Notes:** Use w/ 2–3 other drugs for active TB, based on INH resistance patterns when TB acquired & sensitivity results; prophylaxis usually w/ INH alone. IM rarely used. ↓ Peripheral neuropathy w/ pyridoxine 50–100 mg/d. See CDC guidelines (MMWR) for current recommendations

Isoproterenol (Isuprel) **Uses:** *Shock, cardiac arrest, AV nodal block* **Action:** β_1- & β_2-receptor stimulant **Dose:** *Adults.* 2–10 mcg/min IV Inf; titrate; 2–10 mcg/min titrate (*ECC 2005*) *Peds.* 0.2–2 mcg/kg/min IV Inf; titrate **Caution:** [C, ?] **CI:** Angina, tachyarrhythmias (digitalis-induced or others) **Disp:** 0.02 mcg/mL, 0.2 mg/mL **SE:** Insomnia, arrhythmias, HA, trembling, dizziness **Notes:** Pulse >130 BPM may induce arrhythmias

Isosorbide Dinitrate (Isordil, Sorbitrate, Dilatrate-SR) **Uses:** *Rx & prevent angina,* CHF (w/ hydralazine) **Action:** Relaxes vascular smooth muscle **Dose:** *Acute angina:* 5–10 mg PO (chew tabs) q2–3h or 2.5–10 mg SL PRN q5–10 min; do not give >3 doses in a 15–30-min period. *Angina prophylaxis:* 5–40 mg PO q6h; do not give nitrates on a chronic q6h or qid basis >7–10 d; tolerance may develop; provide 10–12-h drug-free intervals; *dose in CHF:* initial 20 mg 3–4×/d, target 120–160 mg/d **Caution:** [C, ?] **CI:** Severe anemia, NAG, postural ↓ BP, cerebral hemorrhage, head trauma (can ↑ ICP), w/ sildenafil, tadalafil, vardenafil **Disp:** Tabs 5, 10, 20, 30; SR tabs 40 mg; SL tabs 2.5, 5 mg; SR caps 40 mg **SE:** HA, ↓ BP, flushing, tachycardia, dizziness **Notes:** Higher PO dose needed for same results as SL forms

Isosorbide Mononitrate (Ismo, Imdur) **Uses:** *Prevention/Rx of angina pectoris* **Action:** Relaxes vascular smooth muscle **Dose:** 5–10 mg PO bid, w/ the 2 doses 7 h apart or XR (Imdur) 30–60 mg/d PO, max 240 mg **Caution:** [C, ?] **CI:** Head trauma/cerebral hemorrhage (can ICP), w/ sildenafil, tadalafil, vardenafil **Disp:** Tabs 10, 20 mg; XR 30, 60, 120 mg **SE:** HA, dizziness, ↓ BP

Isotretinoin [13-*cis* Retinoic Acid] (Accutane, Amnesteem, Claravis, Sotret) **WARNING:** Must not be used by PRG females; can induce severe birth defects; pt must be capable of complying w/ mandatory contraceptive measures; prescribed according to product-specific risk management system. Because of teratogenicity, is approved for marketing only under a special restricted distribution FDA program called iPLEDGE **Uses:** *Refractory severe acne* **Action:** Retinoic acid derivative **Dose:** 0.5–2 mg/kg/d PO ÷ ; ↓ in hepatic Dz, take w/ food **Caution:** [X, –] Avoid tetracyclines **CI:** Retinoid sensitivity, PRG **Disp:** Caps 10, 20, 30, 40 mg **SE:** Rare: Depression, psychosis, suicidal thoughts; derm sensitivity, xerostomia, photosensitivity, LFTs, triglycerides **Notes:** Risk management program requires 2 (–) PRG tests before Rx & use of 2 forms of contraception 1 mo before, during, & 1 mo after therapy; to prescribe isotretinoin, the prescriber must access the iPLEDGE system via the Internet (www.ipledgeprogram.com); monitor LFTs & lipids

Isradipine (DynaCirc)   Uses: *HTN* Action: CCB Dose: *Adults.* 2.5–5 mg PO bid. Caution: [C, ?] CI: Severe heart block, sinus bradycardia, CHF, dosing w/in several hours of IV β-blockers Disp: Caps 2.5, 5 mg; tabs CR 5, 10 mg SE: HA, edema, flushing, fatigue, dizziness, palpitations

Itraconazole (Sporanox)   WARNING: CI w/ cisapride, pimozide, quinidine, dofetilide, or levacetylmethadol. Serious CV events (eg, ↑ QT, torsade de pointes, ventricular tachycardia, cardiac arrest, and/or sudden death) reported w/ these meds and other CYP3A4 inhibitors. Do not use for onychomycosis w/ ventricular dysfunction Uses: *Fungal Infxns (aspergillosis, blastomycosis, histoplasmosis, candidiasis)* Action: Azole antifungal, ↓ ergosterol synth Dose: 200 mg PO daily-bid (caps w/ meals or cola/grapefruit juice); PO soln on empty stomach; avoid antacids Caution: [C, ?] Numerous interactions CI: See warning; PRG or considering PRG; ventricular dysfunction Disp: Caps 100 mg; soln 10 mg/mL SE: N/V, rash, hepatotoxic, ↓ K+, CHF, ↑ BP, neuropathy Notes: soln & caps not interchangeable; useful in pts who cannot take amphotericin B; follow LFTs

Ixabepilone (Ixempra)   WARNING: CI in combo w/ capecitabine w/ AST/ALT >2.5× ULN or bilirubin >1× ULN due to ↑ tox and neutropenia-related death Uses: *Metastatic/locally advanced breast CA after failure of an anthracycline, a taxane, and capecitabine* Action: Microtubule inhibitor Dose: 40 mg/m² IV over 3 h q3wk Caution: [D, ?/–] CI: Hypersensitivity to Cremophor EL; baseline ANC <1500 cells/mm³ or plt <100,000 cells/mm³; AST or ALT >2.5× ULN, bilirubin >1× ULN Disp: Inj 15, 45 mg SE: neutropenia, leukopenia, anemia, thrombocytopenia, peripheral sensory neuropathy, fatigue/asthenia, myalgia/arthralgia, alopecia, N/V/D, stomatitis/mucositis Notes: Substrate CYP3A4, dose must be adjusted w/ strong CYP3A4 inhibitor/inducers

Ketoconazole (Nizoral)   WARNING: (Oral use) Risk of fatal hepatotox. Concomitant terfenadine, astemizole, and cisapride are CI due to serious cardiovascular adverse events Uses: *Systemic fungal Infxns (Candida, blastomycosis, histoplasmosis, etc); refractory topical dermatophyte Infxn*; PCa when rapid ↓ testosterone needed or hormone refractory Action: Azole, ↓ fungal cell wall synth; high dose blocks P450, ↓ testosterone production Dose: 200 mg PO daily; ↑ to 400 mg PO daily for serious Infxn. PCa: 400 mg PO tid w/hydrocortisone 20–40 mg ÷ bid; best on empty stomach Caution: [C, +/–] Any agent that ↑ gastric pH ↓ absorption; may enhance anticoagulants; w/ EtOH (disulfiram-like Rxn); numerous interactions including statins, niacin CI: CNS fungal Infxns, w/astemizole, triazolam Disp: Tabs 200 mg SE: N, rashes, hair loss, HA, ↑ wgt gain, dizziness, disorientation, fatigue, impotence, hepatox, adrenal suppression, acquired cutaneous adherence ("sticky skin syndrome") Notes: Monitor LFTs; can rapidly ↓ testosterone levels

Ketoconazole, topical (Extina, Kuric, Nizoral AD Shampoo, Xolegel) [Shampoo—OTC]   Uses: *Topical for seborrheic dermatitis, shampoo for dandruff* local fungal Infxns due to dermatophytes & yeast Action:

azole, ↓ fungal cell wall synth **Dose:** *Topical:* Apply q day-bid **Caution:** [C, +/–] **CI:** Broken/inflamed skin **Disp:** Tabs 200 mg; topical cream 2%; (*Xolegel*) gel 2%,(*Extina*) foam 2%, shampoo 1% & 2% **SE:** Irritation, pruritus, stinging **Notes:** Do not dispense foam into hands

Ketoprofen (Orudis, Oruvail) WARNING: May ↑ risk of cv events & GI bleeding; CI for perioperative pain in CABG surgery

Uses: *Arthritis (RA/OA), pain* **Action:** NSAID; ↓ prostaglandins **Dose:** 25–75 mg PO tid-qid, 300 mg/d/max; SR 200 mg/d; w/ food; ↓ w/ hepatic/renal impair, elderly **Caution:** [C(D 3rd tri), –] w/ ACE, diuretics; ↑ warfarin, Li, MTX **CI:** NSAID/ASA sensitivity **Disp:** Caps 50, 75 mg; caps, SR 200 mg **SE:** GI upset, peptic ulcers, dizziness, edema, rash, ↑ BP, ↑ LFTs, renal dysfunction

Ketorolac (Toradol) WARNING: For short-term (≤5 d) Rx of mod–severe acute pain; CI w/ PUD, GI bleed, postcoronary artery bypass graft, anticipated major surgery, severe renal Insuff, bleeding diathesis, labor & delivery, nursing, and w/ ASA/NSAIDs. NSAIDs may cause an increased risk of CV thrombotic events (MI, stroke).

PO CI in peds <16 y **Uses:** *Pain* **Action:** NSAID; ↓ prostaglandins **Dose:** *Adults.* 15–30 mg IV/IM q6h; 10 mg PO qid only as continuation of IM/IV; max IV/IM 120 mg/d, max PO 40 mg/d. *Peds 2–16 y:* 1 mg/kg IM/IV × 1 dose; 30 mg max; IV: 0.5 mg/kg, 15 mg max; do not use for >5 d; ↓ if >65 y, elderly, w/ renal impair, <50 kg **Caution:** [C (D 3rd tri), –] w/ ACE inhibitor, diuretics, BP meds, warfarin **CI:** See Warning **Disp:** Tabs 10 mg; Inj 15 mg/mL, 30 mg/mL **SE:** Bleeding, peptic ulcer Dz, ↑ Cr & LFTs, ↑ BP, edema, dizziness, allergy

Ketorolac Ophthalmic (Acular, Acular LS, Acular PF)
Uses: *Ocular itching* w/ seasonal allergies; inflammation w/ cataract extraction*; pain/photophobia w/ incisional refractive surgery (*Acular PF*); pain w/ corneal refractive surgery (*Acular LS*) **Action:** NSAID **Dose:** 1 gtt qid **Caution:** [C, +] Possible cross-sensitivity to NSAIDs, ASA **CI:** Hypersensitivity **Disp:** *Acular LS:* 0.4% 5 mL; *Acular:* 0.5% 3, 5, 10 mL; *Acular PF:* Soln 0.5% **SE:** Local irritation, ↑ bleeding ocular tissues, hyphemas, slow healing, keratitis **Notes:** Do not use w/ contacts

Ketotifen (Alaway, Zaditor) [OTC]
Uses: *Allergic conjunctivitis* **Action:** Antihistamine H_1-receptor antagonist, mast cell stabilizer **Dose:** *Adults & Peds >3 y:* 1 gtt in eye(s) q8–12h **Caution:** [C, ?/–] **Disp:** Soln 0.025%/5 & 10 mL **SE:** Local irritation, HA, rhinitis, keratitis, mydriasis **Notes:** Wait 10 min before inserting contacts

Kunecatechins [sinecatechins] (Veregen)
Uses: *External genital/perianal warts* **Action:** Unknown; green tea extract **Dose:** Apply 0.5-cm ribbon to each wart 3×/d until all warts clear; not >16 wk **Caution:** [C; ?] **Disp:** Oint 15% **SE:** Erythema, pruritus, burning, pain, erosion/ulceration, edema, induration, rash, phimosis **Notes:** Wash hands before/after use; not necessary to wipe off prior to next use; avoid on open wounds

Labetalol (Trandate)   Uses: *HTN* & hypertensive emergencies (IV
Action: α- & β-Adrenergic blocker Dose: *Adults. HTN:* Initial, 100 mg PO bic
then 200–400 mg PO bid. *Hypertensive emergency:* 20–80 mg IV bolus, the
2 mg/min IV Inf, titrate up to 300 mg; 10 mg IV over 1–2 min; repeat or doubl
dose q10min (150 mg max); or initial bolus, then 2–8 mg/min (*ECC 2005*). **Ped**
PO: 1–3 mg/kg/d in ÷ doses, 1200 mg/d max. *Hypertensive emergency:* 0.4–1.5 m
kg/h IV cont Inf **Caution:** [C (D in 2nd or 3rd tri), +] **CI:** Asthma/COPD, cardio
genic shock, uncompensated CHF, heart block, sinus brady **Disp:** Tabs 100, 20
300 mg; Inj 5 mg/mL **SE:** Dizziness, N, ↓ BP, fatigue, CV effects

**Lactic Acid & Ammonium Hydroxide [Ammonium Lactate
(Lac-Hydrin)**   Uses: *Severe xerosis & ichthyosis* Action: Emollient mois
turizer, humectant **Dose:** Apply bid **Caution:** [B, ?] **Disp:** Cream, lotion, lacti
acid 12% w/ ammonium hydroxide **SE:** Local irritation, photosensitivity **Notes**
Shake well before use

Lactobacillus (Lactinex Granules) [OTC]   Uses: *Control of D,*
especially after antibiotic therapy Action: Replaces nl intestinal flora, lactase production; *Lactobacillus acidophilus* and *Lactobacillus helveticus*. **Dose:** *Adults &*
Peds >3 y: 1 packet, 1–2 caps, or 4 tabs q day-qid **Caution:** [A, +] Some products
may contain whey **CI:** Milk/lactose allergy **Disp:** Tabs, caps; granules in packets
(all OTC) **SE:** Flatulence **Notes:** May take granules on food

Lactulose (Constulose, Generlac, Enulose, others)   Uses:
Hepatic encephalopathy; constipation **Action:** Acidifies the colon, allows
ammonia to diffuse into colon; osmotic effect to ↑ peristalsis **Dose:** *Acute hepatic*
encephalopathy: 30–45 mL PO q1h until soft stools, then tid-qid, adjust 2–3 stool/d.
Constipation: 15–30 mL/d, ↑ to 60 mL/d 1–2 ÷ doses, adjust to 2–3 stools. *Rectally:*
200 g in 700 mL of H₂O PR, retain 30–60 min q4–6h. **Peds Infants:** 2.5–10 mL/
24 h ÷ tid-qid. *Other Peds:* 40–90 mL/24 h ÷ tid-qid. *Peds Constipation:* 5 g
(7.5 mL) PO after breakfast **Caution:** [B, ?] **CI:** Galactosemia **Disp:** Syrup
10 g/15 mL, soln 10 g/15 mL, 10, 20 g/packet **SE:** Severe D, N/V, cramping, flatulence; life-threatening electrolyte disturbances

Lamivudine (Epivir, Epivir-HBV, 3TC [many combo regimens])
WARNING: Lactic acidosis & severe hepatomegaly w/ steatosis reported w/
nucleoside analogs Uses: *HIV Infxn, chronic hep B* Action: NRTI, ↓ HIV RT
& hep B viral polymerase, causes viral DNA chain termination Dose: *HIV: Adults*
& Peds >16 y: 150 mg PO bid or 300 mg PO daily. *Peds able to swallow pills:*
14–21 kg: 75 mg bid; *22–29 kg:* 75 mg q A.M., 150 mg q P.M.; *>30 kg:* 150 mg bid.
Neonates <30 d: 2 mg/kg bid. *Epivir-HBV:* Adults. 100 mg/d PO. Peds 2–17 y: 3
mg/kg/d PO, 100 mg max; ↓ w/ CrCl <50 mL/min **Caution:** [C, –] w/ Inter-
feron-α and ribavirin may cause liver failure; do not use w/ zalcitabine or w/
ganciclovir/valganciclovir **Disp:** Tabs 100 mg (*Epivir*-HBV) 150 mg, 300 mg; soln
5 mg/mL (*Epivir*-HBV), 10 mg/mL **SE:** malaise, fatigue, N/V/D, HA, pancreatitis,

lactic acidosis, peripheral neuropathy, fat redistribution, rhabdomyolysis hyperglycemia, nasal Sxs *Notes:* Differences in formulations; do not use Epivir-HBV for hep in pt with unrecognized HIV due to rapid emergence of HIV resistance

Lamotrigine (Lamictal) **WARNING:** Serious rashes requiring hospitalization & D/C of Rx reported; rash less frequent in adults; ↑ suicidality risk for antiepileptic drug, higher for those w/ epilepsy vs. those using drug for psychological indications **Uses:** *Partial Szs, tonic-clonic Szs, bipolar disorder, Lennox-Gastaut syndrome* **Action:** Phenyltriazine antiepileptic, ↓ glutamate, stabilize neuronal membrane **Dose:** *Adults. Szs:* Initial 50 mg/d PO, then 50 mg PO daily for × 1–2 wk, maint 300–500 mg/d in 2 ÷ doses. *Bipolar:* Initial 25 mg/d PO × 1–2 wk, 50 mg PO daily for 2 wk, 100 mg PO daily for 1 wk, maint 200 mg/d. *Peds.* 0.6 mg/kg in 2 ÷ doses for wk 1 & 2, then 1.2 mg/kg for wk 3 & 4, q1–2wk to maint 5–15 mg/kg/d (max 400 mg/d) 1–2 ÷ doses; ↓ in hepatic Dz or if w/ enzyme inducers or valproic acid **Caution:** [C, –] Interactions w/ other antiepileptics, estrogen, rifampin **Disp:** Tabs 25, 100, 150, 200 mg; chew tabs 2, 5, 25 mg (color-coded for those on interacting meds) **SE:** Photosensitivity, HA, GI upset, dizziness, diplopia, blurred vision, blood dyscrasias, ataxia, rash (may be much more life-threatening to peds than to adults) **Notes:** ? value of therapeutic monitoring, taper w/ D/C

Lansoprazole (Prevacid, Prevacid IV) **Uses:** *Duodenal ulcers, prevent & Rx NSAID gastric ulcers, active gastric ulcers, H. pylori Infxn, erosive esophagitis, & hypersecretory conditions, GERD* **Action:** Proton pump inhibitor **Dose:** 15–30 mg/d PO; *NSAID ulcer prevention:* 15 mg/d PO = 12 wk. *NSAID ulcers:* 30 mg/d PO × 8 wk; *hypersecretory condition:* 60 mg/d before food; 30 mg IV daily = 7 d change to PO for 6–8 wk; ↓ w/ severe hepatic impair **Caution:** [B, ?/–] **Disp:** Caps 15, 30 mg; granules for susp 15, 30 mg, IV 30 mg; once-daily tabs 15, 30 mg **SE:** N/V Abd pain HA, fatigue **Notes:** For IV provided inline filter must be used; do not crush/chew granules

Lanthanum Carbonate (Fosrenol) **Uses:** *Hyperphosphatemia in renal Dz* **Action:** Phosphate binder **Dose:** 750–1500 mg PO daily ÷ doses, w/ or immediately after meal; titrate q2–3wk based on PO_4^{-2} levels **Caution:** [C, ?/–] No data in GI Dz; not for peds **Disp:** Chew tabs 250, 500, 750, 1000 mg **SE:** N/V, graft occlusion, HA, ↓ BP **Notes:** Chew tabs before swallowing; separate from meds that interact with antacids by 2 h

Lapatinib (Tykerb) **Uses:** *Advanced breast CA w/ capecitabine w/ tumors that overexpress HER2 and failed w/ anthracycline, taxane, & trastuzumab* **Action:** TKI **Dose:** Per protocol, 1250 mg PO days 1–21 w/ capecitabine 2000 mg/m²/d divided 2 doses/d days 1–14; ↓ w/ severe cardiac or hepatic impair **Caution:** [D; ?] Avoid CYP3A4 inhibitors/inducers **CI:** w/ Phenothiazines **Disp:** Tabs 250 mg **SE:** N/V/D, anemia, ↓ plt, neutropenia, ↑ QT interval, handfoot syndrome, ↑ LFTs, rash, ↓ left ventricular ejection fraction, interstitial lung Dz and pneumonitis **Notes:** Consider baseline LVEF & periodic ECG

Latanoprost (Xalatan) Uses: *Open-angle glaucoma, ocular HTN* Action: Prostaglandin, ↑ outflow of aqueous humor Dose: 1 gtt eye(s) hs Caution: [C, ?] Disp: 0.005% soln SE: May darken tired irides; blurred vision, ocular stinging, & itching, ↑ number & length of eyelashes Notes: Wait 15 min after before using contacts; separate form other eye products by 5 min

Leflunomide (Arava) WARNING: PRG must be excluded prior to start of Rx Uses: *Active RA, orphan drug for organ rejection* Action: DMARD, ↓ pyrimidine synth Dose: Initial 100 mg/d PO for 3 d, then 10–20 mg/d Caution: [X, –] w/ Bile acid sequestrants, warfarin, rifampin, MTX CI: PRG Disp: Tabs 10, 20, 100 mg SE: D, Infxn, HTN, alopecia, rash, N, joint pain, hep, interstitial lung Dz, immunosuppression Notes: Monitor LFTs, CBC PO₄ during initial therapy; vaccine should be up-to-date, do not give w/ live vaccines

Lenalidomide (Revlimid) WARNING: Significant teratogen; patient must be enrolled in RevAssist risk-reduction program; hematologic tox, DVT & PE risk Uses: *MDS, combo w/ dexamethasone in multiple myeloma in pt failing one prior therapy* Action: Thalidomide analog, immune modulator Dose: *Adults.* 10 mg PO daily; swallow whole w/ water; multiple myeloma 25 mg/d days 1–21 of 28-d cycle w/ appropriate dose of dexamethasone Caution: [X, –] w/ Renal impair Disp: Caps 5, 10, 15, 25 mg SE: D, pruritus, rash, fatigue, night sweats, edema, nasopharyngitis, ↓ BM (plt, WBC), ↑ K⁺, ↑ LFTs, thromboembolism Notes: Monitor CBC and for thromboembolism, hepatotox; routine PRG tests required; Rx only in 1-mo increments; limited distribution network; males must use condom and not donate sperm; use at least 2 forms contraception at least 4 wk beyond D/C

Lepirudin (Refludan) Uses: *HIT* Action: Direct thrombin inhibitor Dose: *Bolus:* 0.4 mg/kg IV, then 0.15 mg/kg/h Inf; if >110 kg 44 mg of Inf 16.5 mg/h max; ↓ dose & Inf rate if CrCl <60 mL/min or if used w/ thrombolytics Caution: [B, ?/–] Hemorrhagic event or severe HTN CI: Active bleeding Disp: Inj 50 mg SE: Bleeding, anemia, hematoma, anaphylaxis Notes: Adjust based on aPTT ratio, maintain aPTT 1.5–2 × control

Letrozole (Femara) Uses: *Advanced breast CA in postmenopausal; adjuvant early breast CA in postmenopausal* Action: Nonsteroidal aromatase inhibitor Dose: 2.5 mg/d PO; q other day w/ severe liver Dz or cirrhosis Caution: [D, ?] CI: PRG, premenopausal Disp: Tabs 2.5 mg SE: Anemia, N, hot flashes, arthralgia Notes: Monitor CBC, thyroid Fxn, lytes, LFTs, & SCr

Leucovorin (Wellcovorin) Uses: *OD of folic acid antagonist; megaloblastic anemia, augment 5-FU impaired MTX elimination; w/ 5-FU in colon CA* Action: Reduced folate source; circumvents action of folate reductase inhibitors (eg, MTX) Dose: *Leucovorin rescue:* 10 mg/m² PO/IM/IV q6h; start w/in 24 h after dose or 15 mg PO/IM/IV q6h, 25 mg/dose max PO; *Folate antagonist OD (eg, Pemetrexed)* 100 mg/m² IM/IV × 1 then 50 mg/m² IM/IV q6h × 8 d 100 mg/m² × 1; *5-FU adjuvant tx, colon CA per protocol; low dose:* 20 mg/m² IV × 5 d w/ 5-FU 425 mg/m²/d IV × 5 d, repeat q4–5wk × 6; *high dose:* 500 mg/m²

IV q wk × 6, w/ 5-FU 500 mg/m² IV q wk × 6 wk, repeat after 2 wk off × 4; *Megaloblastic anemia*: 1 mg IM/IV daily **Caution:** [C, ?/–] **CI:** Pernicious anemia **Disp:** Tabs 5, 10, 15, 25 mg; Inj 50 mg, 100 mg, 200 mg, 350 mg, 500 mg **SE:** Allergic Rxn, N/V/D, fatigue, wheezing, ↑ plt **Notes:** Monitor Cr, methotrexate levels q24h w/ leucovorin rescue; do not use intrathecally/intraventricularly; w/ 5-FU CBC w/ diff, plt, LFTs, lytes

Leuprolide (Lupron, Lupron DEPOT, Lupron DEPOT-Ped, Viadur, Eligard) **Uses:** *Advanced PCa (all except Depot-Ped), endometriosis (Lupron), uterine fibroids (Lupron), & precocious puberty (Lupron-Ped)* **Action:** LHRH agonist; paradoxically ↓ release of GnRH w/ ↓ LH from anterior pituitary; in men ↓ testosterone **Dose:** *Adults. PCa: Lupron DEPOT:* 7.5 mg IM q28d or 22.5 mg IM q3mo or 30 mg IM q4mo. *Eligard:* 7.5 mg SQ q28d or 22.5 mg SQ q3mo or 30 mg SQ q4mo or 45 mg SQ q 6 mo. *Endometriosis (Lupron DEPOT):* 3.75 mg IM q mo × 6 or 11.25 mg IM q3mo × 2. *Fibroids:* 3.75 mg IM q mo × 3 or 11.25 mg IM × 1. *Peds. CPP (Lupron DEPOT-Ped):* 50 mcg/kg/d SQ Inj; ↑ by 10 mcg/kg/d until total downregulation achieved. *Lupron DEPOT: <25 kg:* 7.5 mg IM q4wk; *>25–37.5 kg:* 11.25 mg IM q4wk; *>37.5 kg:* 15 mg IM q4wk, ↑ by 3.75 mg q4wk until response **Caution:** [X, –] w/ Impending cord compression in PCa **CI:** AUB, implant in women/peds; PRG **Disp:** Inj 5 mg/mL; *Lupron DEPOT* 3.75 (1 mo for fibroids, endometriosis); *Lupron DEPOT* for PCa: 7.5 mg (1 mo), 11.25 (3 mo), 22.5 (3 mo), 30 mg (4 mo); *Eligard depot* for PCA: 7.5 (1 mo); 22.5 (3 mo), 30 (4 mo), 45 mg (6 mo); *Viadur* 65 mg 12-mo SQ implant (unavailable to new Rx after April 2008), *Lupron DEPOT-Ped* 7.5, 11.25, 15 mg **SE:** Hot flashes, gynecomastia, N/V, alopecia, anorexia, dizziness, HA, insomnia, paresthesias, depression exacerbation, peripheral edema, & bone pain (transient "flare Rxn" at 7–14 d after the 1st dose [LH/testosterone surge before suppression]); ↓ BMD w/ >6 mo use, bone loss possible **Notes:** Nonsteroidal antiandrogen (eg, bicalutamide) may block flare in men w/ PCa

Levalbuterol (Xopenex, Xopenex HFA) **Uses:** *Asthma (Rx & prevention of bronchospasm)* **Action:** Sympathomimetic bronchodilator; *R*-isomer of albuterol **Dose:** Based on NIH Guidelines 2007 *Adults.* Acute–severe exacerbation Xopenex HFA 4–8 puffs q20min up to 4 h, the q1–4h PRN or nebulizer 1/25–2.5 mg q20min × 3, then 1.25–5 mg q1–4h PRN; *Peds <4 y:* Quick relief 0.31–1.25 mg q4–6h PRN, severe 1.25 mg q20min × 3, then 0.075–0.15 mg/kg q1–4h PRN, 5 mg max. *5–11 y:* Acute–severe exacerbation 1.25 mg q20min × 3, then 0.075–0.15 mg/kg q1–4h PRN, 5 mg max. *>11 y:* 0.63–1.25 mg nebulizer q6–8h **Caution:** [C, ?] w/ Non–K⁺-sparing diuretics, CAD, HTN, arrhythmias, ↓ K⁺ **CI:** w/ Phenothiazines 7 TCAs, MAOI w/in 14 d **Disp:** Multidose inhaler (Xopenex HFA) 45 mcg/puff (15 g); soln nebulizer Inh 0.31, 0.63, 1.25 mg/3 mL; concentrate 1.25 mg/0.5 mL **SE:** Paradox bronchospasm, anaphylaxis, angioedema, tachycardia, nervousness, V, ↓ K⁺ **Notes:** May ↓ CV side effects compared w/ albuterol; do not mix w/ other nebs or dilute

Levetiracetam (Keppra)   Uses: *Adjunctive PO Rx in partial onset Sz (adults & peds ≥4 y), myoclonic Szs (adults & peds ≥12 y) w/ juvenile myoclonic epilepsy (JME), primary generalized tonic-clonic (PGTC) Szs (adults & peds ≥6 y) w/ idiopathic generalized epilepsy. Adjunctive Inj Rx partial-onset Szs in adults w/ epilepsy; and myoclonic Szs in adults w/ JME. Inj alternative for adults (≥16 y) when PO not possible* **Action:** Unknown **Dose:** *Adults & Peds >16 y:* 500 mg PO bid, titrate q2wk, may ↑ 3000 mg/d max. *Peds 4–15 y:* 10–20 mg/kg/d ÷ in 2 doses, 60 mg/kg/d max (↓ in renal Insuff) **Caution:** [C, ?/–] Elderly, w/ renal impair, psychological disorders; ↑ suicidality risk for antiepileptic drugs, higher for those w/ epilepsy vs. those using drug for psychological indications; Inj not for <16 y **CI:** Component allergy **Disp:** Tabs 250, 500, 750, 1000 mg, soln 100 mg/mL; Inj 100 mg/mL **SE:** Dizziness, somnolence, HA,N/V hostility, aggression, hallucinations, myelosuppression, impaired coordination **Notes:** Do not D/C abruptly; post-market hepatic failure and pancytopenia reported

Levobunolol (A-K Beta, Betagan)   Uses: *Open-angle glaucoma, ocular HTN* **Action:** β-Adrenergic blocker **Dose:** 1 gtt daily-bid **Caution:** [C, ?] w/ Verapamil or systemic β-blockers **CI:** Asthma, COPD sinus bradycardia, heart block (2nd-, 3rd-degree) CHF **Disp:** Soln 0.25, 0.5% **SE:** Ocular stinging/burning, bradycardia, ↓ BP **Notes:** Possible systemic effects if absorbed

Levocetirizine (Xyzal)   Uses: *Perennial/seasonal allergic rhinitis, chronic urticaria* **Action:** Antihistamine **Dose:** *Adults.* 5 mg q day *Peds 6–11 y:* 2.5 mg q day **Caution:** [B, ?] ↓ Adult dose w/renal impair, CrCl 50–80 mL/min 2.5 mg daily, 30–50 mL/min 2.5 mg q other day 10–30 mL/min 2.5 mg 2×/wk **CI:** Peds 6–11 y w/ renal impair, adults w/ ESRD **Disp:** Tab 5 mg, soln 0.5 mL/mL (150 mL) **SE:** CNS depression, drowsiness, fatigue, xerostomia **Notes:** Take in evening

Levofloxacin (Levaquin)   **WARNING:** ↑ Risk Achilles tendon rupture and tendonitis Uses: *Skin/skin structure Infxn(SSSI), UTI, chronic bacterial prostatitis, acute pyelo, acute bacterial sinusitis, acute bacterial exacerbation of chronic bronchitis, CAP, including multidrug-resistant S. pneumoniae, nosocomial pneumonia; Rx inhalational anthrax in adults & peds ≥6 mo* **Action:** Quinolone, ↓ DNA gyrase. *Spectrum:* Excellent gram(+) except MRSA & E. faecium; excellent gram(–) except Stenotrophomonas maltophilia & Acinetobacter sp; poor anaerobic **Dose:** *Adults ≥18 y:* IV/PO: *Bronchitis:* 500 mg q day × 7 d. *CAP:* 500 mg q day × 7–14 d or 750 mg q day × 5 d. *Sinusitis:* 500 mg q day × 10–14 d or 750 mg q day × 5 d. *Prostatitis:* 500 mg q day × 28 d. *Uncomp SSSI:* 500 mg q day × 7–10 d. *Comp SSSI/Nosocomial Pneumonia:* 750 mg q day × 7–14 d. *Anthrax:* 500 mg q day × 60 d; *Uncomp UTI:* 250 mg q day × 3 d. *Comp UTI/Acute Pyelo:* 250 mg q day × 10 d or 750 mg q day × 5 d. CrCl 10–19 mL/min: 250 mg, then 250 mg q48h or 750 mg, then 500 mg q48h. *Hemodialysis:* 750 mg, then 500 mg q48h. *Peds ≥6 mo:* Anthrax only >50 kg: 500 mg q 24h × 60 d, <50 kg 8 mg/kg (250 mg/dose max) q12h for 60 d ↓ w/ renal impair avoid antacids w/ PO; oral soln 1 h before, 2 h after meals **Caution:** [C, –] w/ Cation-containing products (eg, antacids), w/ drugs that ↑ QT interval **CI:** Quinolone sensitivity **Disp:** Tabs 250, 500, 750 mg; premixed IV 250, 500, 750 mg, Inj 25 mg/mL; Leva-Pak 750 mg × 5 d **SE:** N/D, dizziness, rash, GI upset, photosensitivity, CNS stimulant w/ IV use, *C. difficile* enterocolitis; rare fatal hepatox **Notes:** Use w/ steroids ↑ tendon risk; only for anthrax in peds

Levofloxacin ophthalmic (Quixin, Iquix) Uses: *Bacterial conjunctivitis* **Action:** See levofloxacin **Dose:** *Ophthal* 1–2 gtt in eye(s) q2h while awake × 2 d, then q4h while awake × 5 d **Caution:** [C, –] **CI:** Quinolone sensitivity **Disp:** 25 mg/mL ophthal soln 0.5% (Quixin), 1.5% (Iquix) **SE:** Ocular burning/pain, ↓ vision, fever, foreign body sensation, HA, pharyngitis, photophobia

Levonorgestrel (Plan B) Uses: *Emergency contraceptive ("morning-after pill")*; prevents PRG if taken <72 h after unprotected sex/contraceptive failure **Action:** Progestin, alters tubal transport & endometrium to implantation **Dose:** *Adults & Peds (postmenarche females):* 0.75 mg q12h × 2 **Caution:** [X, +] **CI:** Known/suspected PRG, AUB **Disp:** Tab, 0.75 mg, 2 blister pack **SE:** N/V, Abd pain, fatigue, HA, menstrual changes. **Notes:** Will not induce abortion; ↑ risk of ectopic PRG; OTC ("behind the counter") if >18 y, RX if <18 y varies by state

Levonorgestrel IUD (Mirena) Uses: *Contraception, long-term* **Action:** Progestin, alters endometrium, thicken cervical mucus, inhibits ovulation and implantation **Dose:** Up to 5 y, insert w/in 7 d menses onset or immediately after 1st tri abortion; wait 6 wk if postpartum; replace any time during menstrual cycle **Caution:** [C, ?] **CI:** PRG, w/ active hepatic Dz or tumor, uterine anomaly, breast CA, acute/Hx of PID, postpartum endometriosis, infected abortion last 3 mo, gynecological neoplasia, abnormal Pap, AUB, untreated cervicitis/vaginitis, multiple sex partners, ↑ increased susceptibility to Infxn **Disp:** 52 mg IUD **SE:** Failed insertion, ectopic pregnancy, sepsis, PID, infertility, PRG comps w/ IUD left in place, abortion, embedment, ovarian cysts, perforation uterus/cervix, intestinal obst/perforation, peritonitis, N, Abd pain, ↑ BP, acne, HA **Notes:** Inform pt does not protect against STD/HIV; see insert for insertion instructions; reexamine placement after 1st menses; 80% PRG w/in 12 mo of removal

Levorphanol (Levo-Dromoran) [C-II] Uses: *Mod–severe pain; chronic pain* **Action:** Narcotic analgesic, morphine derivative **Dose:** 2–4 mg PO PRN q6–8h; ↓ in hepatic impair **Caution:** [B/D (prolonged use/high doses at term), ?/–] w/ ↑ ICP, head trauma, adrenal Insuff **CI:** Component allergy **Disp:** Tabs 2 mg **SE:** Tachycardia, ↓ BP, drowsiness, GI upset, constipation, resp depression, pruritus

Levothyroxine (Synthroid, Levoxyl, others) WARNING: Not for obesity or wgt loss; tox with high doses, especially when combined with sympathomimetic amines Uses: *Hypothyroidism, pituitary thyroid-stimulating hormone (TSH) suppression, myxedema coma* **Action:** T_4 supl L-thyroxine **Dose:** **Adults.** *Hypothyroid* titrate until euthyroid >50 y w/ heart Dz or <50 w/ heart Dz 25–50 mcg/d, ↑ q6–8wk; >50 y w/ heart Dz 12.5–25 mcg/d, ↑ q6–8wk;

usual 100–200 mcg/d. *Myxedema*: 200–500 mcg IV, then 100–300 mcg/d. *Peds. Hypothyroid*: **0–3 mo:** 10–15 mcg/kg/24 h PO; **3–6 mo:** 8–10 mcg/kg/d PO; **6–12 mo:** 6–8 mcg/kg/d PO; **1–5 y:** 5–6 mcg/kg/d PO; **6–12 y:** 4–5 mcg/kg/d PO; **>12 y:** 2–3 mcg/kg/d PO; if growth and puberty complete 1.7 mcg/kg/d; ↓ dose by 50% if IV; titrate based on response & thyroid tests; dose can ↑ rapidly in young/middle-aged; best on empty stomach **Caution:** [A, +] **CI:** Recent MI, uncorrected adrenal Insuff; many drug interactions; in elderly w/ CV Dz **Disp:** Tabs 25, 50, 75, 88, 100, 112, 125, 137, 150, 175, 200, 300 mcg; Inj 200, 500 mcg **SE:** Insomnia, wgt loss, N/V/D, ↑ LFTs, irregular periods, ↓ BMD, alopecia, arrhythmia **Notes:** Take w/ full glass of water (prevents choking); PRG may ↑ need for higher doses; takes 6 wk to see effect on TSH; wait 6 wk before checking TSH after dose change

Lidocaine, systemic (Xylocaine, others) Uses: **Rx cardiac arrhythmias** **Action:** Class IB antiarrhythmic **Dose:** *Adults. Antiarrhythmic, ET:* 5 mg/kg; follow w/ 0.5 mg/kg in 10 min if effective. *IV load:* 1 mg/kg/dose bolus over 2–3 min; repeat in 5–10 min; 200–300 mg/h max; cont Inf 20–50 mcg/kg/min or 1–4 mg/min; *Cardiac arrest from VF/VT: Initial:* 1.0–1.5 mg/kg IV. *Refractory VF:* Additional 0.5–0.75 mg/kg IV push, repeat in 5–10 min, max total 3 mg/kg. ET: 2–4 mg/kg. *Perfusing stable VT, wide complex tachycardia or ectopy:* 1.0–1.5 mg/kg IV push; repeat 0.5–0.75 mg/kg q 5–10 min; max total 3 mg/kg; Maint 1–4 mg/min (30–50 mcg/min) *(ECC 2005).* *Peds. Antiarrhythmic, ET, load:* 1 mg/kg; repeat in 10–15 min 5 mg/kg max total, then IV Inf 20–50 mcg/kg/min **Caution:** [B, +] Corn allergy **CI:** Adams-Stokes syndrome; heart block **Disp:** *Inj IV:* 1% (10 mg/mL), 2% (20 mg/mL); admixture 4, 10, 20%. *IV Inf:* 0.2, 0.4% **SE:** Dizziness, paresthesias, & convulsions associated w/ tox **Notes:** 2nd line to amiodarone in ECC; dilute ET dose 1–2 mL w/ NS; for IV forms, ↓ w/ liver Dz or CHF; systemic levels: steady state 6–12 h: *Therapeutic:* 1.2–5 mcg/mL; *Toxic:* >6 mcg/mL; half-life: 1.5 h

Lidocaine; Lidocaine with Epinephrine (Anestacon Topical, Xylocaine, Xylocaine Viscous, Xylocaine MPF others) Uses: **Local anesthetic, epidural/caudal anesthesia, regional nerve blocks, topical on mucous membranes (mouth/pharynx/urethra)** **Action:** Anesthetic; stabilizes neuronal membranes; inhibits ionic fluxes required for initiation and conduction **Dose:** *Adults. Local Inj anesthetic:* 4.5 mg/kg max total dose or 300 mg; w/ epi 7 mg/kg or total 500 mg max dose. *Oral:* 15 mL viscous swish and spit or *pharyngeal* gargle and swallow, do not use <3-h intervals or >8 × in 24 h. *Urethra:* 10–15 mL (200–300 mg) jelly in men, 5 mL female urethra; 600 mg/24 h max. *Peds. Topical:* Apply max 3 mg/kg/dose. *Local Inj anesthetic:* Max 4.5 mg/kg (Table 2) **Caution:** [B, +] Corn allergy; epi-containing soln may interact w/ TCA or MAOI and cause severe ↑ BP **CI:** Do not use lidocaine w/ epi on digits, ears, or nose (vasoconstriction & necrosis) **Disp:** *Inj local:* 0.5, 1, 1.5, 2, 4, 10, 20%; Inj w/ epi 0.5%/1:200,000, 1%/1:100,000, 2%/1:100,000; (MPF) 1%/1:200,000, 1.5%/1:200,000, 2%/1:200,000; (*Dental formulations*) 2%/1:50,000, 2%/1:100,000; cream 2%; gel 2,

2.5%; oint 2.5, 5%; liq 2.5%; soln 2, 4%; viscous 2% **SE:** Dizziness, paresthesias, & convulsions associated w/ tox **Notes:** See Table 2

Lidocaine powder intradermal injection system (Zingo)

Uses: *Local anesthesia before venipuncture or IV in peds 3–18 y* **Action:** Local amide anesthetic **Dose:** Apply 3 min before procedure **Caution:** [N/A, N/A] only on intact skin **CI:** Lidocaine allergy **Disp:** 6.5-Inch device to administer under pressure 0.5 mg lidocaine powder in 2-cm area, single use **SE:** Skin Rxn, edema, petechiae

Lidocaine/Prilocaine (EMLA, LMX)

Uses: *Topical anesthetic for intact skin or genital mucous membranes*; adjunct to phlebotomy or dermal procedures **Action:** Amide local anesthetics **Dose:** *Adults. EMLA cream, anesthetic disc (1 g/10 cm²):* Thick layer 2–2.5 g to intact skin, cover w/ occlusive dressing (eg, Tegaderm) for at least 1 h. *Anesthetic disc:* 1 g/10 cm² for at least 1 h. *Peds. Max dose: <3 mo or <5 kg:* 1 g/10 cm² for 1 h. *3–12 mo & >5 kg:* 2 g/20 cm² for 4 h. *1–6 y & >10 kg:* 10 g/100 cm² for 4 h. *7–12 y & >20 kg:* 20 g/200 cm² for 4 h **Caution:** [B, +] Methemoglobinemia **CI:** Use on mucous membranes, broken skin, eyes; allergy to amide-type anesthetics **Disp:** Cream 2.5% lidocaine/2.5% prilocaine; anesthetic disc (1 g); periodontal gel 2.5/2.5% **SE:** Burning, stinging, methemoglobinemia **Notes:** Longer contact time ↑ effect

Lindane (Kwell, others)

WARNING: Only for pts intolerant/failed first-line therapy w/ safer agents. Szs and deaths reported w/ repeat/prolonged use. Caution due to increased risk of neurotox in infants, children, elderly, w/ other skin conditions, and if <50kg. Instruct pts on proper use and inform that itching occurs after successful killing of scabies or lice **Uses:** *Head lice, pubic "crab" lice, body lice, scabies* **Action:** Ectoparasiticide & ovicide **Dose:** *Adults & Peds. Cream or lotion:* Thin layer to dry skin after bathing, leave for 8–12 h, pour on laundry. *Shampoo:* Apply 30 mL to dry hair, develop a lather w/ warm water for 4 min, comb out nits **Caution:** [C, +/–] **CI:** Premature infants, uncontrolled Szs disorders open wounds **Disp:** Lotion 1%; shampoo 1% **SE:** Arrhythmias, Szs, local irritation, GI upset, ataxia, alopecia, N/V, aplastic anemia **Notes:** Caution w/ overuse (may be absorbed); may repeat Rx in 7 d; try OTC first w/ pyrethrins (Pronto, Rid, others)

Linezolid (Zyvox)

Uses: *Infxns caused by gram(+) bacteria (including VRE), pneumonia, skin Infxns* **Action:** Unique, inhib ribosomal bacterial RNA; bacteriocidal for streptococci, bacteriostatic for enterococci & staphylococci. **Spectrum:** Excellent gram(+) including VRE & MRSA **Dose:** *Adults.* 400–600 mg IV or PO q12h. *Peds.* 10 mg/kg IV or PO q8h (q12h in preterm neonates) **Caution:** [C, ?/–] w/ Reversible MAOI, avoid foods w/ tyramine & cough/cold products w/ pseudoephedrine; w/ ↓ BM **Disp:** Inj 200, 600 mg; tabs 600 mg; susp 100 mg/5 mL **SE:** Lactic acidosis, peripheral/optic neuropathy, HTN, N/D, HA, insomnia, GI upset, ↓ BM, tongue discoloration **Notes:** ✓ weekly CBC; not for gram(−) Infxn, ↑ deaths in catheter-related Infxns

Liothyronine (Cytomel, Triostat, T₃) **WARNING:** Not for obesity or wgt loss **Uses:** *Hypothyroidism, nontoxic goiter, myxedema coma, thyroid suppression therapy* **Action:** T_3 replacement **Dose:** *Adults.* Initial 25 mcg/24 h, titrate by response & TFT; maint of 25–100 mcg/d PO. *Myxedema coma:* 25–50 mcg IV. *Myxedema:* 5 mcg/d, PO ↑ 5–10 mcg/d q1–2wk; maint 50–100 mcg/d. *Nontoxic goiter:* 5 mcg/d PO, ↑ 5–10 mcg/d q1–2wk; usual dose 75 mcg/d. *T₃ suppression test:* 75–100 mcg/d × 7d. **Peds.** Initial 5 mcg/24 h, titrate by 5-mcg/ 24-h increments at q3–4d intervals; maint peds 1–3 yrs: 50 mcg/d. *Infants–12 mo:* 20 mcg/d. *>3 y:* adult dose; ↓ in elderly & CV Dz **Caution:** [A, +] **CI:** Recent MI, uncorrected adrenal Insuff, uncontrolled HTN, thyrotoxicosis, artificial rewarming **Disp:** Tabs 5, 25, 50 mcg; Inj 10 mcg/mL **SE:** Alopecia, arrhythmias, CP, HA, sweating, twitching, ↑ HR, ↑ BP, MI, CHF, fever **Notes:** Monitor TFT; separate antacids by 4 h; monitor glucose w/ DM meds; when switching from IV to PO, taper IV slowly

Lisdexamfetamine dimesylate (Vyvanse) [C-II] **WARNING:** Amphetamines have high potential for abuse; prolonged administration may lead to dependence; misuse may cause sudden death and serious CV events **Uses:** *ADHD* **Action:** CNS stimulant **Dose:** *Adults & Peds 6–12 y:* 30 mg daily, ↑ q wk 10–20 mg/d, 70 mg/d max **Caution:** [C, ?/–] w/ Potential for drug dependency in pt w/ psychological or Sz disorder, Tourette, HTN **CI:** Severe arteriosclerotic CV Dz, mod–severe ↑ BP, ↑ thyroid, sensitivity to sympathomimetic amines, NAG, agitated states, Hx drug abuse, w/ or w/in 14 d of MAOI **Disp:** Caps 30, 50, 70 mg **SE:** Headache, insomnia, decreased appetite **Notes:** AHA statement April 2008: All children diagnosed with ADHD who are candidates for stimulant meds should undergo CV assessment prior to use

Lisinopril (Prinivil, Zestril) **WARNING:** ACE inhibitors can cause fetal injury/death in 2nd/3rd tri; D/C w/ PRG **Uses:** *HTN, CHF, prevent DN & AMI* **Action:** ACE inhibitor **Dose:** 5–40 mg/24 h PO daily-bid, CHF target 40 mg/d. *AMI:* 5 mg w/in 24 h of MI, then 5 mg after 24 h, 10 mg after 48 h, then 10 mg/d; ↓ in renal Insuff; use low dose, ↑ slowly in elderly **Caution:** [D, –] **CI:** Bilateral RAS, PRG ACE inhibitor sensitivity (angioedema) **Disp:** Tabs 2.5, 5, 10, 20, 30, 40 mg **SE:** Dizziness, HA, cough, ↓ BP, angioedema, ↑ K⁺, ↑ Cr, rare ↓ BM **Notes:** To prevent DN, start when urinary microalbuminemia begins; ✓ K, BUN, Cr, K⁺, WBC

Lithium Carbonate (Eskalith, Lithobid, others) **WARNING:** Li tox related to serum levels and can be seen at close to therapeutic levels **Uses:** *Manic episodes of bipolar Dz,* augment antidepressants, aggression, post-traumatic stress disorder **Action:** ?, Effects shift toward intraneuronal metabolism of catecholamines **Dose:** *Adults.* Bipolar, acute mania: 1800 mg/d PO in 2–3 ÷ doses (target serum 1–1.5 mEq/L ✓ 2×/wk until stable). *Bipolar maint:* 900–1200 /d PO in 2–3 ÷ doses (target serum 0.6–1.2 mEq/L). *Peds ≥12 y:* See adult; ↓ in renal Insuff, elderly **Caution:** [D, –] Many drug interactions; avoid ACE inhibitor or diuretics; thyroid Dz **CI:** Severe renal impair or CV Dz, lactation **Disp:** Caps 150, 300, 600 mg; tabs 300 mg; SR tabs 300 mg, CR tabs 450 mg; syrup & soln 300 mg/5 mL **SE:** Polyuria, polydipsia, nephrogenic DI, long-term may affect renal conc ability and cause fibrosis; tremor; Na retention or diuretic use may ↑ tox; arrhythmias, dizziness, alopecia, goiter ↓ thyroid, N/V/D, ataxia, nystagmus, ↓ BP **Notes:** Levels: *Trough:* just before next dose; *Therapeutic:* 0.8–1.2 mEq/mL; *Toxic:* >1.5 mEq/mL. *Half-life:* 18–20h. Follow levels q1–2mo on maint

Lodoxamide (Alomide) Uses: *Vernal conjunctivitis/keratitis* **Action:** Stabilizes mast cells **Dose:** *Adults & Peds >2 y:* 1–2 gtt in eye(s) qid ≈ 3 mo **Caution:** [B, ?] **Disp:** Soln 0.1% **SE:** Ocular burning, stinging, HA **Notes:** Do not use soft contacts during use

Lomefloxacin (Maxaquin) Uses: *UTI, acute exacerbation of chronic bronchitis; prophylaxis in transurethral procedures* **Action:** Quinolone antibiotic; ↓ DNA gyrase *Spectrum:* Good gram(–) including *H. influenzae* except *Stenotrophomonas maltophilia, Acinetobacter* & some *P. aeruginosa* **Dose:** 400 mg/d PO; ↓ w/ renal Insuff; separate antacids **Caution:** [C, –] Interactions w/ cation-containing meds **CI:** Quinolone allergy, children <18 y, ↑ Qt interval, ↓ K+ **Disp:** Tab 400 mg **SE:** N/V/D, Abd pain, photosensitivity, Szs, HA, dizziness, tendon rupture, peripheral neuropathy, pseudomembranous colitis, anaphylaxis

Loperamide (Diamode, Imodium) [OTC] Uses: *Diarrhea* **Action:** Slows intestinal motility **Dose:** *Adults.* Initial 4 mg PO, then 2 mg after each loose stool, up to 16 mg/d. *Peds 2–5 y, 13–20 kg:* 1 mg PO tid; *6–8 y, 20–30 kg:* 2 mg PO bid; *8–12 y, >30 kg:* 2 mg PO tid **Caution:** [C, –] Not for acute D caused by *Salmonella, Shigella,* or *C. difficile;* w/ HIV may cause toxic megacolon **CI:** Pseudomembranous colitis, bloody D, Abd pain w/o D, <2 y **Disp:** Caps 2 mg; tabs 2 mg; liq 1 mg/5 mL, 1 mg/7.5 mL (OTC) **SE:** Constipation, sedation, dizziness, Abd cramp, N

Lopinavir/Ritonavir (Kaletra) Uses: *HIV Infxn* **Action:** Protease inhibitor **Dose:** *Adults.* TX naïve: 800/200 mg PO daily or 400/100 mg PO bid; *TX experienced pt:* 400/100 mg PO bid (↑ dose if w/ amprenavir, efavirenz, fosamprenavir, nelfinavir, nevirapine); do not use q day dosing w/ concomitant therapy. *Peds 7–15 kg:* 12/3 mg/kg PO bid. *15–40 kg:* 10/2.5 mg/kg PO bid. *>40 kg:* adult dose; w/ food **Caution:** [C, ?/–] Numerous interactions, w/ hepatic impair **CI:** w/ Drugs dependent on CYP3A/CYP2D6 (Table 11), statins, St. John's wort, fluconazole **Disp:** (mg lopinavir/ritonavir) Tab 100/25 mg, 200/50 mg, soln 400/100/5 mL **SE:** Avoid disulfiram (soln has EtOH), metronidazole; GI upset, asthenia, ↑ cholesterol/triglycerides, pancreatitis; protease metabolic syndrome

Loratadine (Claritin, Alavert) Uses: *Allergic rhinitis, chronic idiopathic urticaria* **Action:** Nonsedating antihistamine **Dose:** *Adults.* 10 mg/d PO. *Peds 2–5 y:* 5 mg PO daily. *>6 y:* adult dose; on empty stomach; ↓ in hepatic Insuff; q other day dose w/ CrCl <30 mL/min **Caution:** [B, +/–] **CI:** Component allergy **Disp:** Tabs 10 mg (OTC); rapidly disintegrating RediTabs 10 mg; chew tabs 5 mg; syrup 1 mg/mL **SE:** HA, somnolence, xerostomia, hyperkinesis in peds

Lorazepam (Ativan, others) [C-IV] Uses: *Anxiety & anxiety w/ depression; sedation; control status epilepticus*; EtOH withdrawal; antiemetic **Action:** Benzodiazepine; antianxiety agent; works via postsynaptic GABA receptors **Dose:** *Adults. Anxiety:* 1–10 mg PO in 2–3 ÷ doses. *Pre-op:* 0.05 mg/kg to 4 mg max IM 2 h before or 0.044 mg/kg-2mg max IV 15–20 min before surgery. *Insomnia:* 2–4 mg PO hs. *Status epilepticus:* 4 mg/dose slow over 2–5 min IV PRN q10–15min; usual total dose 8 mg. *Antiemetic:* 0.5–2 mg IV or PO q4–6h PRN. *EtOH withdrawal:* 2–5 mg IV or 1–2 mg PO initial depending on severity; titrate. *Peds. Status epilepticus:* 0.05–0.1 mg/kg/dose IV over 2–5 min, repeat at 1–20-min intervals × 2 PRN. *Antiemetic, 2–15 y:* 0.05 mg/kg (to 2 mg/dose) prechemotherapy; ↓ in elderly; do not administer IV >2 mg/min or 0.05 mg/kg/min **Caution:** [D, ?/–] w/ Hepatic impair, other CNS depression, COPD; ↓ dose by 50% w/ valproic acid and probenecid **CI:** Severe pain, severe ↓ BP, sleep apnea, NAG, allergy to propylene glycol or benzyl alcohol **Disp:** Tabs 0.5, 1, 2 mg; soln, PO conc 2 mg/mL; Inj 2, 4 mg/mL **SE:** Sedation, memory impair, EPS, dizziness, ataxia, tachycardia, ↓ BP constipation, resp depression **Notes:** ~ 10 min for effect if IV; IV Inf requires inline filter

Losartan (Cozaar) **WARNING:** Can cause fatal injury and death if used in 2nd & 3rd trimesters. D/C therapy if PRG detected **Uses:** *HTN, DN, prevent CVA in HTN & LVH* **Action:** Angiotensin II receptor antagonist **Dose:** *Adults.* 25–50 mg PO daily-bid, max 100 mg; ↓ in elderly/hepatic impair. *Peds ≥6 y: HTN:* Initial 0.7 mg/kg q day, ↑ to 50 mg/d PRN; 1.4 mg/kg/d or 100 mg/d max **Caution:** [C (1st tri, D 2nd & 3rd tri), ?/–] w/ NSAIDs; w/ K⁺-sparing diuretics, supl may cause ↑ K⁺; w/ RAS, hepatic impair **CI:** PRG, component sensitivity **Disp:** Tabs 25, 50, 100 mg **SE:** ↓ BP in pts on diuretics; ↑ K⁺; GI upset, facial/angioedema, dizziness, cough, weakness, ↓ renal fxn

Lovastatin (Mevacor, Altoprev) Uses: *Hypercholesterolemia to ↓ risk of MI, angina* **Action:** HMG-CoA reductase inhibitor **Dose:** *Adults.* 20 mg/d PO w/ P.M. meal; may ↑ at 4-wk intervals to 80 mg/d max or 60 mg ER tab; take w/ meals. *Peds 10–17 y (at least 1-y postmenarchal): Familial ↑ cholesterol:* 10 mg PO q day, ↑ q4wk PRN to 40 mg/d max (immediate release w/ P.M. meal) **Caution:** [X, –] Avoid w/ grapefruit juice, gemfibrozil, Dosing escalation w/ renal impair **CI:** Active liver Dz, PRG, lactation **Disp:** Tabs 10, 20, 40 mg; ER tabs 20, 40, 60 mg **SE:** HA & GI intolerance common; promptly report any unexplained muscle pain, tenderness, or weakness (myopathy) **Notes:** Maintain cholesterol-lowering diet; LFTs q12wk × 1 y, then q6mo; may alter TFT

Lubiprostone (Amitiza) Uses: *Chronic idiopathic constipation in adults, IBS w/ constipation in females >18 y* **Action:** Selective Cl⁻ channel activator; ↑ intestinal motility **Dose:** *Adults. Constipation:* 24 mcg PO bid w/ food. *IBS:* 8 mcg bid; w/ food **CI:** Mechanical GI obst **Caution:** [C, ?/–] Severe D, severe renal or mod–severe hepatic impair **Disp:** Gelcaps 8, 24 mcg **SE:** N/D, HA, GI distention, Abd pain **Notes:** Not approved in males; requires (–) PRG test before; use contraception; periodically reassess drug need; not for chronic use; may experience severe dyspnea w/in 1 h of dose, usually resolves w/in 3 h

Lutropin Alfa (Luveris) **Uses:** *Infertility w/ profound LH deficiency* **Action:** Recombinant LH **Dose:** 75 units SQ w/ 75–150 units FSH, 2 separate Inj max 14 d **Caution:** [X, ?/M] Potential for arterial thromboembolism **CI:** Primary ovarian failure, uncontrolled thyroid/adrenal dysfunction, intracranial lesion, AUB, hormone-dependent GU tumor, ovarian cyst, PRG **Disp:** Inj 75 units **SE:** HA, N, ovarian hyperstimulation syndrome, ovarian torsion, Abd pain due to ovarian enlargement, breast pain, ovarian cysts; ↑ risk of multiple births **Notes:** Rotate Inj sites; do not exceed 14 d duration unless signs of imminent follicular development; monitor ovarian ultrasound and serum estradiol; specific pt information packets given

Lymphocyte Immune Globulin [Antithymocyte Globulin, ATG] (Atgam) **WARNING:** Should only be used by physician experienced in immunosuppressive TX or management of solid-organ and/or bone marrow transplant pts. Adequate lab and supportive medical resources must be readily available in the facility for pt management **Uses:** *Allograft rejection in renal transplant pts; aplastic anemia if not candidates for BMT,* prevent rejection of other solid-organ transplants, GVHD after BMT **Action:** ↓ Circulating T lymphocytes, human, & equine product **Dose:** *Adults.* *Prevent rejection:* 15 mg/kg/d IV × 14 d, then q other day × 14 d; initial dose w/in 24 h before/after transplant. *Rx rejection:* Same except use 10–15 mg/kg/d; max 21 doses in 28 d. *Aplastic anemia:* 10–20 mg/kg/d × 8–14 d, then q other day × 7 doses for total 21 doses in 28 d. *Peds.* *Prevent rejection:* 5–25 mg/kg/d IV **Caution:** [C, –] **CI:** Hx Rxn to other equine γ-globulin preparation, leukopenia, thrombocytopenia **Disp:** Inj 50 mg/mL **SE:** D/C w/ severe thrombocytopenia/leukopenia; rash, fever, chills, ↓ BP, HA, ↑ K+, CP, edema, N/V/D, lightheadedness **Notes:** Test dose: 0.1 mL 1:1000 dilution in NS, a systemic Rxn precludes use; give via central line; consider pretreatment w/ antipyretic, antihistamine, and/or corticosteroids

Magaldrate (Riopan-Plus) [OTC] **Uses:** *Hyperacidity associated w/ peptic ulcer, gastritis, & hiatal hernia* **Action:** Low-Na antacid **Dose:** 5–10 mL PO between meals & hs, on empty stomach **Caution:** [C, ?/+] **CI:** Ulcerative colitis, diverticulitis, appendicitis, ileostomy/colostomy, renal Insuff (Mg content) **Disp:** Susp magaldrate/simethicone 540/20 mg & 1080/40 mg/5 mL **SE:** ↑ Mg2+, ↓ PO4, white flecked feces, constipation, N/V/D **Notes:** <0.3 mg Na/tab or tsp

Magnesium Citrate (Citroma, others) [OTC] **Uses:** *Vigorous bowel preparation*; constipation **Action:** Cathartic laxative **Dose:** *Adults.* 120–300 mL PO PRN. *Peds.* 0.5 mL/kg/dose, q4–6h to 200 mL PO max; w/ a beverage **Caution:** [B, +] w/ Neuromuscular Dz **CI:** Severe renal Dz, heart block, N/V, rectal bleeding intestinal obst/perforation/impaction, colostomy, ileostomy, ulcerative volitis, diverticulitis **Disp:** soln 290 mg/5 mL (300 mL); 100 mg tabs **SE:** Abd cramps, gas, ↓ BP, ↑ Mg, resp depression **Notes:** Only for occasional use w/ constipation

Magnesium Hydroxide (Milk of Magnesia) [OTC]   **Uses:**
Constipation, hyperacidity, Mg replacement **Action:** NS laxative **Dose:** *Adults. Antacid:* 5–15 mL (400 mg/5 mL) or 2–4 (311 mg) tabs PO PRN qid. *Mg²⁺ replacement:* 2–4 (500 mg) tabs PO qhs or ÷ doses. *Laxative:* 30–60 mL (400 mg/5 mL) or 15–30 mL (800 mg/5 mL) or 8 (311 mg) tabs PO qhs or ÷ doses. *Peds. Antacid and Mg²⁺ replacement:* <12 y not ok. *Laxative: <2 y:* 5–15 mL (400 mg/5 mL) PO qhs or ÷ doses. *2–5 y:* 5–15 mL (400 mg/5 mL) PO qhs or ÷ doses. *6–11 y:* 15–30 mL (400 mg/5 mL) or 7.5–15 mL (800 mg/5 mL) PO qhs or ÷ doses. *3–5 y:* 2 (311-mg) tabs PO qhs or ÷ doses. *6–11 y:* 4 (311-mg) tabs PO qhs or ÷ doses **Caution:** [B, +] w/ Neuromuscular Dz or renal impair **CI:** Renal Insuff, intestinal obst, ileostomy/colostomy **Disp:** Chew tabs 311, 500 mg; liq 400, 800 mg/5 mL (OTC) **SE:** D, Abd cramps **Notes:** For occasional use in constipation

Magnesium Oxide (Mag-Ox 400, others) [OTC]   **Uses:**
Replace low Mg levels **Action:** Mg supl **Dose:** 400–800 mg/d or ÷ w/ food in full glass of H₂O; ↓ w/ renal impair **Caution:** [B, +] w/ Neuromuscular Dz & renal impair, w/ bisphosphonates, calcitriol, CCBs, neuromuscular blockers, tetracyclines, quinolones **CI:** Ulcerative colitis, diverticulitis, ileostomy/colostomy, heart block **Disp:** Caps 140 250, 500, 600 mg; tabs 400 mg (OTC) **SE:** D, N

Magnesium Sulfate (various)   **Uses:** *Replace low Mg²⁺;* preeclampsia, eclampsia, & premature labor, cardiac arrest, AMI arrhythmias, cerebral edema, barium poisoning, Szs, pediatric acute nephritis*; refractory ↓ K⁺ & ↓ Ca²⁺ **Action:** Mg²⁺ supl, bowel evacuation, ↓ acetylcholine in nerve terminals, ↑ rate of sinoatrial node firing **Dose:** *Adults.* 3 g IM/IV q6h × 4 PRN; *Supl:* 1–2 g IM or IV; repeat PRN. *Preeclampsia/premature labor:* 4-g load then 1–4 g/h IV Inf. *Cardiac arrest:* 1–2 g IV push (2–4 mL 50% soln) in 10 mL D₅W. *AMI:* Load 1–2 g in 50–100 mL D₅W over 5–60 min IV; then 0.5–1.0 g/h IV up to 24 h *(ECC 2005)*. *Peds.* 25–50 mg/kg/dose IM, IV, IO q4–6h for 3–4 doses; repeat PRN; q8–12h in neonates; max 2 g single dose; ↓ dose w/ low urinary output or renal Insuff **Caution:** [A/C (manufacturer specific), +] w/ Neuromuscular Dz; interactions see Magnesium Oxide and aminoglycosides **CI:** Heart block, renal failure **Disp:** Premix Inj: 10, 20, 40, 80 mg/mL; Inj 125, 500 mg/mL; oral/topical powder 227, 454, 480, 1810, 1920, 2721 g **SE:** CNS depression, D, flushing, heart block, ↓ BP, vasodilation **Notes:** different formulation may contain Al²⁺

Mannitol (various)   **Uses:** *Cerebral edema, ↑ intraocular pressure, renal impair, poisonings, GU irrigation* **Action:** Osmotic diuretic **Dose:** *Test dose:* 0.2 g/kg/dose IV over 3–5 min; if no diuresis w/in 2 h, D/C. *Oliguria:* 50–100 g IV over 90 min; ↑ IOP: 0.5–2 g/kg IV over 30 min. *Cerebral edema:* 0.25–1.5 g/kg/dose IV >30 min **Caution:** [C, ?/M] w/ CHF or vol overload, w/ nephrotoxic drugs & lithium **CI:** Anuria, dehydration, heart failure, PE **Disp:** Inj 5, 10, 15, 20, 25%; GU soln 5% **SE:** May exacerbate CHF, N/V/D, ↓/↑ BP, ↑ HR **Notes:** Monitor for vol depletion

Maraviroc (Selzentry)   WARNING: Possible drug-induced hepatotox
Uses: *Tx of CCR5-tropic HIV Infxn* Action: Antiretroviral, CCR5 corecep-
tor antagonist Dose: 300 mg bid Caution: [B, –] w/ Concomitant CYP3A induc-
ers/inhibitors CI: None Disp: Tab 150, 300 mg SE: Fever, URI, cough, rash

**Measles, Mumps, Rubella, & Varicella Virus Vaccine Live
[MMRV] (ProQuad)**   Uses: *Vaccination against measles, mumps, rubella,
& varicella 12 mo–12 y or for 2nd dose of measles, mumps, & rubella (MMR)*
Action: Active immunization, live attenuated viruses Dose: 1 (0.5 mL) vial SQ Inj
Caution: [C,?/M] Hx of cerebral injury or Szs (febrile Rxn), w/ ↓ plt CI: Hx anaphylaxis to neomycin, blood dyscrasia, lymphoma, leukemia, malignant neoplasias
affecting BM, w/ immunosuppression, febrile illness, untreated TB, temp
>101.3°F, PRG Disp: Inj SE: Fever, Inj site Rxn, rash Notes: Per FDA, CDC ↑ of
febrile Sz in combo vaccine vs. MMR and varicella separately; preferable to use 2
separate vaccines; allow 1 mo between Inj & any other measles vaccine or 3 mo
between any other varicella vaccine; limited avail of MMRV; substitute MMR II or
Varivax; avoid those who have not been exposed to varicella for 6 wk post-Inj; avoid
contain albumin or trace egg antigen; avoid salicylates

Mecasermin (Increlex, Iplex)   Uses: *Growth failure in severe primary IGF-1 deficiency or human growth hormone (HGH) antibodies* Action:
Human IGF-1(recombinant DNA origin) Dose: Peds. 0.04–0.08 mg/kg SQ bid;
may ↑ by 0.04 mg/kg per dose to 0.12 mg/kg bid; take w/in 20 min of meal due to
insulin-like hypoglycemic effect Caution: [C,?/M] Contains benzyl alcohol CI:
Closed epiphysis, neoplasia, not for IV Disp: Vial 40 mg SE: Tonsillar hypertro-
phy, ↑ AST, ↑ LDH, HA, Inj site Rxn, V, hypoglycemia Notes: Rapid dose ↑ may
cause hypoglycemia; initial funduscopic exam and during treatment; consider
monitoring glucose until dose stable; limited distribution; rotate Inj site

Mechlorethamine (Mustargen)   WARNING: Highly toxic, handle
w/ care, limit use to experienced physicians; avoid exposure during PRG; vesicant
Uses: *Hodgkin Dz (stages III, IV), cutaneous T-cell lymphoma (mycosis fungoides), lung CA, CML, malignant pleural effusions, CLL, polycythemia vera,*
psoriasis Action: Alkylating agent, nitrogen analog of sulfur mustard Dose: Per
protocol; 0.4 mg/kg single dose or 0.1 mg/kg/d for 4 d, repeat at 4–6-wk intervals;
6 mg/m² IV on days 1 & 8 of 28-d cycle; Intracavitary: 0.2–0.4 mg/kg × 1, may
repeat PRN; Topical: 0.01–0.02% soln, lotion, oint Caution: [D, ?/–] CI: PRG,
known infect Dz, severe myelosuppression Disp: Inj 10 mg; topical soln, lotion,
oint SE: ↓ BM, thrombosis, thrombophlebitis at site; tissue damage w/ extrav (Na
thiosulfate used topically to Rx); N/V/D, skin rash/allergic dermatitis w/ contact,
amenorrhea, sterility (especially in men), secondary leukemia if treated for
Hodgkin Dz, chromosomal alterations, hepatotox, peripheral neuropathy Notes:
Highly volatile and emetogenic; give w/in 30–60 min of preparation

Meclizine (Antivert)(Bonine, Dramamine [OTC])   Uses: *Motion
sickness, vertigo* Action: Antiemetic, anticholinergic, & antihistaminic properties

Dose: *Adults & Peds >12 y: Motion Sickness:* 12.5–25 mg PO 1 h before travel, repeat PRN q12–24h. *Vertigo:* 25–100 mg/d ÷ doses **Caution:** [B, ?/–] NAG, BPH, BOO, elderly, asthma **Disp:** Tabs 12.5, 25, 50 mg; chew tabs 25 mg; caps 25, 30 mg (OTC) **SE:** Drowsiness, xerostomia, blurred vision, thickens bronchial secretions

Medroxyprogesterone (Provera, Depo Provera, Depo-Sub Q Provera)
WARNING: Do not use in the prevention of CV Dz or dementia; ↑ risk MI, stroke, breast CA, PE, & DVT in postmenopausal women (50–79 y). ↑ Dementia risk in postmenopausal women (≥65 y). Risk of significant bone loss **Uses:** *Contraception; secondary amenorrhea; endometrial CA, ↓ endometrial hyperplasia* AUB caused by hormonal imbalance **Action:** Progestin supl **Dose:** *Contraception:* 150 mg IM q3mo depo or 104 mg SQ q3mo (depo SQ). *Secondary amenorrhea:* 5–10 mg/d PO for 5–10 d. *AUB:* 5–10 mg/d PO for 5–10 d beginning on the 16th or 21st d of menstrual cycle. *Endometrial CA:* 400–1000 mg/wk IM. *Endometrial hyperplasia:* 5–10 mg/d × 12–14 d on day 1 or 16 of cycle; ↓ in hepatic Insuff **Caution:** *Provera* [X, –] *Depo Provera* [X, +] **CI:** Thrombophlebitis/embolic disorders, cerebral apoplexy, ↑ LFTs, CA breast/genital organs, undiagnosed Vag bleeding, missed abortion, PRG, as a diagnostic test for PRG **Disp:** *Provera* tabs 2.5, 5, 10 mg; depot Inj 150, 400 mg/mL; depo SQ Inj 104 mg/10.65 mL **SE:** Breakthrough bleeding, spotting, altered menstrual flow, breast tenderness, galactorrhea, depression, insomnia, jaundice, N, wgt gain, acne, hirsutism, vision changes **Notes:** Perform breast exam & Pap smear before contraceptive therapy; obtain PRG test if last Inj >3 mo

Megestrol Acetate (Megace, Megace-ES)
Uses: *Breast/endometrial CAs; appetite stimulant in cachexia (CA & HIV)* **Action:** Hormone; antileuteinizing; progesterone analog **Dose:** *CA:* 40–320 mg/d PO in ÷ doses. *Appetite:* 800 mg/d PO ÷ dose or Megace ES 625 mg/d **Caution:** [X, –] Thromboembolism; handle w/ care **CI:** PRG **Disp:** Tabs 20, 40 mg; susp 40 mg/mL, Megace ES 125 mg/mL **SE:** DVT, edema, menstrual bleeding, photosensitivity, N/V/D, HA, mastodynia, ↑ CA, ↑ glucose, insomnia, rash, ↓ BM, ↑ BP, CP, palpitations, **Notes:** Do not D/C abruptly; Megace ES not equivalent to others mg/mg; Megace ES approved only for anorexia

Meloxicam (Mobic)
WARNING: May ↑ risk of cardiovascular events & GI bleeding; CI in post-op CABG **Uses:** *Osteoarthritis, RA, JRA* **Action:** NSAID w/ ↑ COX-2 activity **Dose:** *Adults.* 7.5–15 mg/d PO. *Peds >2 y:* 0.125 mg/kg/d, max 7.5 mg; take w/ food **Caution:** [C, D (3rd tri) ?/–] w/ Severe renal Insuff, CHF, ACE inhibitor, diuretics, Li²⁺, MTX, warfarin **CI:** Peptic ulcer, NSAID, or ASA sensitivity, PRG, post-op coronary artery bypass graft **Disp:** Tabs 7.5, 15 mg; susp 7.5 mg/5 mL **SE:** HA, dizziness, GI upset, GI bleeding, edema, ↑ BP, renal impair, rash (Stevens-Johnson syndrome), ↑ LFTs

Melphalan [L-PAM] (Alkeran)
WARNING: Administer under the supervision of a qualified physician experienced in the use of chemotherapy; severe BM depression, leukemogenic & mutagenic **Uses:** *Multiple myeloma,

ovarian CAs,* breast & testicular CA, melanoma; allogenic & ABMT (high dose); neuroblastoma, rhabdomyosarcoma **Action:** Alkylating agent, nitrogen mustard **Dose:** *Adults. Multiple myeloma:* 16 mg/m^2 IV q2wk × 4 doses then at 4-wk intervals after tox resolves; w/ renal impair ↓ IV dose 50% or 6 mg PO q day ×2–3 wk, then D/C up to 4 wk, follow counts then 2 mg q day. *Ovarian CA:* 0.2 mg/kg q day × 5 d, repeat q4–5wk based on counts. **Peds.** *Off-label rhabdomyosarcoma:* 10–35 mg/ m^2/dose IV q21–28d. *w/ BMT for Neuroblastoma:* 100–220 mg/m^2/dose IV × 1 or ÷ 2–5 daily doses; Inf over 60 min; ↓ in renal Insuff **Caution:** [D, ?/–] w/ Cisplatin, digitalis, live vaccines **CI:** Allergy or resistance **Disp:** Tabs 2 mg; Inj 50 mg **SE:** N/V, secondary malignancy, a-fib, ↓ LVEF, ↓ BM, secondary leukemia, alopecia, dermatitis, stomatitis, pulm fibrosis; rare allergic Rxns **Notes:** Take PO on empty stomach, false (+) direct Coombs test

Memantine (Namenda)
Uses: *Mod/severe Alzheimer Dz,* mild–mod vascular dementia, mild cognitive impair **Action:** *N*-methyl-D-aspartate receptor antagonist **Dose:** Target 20 mg/d, start 5 mg/d, ↑ to 10 mg/d to 20 mg/d, wait >1 wk before ↑ dose; use ÷ doses if >5 mg/d. *Vascular dementia:* 10 mg PO bid; w/ severe renal impair **Caution:** [B, ?/–] Hepatic/mild–mod renal impair; Sx disorders **Disp:** Tabs 5, 10 mg, combo pak: 5 mg × 28 + 10 mg × 21; sol 2 mg/mL **SE:** Dizziness, confusion, HA, V, constipation, coughing, ↑ BP, pain, somnolence, hallucinations **Notes:** Renal clearance ↓ by alkaline urine (↓ 80% at pH 8)

Meningococcal conjugate vaccine (Menactra, MCV4)
Uses: *Immunize against Neisseria meningitidis* (meningococcus) 2–55 y* **Action:** Active immunization; diphtheria toxoid conjugate of *N. meningitidis* A, C, Y, W-135 **Dose:** *Adults 18–55 y & Peds ≥2 y:* 0.5 mL IM × 1 **Caution:** [C, ?/–] w/ Immunosuppression **CI:** Allergy to class/compound/latex; Guillain-Barré **Disp:** Inj **SE:** Local Inj site Rxns, HA, N/V, anorexia, fatigue, arthralgia, Guillain-Barré **Notes:** IM only; keep epi available for Rxns; use polysaccharide vaccine if >55 y; do not confuse w/ Menomune (MPSV4); ACIP recommends MCV4 for 2–55 y, but 2–10 may have ↑ Rxn compared to Menomune; peds 2–10 previously vaccinated w/ MPSV4 remain at ↑ risk for meningococcal Dz; ACIP recommends vaccinate w/ MCV4 3–5 y after MPSV4

Meningococcal Polysaccharide Vaccine [MPSV4] (Menomune A/C/Y/ W-135)
Uses: *Immunize against Neisseria meningitidis* (meningococcus)* **Action:** Active immunization **Dose:** *Adults & Peds >2 y:* 0.5 mL SQ (not IM, intradermally, IV); may repeat 3–5 y if high risk **Caution:** [C, ?/–] w/ Immunocompromised **CI:** Thimerosal/latex/sensitivity; w/ pertussis or typhoid vaccine, <2 y **Disp:** Inj **SE:** SQ only; local Inj site Rxns, HA **Notes:** Keep epi (1:1000) available for Rxns. OK in 2–10 y, but considered alternative to MCV4 in 11–54 y. Preferred in >55 y; active against serotypes A, C, Y, & W-135 but not group B; high risk need revaccination q3–5y (use MCV4)

Meperidine (Demerol, Meperitab) [C–II]
Uses: *Mod–severe pain,* postoperative shivering, rigors form amphotericin B **Action:** Narcotic analgesic

Dose: *Adults.* 50–150 mg PO or IV/IM/SQ q3–4h PRN. *Peds.* 1–1.5 mg/kg/dose PO or IM/SQ q3–4h PRN, up to 100 mg/dose; ↓ in elderly/hepatic impair, avoid in renal impair **Caution:** [C/D] (prolonged use or high dose at term), +] ↓ Sz threshold, adrenal Insuff, head injury, ↑ ICP, hepatic impair, not ok in sickle cell Dz **CI:** w/ MAOIs, renal failure, PRG **Disp:** Tabs 50, 100 mg; syrup/soln 50 mg/5 mL; Inj 10, 25, 50, 75, 100 mg/mL **SE:** Resp/CNS depression, Szs, sedation, constipation, ↓ BP, rash N/V, biliary and urethral spasms, dyspnea **Notes:** Analgesic effects potentiated w/ hydroxyzine; 75 mg IM = 10 mg morphine IM; not best in elderly; do not use oral for acute pain; not ok for repetitive use in ICU setting

Meprobamate (various) [C-IV]
Uses: *Short-term relief of anxiety* muscle spasm, TMJ relief **Action:** Mild tranquilizer; antianxiety **Dose:** *Adults.* 400 mg PO tid-qid, max 2400 mg/d. *Peds 6–12 y:* 100–200 mg PO bid-tid; ↓ in renal/liver impair **Caution:** [D, +/–] Elderly, Sz Dz **CI:** NAG, porphyria, PRG **Disp:** Tabs 200, 400 mg **SE:** Drowsiness, syncope, tachycardia, edema, rash (Stevens-Johnson syndrome), N/V/D, ↓ WBC, agranulocytosis **Notes:** Do not abruptly D/C

Mercaptopurine [6-MP] (Purinethol)
Uses: *ALL* 2nd-line Rx for CML & NHL, maint ALL in children, immunosuppressant w/ autoimmune Dzs (Crohn Dz, ulcerative colitis) **Action:** Antimetabolite, mimics hypoxanthine **Dose:** *Adults.* ALL induction: 1.5–2.5 mg/kg/d; *maint* 80–100 mg/m²/d or 2.5–5 mg/kg/d; w/ allopurinol use 67–75% ↓ dose of 6-MP (interference w/ xanthine oxidase metabolism). *Peds.* ALL induction: 2.5–5 mg/kg/d PO or 70–100 mg/m²/d *maint* 1.5–2.5 mg/kg/d PO or 50–75 mg/m²/d q day; ↓ w/ renal/hepatic Insuff; take on empty stomach **Caution:** [D, ?] w/ Allopurinol, immunosuppression, TMP-SMX, warfarin, salicylates **CI:** Prior resistance, severe hepatic Dz, BM suppression, PRG **Disp:** Tabs 50 mg **SE:** Mild hematotox, mucositis, stomatitis, D rash, fever, eosinophilia, jaundice, hep, hyperuricemia, hyperpigmentation, alopecia **Notes:** Handle properly; limit use to experienced physicians; ensure adequate hydration; for ALL, evening dosing may ↓ risk of relapse; low emetogenicity

Meropenem (Merrem)
Uses: *Intra-Abd Infxns, bacterial meningitis, skin Infxn* **Action:** Carbapenem; ↓ cell wall synth. *Spectrum:* Excellent gram(+) (except MRSA, methicillin-resistant *S. epidermidis* [MRSE] & *E. faecium*); excellent gram(–) including extended-spectrum β-lactamase producers; good anaerobic **Dose:** *Adults. Abd Infxn:* 1 to 2 g IV q8h. *Skin Infxn:* 50 mg IV q8h. *Meningitis:* 2 g IV q8h. *Peds ≥3 mo, <50 kg: Abd Infxn:* 20 mg/kg IV q8h. *Skin Infxn:* 20 mg/kg IV q8h. *Meningitis:* 40 mg/kg IV q8h; *Peds >50 kg:* Use adult dose; max 2 g IV q8h; ↓ in renal Insuff (see insert) **Caution:** [B, ?] w/ Probenecid, VPA **CI:** β-Lactam sensitivity **Disp:** Inj 1 g, 500 mg **SE:** Less Sz potential than imipenem; *C. difficile* enterocolitis, D, ↓ plt **Notes:** Overuse ↑ bacterial resistance

Mesalamine (Asacol, Canasa, Lialda, Pentasa, Rowasa)
Uses: *Rectal: mild–mod distal ulcerative colitis, proctosigmoiditis, proctitis; oral:

treat/maint of mild-mod ulcerative colitis* **Action:** 5-ASA derivative, may inhibit prostaglandins, may ↓ leukotrienes and TNF-α **Dose:** *Rectal:* 60 mL qhs, retain 8 h (enema), 500 mg bid-tid or 1000 mg qhs (supp) *PO:* Caps: 1 g PO qid; tab: 1.6–2.4 g/d ÷ doses (tid-qid); DR 2.4–4.8 g PO daily 8 wk max, do not cut/crush/chew w/food; ↓ initial dose in elderly **Caution:** [B, M] W/ Digitalis, PUD, pyloric stenosis, renal Insuff, elderly **CI:** Salicylate sensitivity **Disp:** Tabs ER (*Asacol*) 400, 800 mg; ER caps (*Pentasa*) 250, 500 mg; DR tab (*Lialda*) 1.2 g; supp 500, (*Canasa*) 1000 mg; (*Rowasa*) rectal-susp 4 g/60 mL **SE:** Yellow-brown urine, HA, malaise, Abd pain, flatulence, rash, pancreatitis, pericarditis, dizziness, rectal pain, hair loss, intolerance syndrome (bloody D) **Notes:** retain rectally 1–3 h; ✓ CBC, Cr, BUN; Sx may ↑ when starting

Mesna (Mesnex) **Uses:** *Prevent hemorrhagic cystitis due to ifosfamide or cyclophosphamide* **Action:** Antidote, reacts with acrolein and other metabolites to form stable compounds **Dose:** Per protocol; dose as % of ifosfamide or cyclophosphamide dose. *IV bolus:* 20% (eg, 10–12 mg/kg) IV at 0, 4, & 8 h, then 40% at 0, 1, 4, & 7 h; *IV Inf:* 20% prechemotherapy, 50–100% w/ chemotherapy, then 25–50% for 12 h following chemotherapy; *Oral:* 100% ifosfamide dose given as 20% IV at hour 0 then 40% PO at hours 4 & 8; if PO dose vomited repeat or give dose IV; mix PO w/ juice **Caution:** [B; ?/–] **CI:** Thiol sensitivity **Disp:** Inj 100 mg/mL; tabs 400 mg **SE:** ↓ BP, ↓ plt, ↑ HR, ↑ RR allergic Rxns, HA, GI upset, taste perversion **Notes:** Hydration helps ↓ hemorrhagic cystitis; higher dose for BMT; IV contains benzyl alcohol

Metaproterenol (Alupent, Metaprel) **Uses:** *Asthma & reversible bronchospasm, COPD* **Action:** Sympathomimetic bronchodilator **Dose:** *Adults.* *Nebulized:* 5% 2.5 mL q4–6h or PRN. *MDI:* 1–3 Inh q3–4h, 12 Inh max/24 h; wait 2 min between Inh. *PO:* 20 mg q6–8h. *Peds ≥12 y:* MDI: 2–3 Inh q3–4h, 12 Inh/d max. *Nebulizer:* 2.5 mL (soln 0.4%, 0.6%) tid-qid, up to q4h. *Peds >9 y or <60 lbs:* 20 mg PO tid-qid; *6–9 yo or <60 lbs:* 10 mg PO tid-qid; ↓ in elderly **Caution:** [C, ?/–] w/ MAOI, TCA, sympathomimetics; avoid w/ β-blockers **CI:** Tachycardia, other arrhythmias **Disp:** Aerosol 0.65 mg/Inh; soln for Inh 0.4%, 0.6%; tabs 10, 20 mg; syrup 10 mg/5 mL **SE:** Nervousness, tremor, tachycardia, HTN, ↑ glucose, ↓ K⁺, ↑ IOP **Notes:** Fewer β₁ effects than isoproterenol & longer acting, but not a 1st-line β-agonist. Use w/ face mask <4 y; oral ↑ ADR

Metaxalone (Skelaxin) **Uses:** *Painful musculoskeletal conditions* **Action:** Centrally acting skeletal muscle relaxant **Dose:** 800 mg PO tid-qid **Caution:** [C, ?/–] w/ Elderly, EtOH & CNS depression anemia **CI:** Severe hepatic/renal impair; drug-induced, hemolytic, or other anemias **Disp:** Tabs 800 mg **SE:** N/V, HA, drowsiness, hep

Metformin (Glucophage, Glucophage XR) **WARNING:** Associated w/ lactic acidosis **Uses:** *Type 2 DM,* polycystic ovary syndrome (PCOS) HIV lipodystrophy **Action:** Biguanide; ↓ hepatic glucose production & intestinal absorption of glucose; ↑ insulin sensitivity **Dose:** *Adults.* Initial: 500 mg PO bid;

or 850 mg daily, titrate 1–2-wk intervals may ↑ to 2550 mg/d max; take w/ A.M. & P.M. meals; can convert total daily dose to daily dose of XR. *Peds 10–16 y:* 500 mg PO bid, ↑ 500 mg/wk to 2000 mg/d max in ÷ doses; do not use XR formulation in peds **Caution:** [B, +/–] Avoid EtOH; hold dose before & 48 h after ionic contrast; hepatic impair, elderly **CI:** SCr >1.4 in females or >1.5 in males; hypoxemic conditions (eg, acute CHF/sepsis); metabolic acidosis **Disp:** Tabs 500, 850, 1000 mg; XR tabs 500, 750, 1000 mg; soln 100 mg/mL **SE:** Anorexia, N/V/D, flatulence, weakness, myalgia, rash

Methadone (Dolophine, Methadose) [C-II]   WARNING: Deaths
reported during initiation and conversion of pain pts to methadone Rx from Rx w/other opioids. Resp depression and QT prolongation, arrhythmias observed. Only dispensed by certified opioid treatment programs for addiction. Analgesic use must outweigh risks **Uses:** *Severe pain not responsive to nonnarcotics; detox w/ maint of narcotic addiction* **Action:** Narcotic analgesic **Dose:** *Adults.* 2.5–10 mg IM/IV/SQ q8–12h or 5–15 mg PO q8h; titrate as needed; see insert for conversion from other opioids. *Peds.*(Not FDA approved) 0.1 mg/kg q4–12h IV; ↑ slowly to avoid resp depression; ↓ in renal impair **Caution:** [C, –] Avoid w/ severe liver Dz **CI:** Resp depression, acute asthma, ileus **Disp:** Tabs 5, 10 mg; tab dispersible 40 mg; PO soln 5, 10 mg/5 mL; PO conc 10 mg/mL; Inj 10 mg/mL **SE:** Resp depression, sedation, constipation, urinary retention, ↑ QT interval, arrhythmias, ↓ HR, syncope, ↓ K+, ↓ Mg2+ **Notes:** Parenteral:oral 1:2; Equianalgesic w/ parenteral morphine; longer half-life; resp depression occurs later an lasts longer than analgesic effect, use w/caution to avoid iatrogenic OD

Methenamine Hippurate (Hiprex) Methenamine Mandelate (UROQUID-Acid No. 2)   **Uses:** *Suppress recurrent UTI long-term. Use
only after infxn cleared by antibiotics* **Action:** Converted to formaldehyde & ammonia in acidic urine; nonspecific bactericidal action **Dose:** *Adults.* Hippurate: 1 g PO bid. *Mandelate:* initial 1 g qid PO pc & hs, maint 1–2 g/d. *Peds 6–12 y: Hippurate:* 0.5–1 g PO bid PO ÷ bid. *>2 y: Mandelate:* 50–75 mg/kg/d PO ÷ qid; take w/ food, ascorbic acid w/hydration **Caution:** [C, +] **CI:** Renal Insuff, severe hepatic Dz, & severe dehydration **Disp:** *Methenamine hippurate* (Hiprex, Urex): Tabs 1 g. *Methenamine mandelate:* 500 mg, 1 g EC tabs **SE:** Rash, GI upset, dysuria, ↑ LFTs, superinfection w/ prolonged use, *C. difficile*-associated diarrhea. **Notes:** Use w/ sulfonamides may precipitate in urine. Hippurate not indicated in peds <6 y. Not for pts w/ indwelling catheters as dwell time required for action

Methimazole (Tapazole)   **Uses:** *Hyperthyroidism, thyrotoxicosis,*
preparation for thyroid surgery or radiation **Action:** Blocks T_3 & T_4 formation, but does not inactivate circulating T_3, T_4 **Dose:** *Adults.* Initial based on severity: 15–60 mg/d PO q8h. *Maint:* 5–15 mg PO daily. *Peds.* Initial: 0.4–0.7 mg/kg/24 h PO q8h. *Maint:* 1/3–2/3 of initial dose PO daily; take w/ food **Caution:** [D, –] w/ Other meds **CI:** Breast-feeding **Disp:** Tabs 5, 10, 20 mg **SE:** GI upset, dizziness,

blood dyscrasias, dermatitis, fever, hepatic Rxns, lupus-like syndrome **Notes:** Follow clinically & w/ TFT, CBC w/ diff

Methocarbamol (Robaxin)

Uses: *Relief of discomfort associated w/ painful musculoskeletal conditions* **Action:** Centrally acting skeletal muscle relaxant **Dose:** *Adults & Peds >16 y:* 1.5 g PO qid for 2–3 d, then 1-g PO qid maint. *Tetanus:* 1–2 g IV q6h × 3 d, then use PO. *<16 y:* 15 mg/kg/dose or 500 mg/m² IV, may repeat PRN (tetanus only), max 1.8 g/m²/d × 3 d **Caution:** Sz disorders [C, +] **CI:** MyG, renal impair w/IV **Disp:** Tabs 500, 750 mg; Inj 100 mg/mL **SE:** Can discolor urine, lightheadedness, drowsiness, GI upset, ↓ HR, ↓ BP **Note:** Tabs can be crushed and added to NG, do not operate heavy machinery

Methotrexate (Rheumatrex Dose Pack, Trexall) WARNING:

Administration only by experienced physician; do not use in women of childbearing age unless absolutely necessary (teratogenic); impaired elimination w/ impaired renal Fxn, ascites, pleural effusion; severe ↓ BM w/ NSAIDs; hepatotoxic, occasionally fatal; can induce life-threatening pneumonitis; D and ulcerative stomatitis require D/C; lymphoma risk; may cause tumor lysis syndrome; can cause severe skin Rxn, opportunistic Infxns; w/ RT can ↑ tissue necrosis risk. Preservatives make this agent unsuitable for intrathecal or higher dose use **Uses:** *ALL, AML, leukemic meningitis, trophoblastic tumors (choriocarcinoma, hydatidiform mole), breast, lung, head, & neck CAs, Burkitt lymphoma, mycosis fungoides, osteosarcoma, Hodgkin Dz & NHL, psoriasis; RA, JRA,* chronic Dz **Action:** ↓ Dihydrofolate reductase-mediated prod of tetrahydrofolate, causes ↓ DNA synth **Dose:** *Adults. CA:* Per protocol. *RA:* 7.5 mg/wk PO 1/wk 1 or 2.5 mg q12h PO for 3 doses/wk. *Psoriasis:* 2.5–5 mg PO q12h × 3d/wk or 10–25 mg PO/IM q wk. *Chronic:* 15–25 mg IM/SQ q wk, then 15 mg/wk. *Peds.* 10 mg/m² PO/IM q wk, then 5–14 mg/m² × 1 or as 3 ÷ divided doses 12 h apart; ↓ elderly, w/ renal/hepatic impair **Caution:** [D, –] w/ Other nephro-/hepatotoxic meds, multiple interactions, w/Sz, profound ↓ BM w/ CA related **CI:** Severe renal/hepatic impair, PRG/lactation **Disp:** Dose pack 2.5 mg in 8, 12, 16, 20, or 24 doses; tabs 2.5, 5, 7.5, 10, 15 mg; Inj 25 mg/mL; Inj powder 20 mg, 1 g **SE:** ↓ BM, N/V/D, anorexia, mucositis, hepatotox (transient & reversible; may progress to atrophy, necrosis, fibrosis, cirrhosis), rashes, dizziness, malaise, blurred vision, alopecia, photosensitivity, renal failure, pneumonitis; rare pulm fibrosis; chemical arachnoiditis & HA w/ IT delivery **Notes:** Monitor CBC, LFTs, Cr, MTX levels & chest x-ray (CXR); "high dose" >500 mg/m² require leucovorin rescue to ↓ tox; w/ intrathecal, use preservative-/alcohol-free soln; systemic levels: *Therapeutic:* >0.01 micromole; *Toxic* >10 micromoles over 24 h

Methyldopa (Aldomet)

Uses: *HTN* **Action:** Centrally acting antihypertensive, ↓ sympathetic outflow **Dose:** *Adults.* 250–500 mg PO bid-tid (max 2–3 g/d) or 250 mg–1 g IV q6–8h. *Peds Neonates:* 2.5–5 mg/kg PO q8h. *Other peds:* 10 mg/kg/24 h PO in 2–3 ÷ doses or 5–10 mg/kg/dose IV q6–8h to max 65 mg/kg/24 h; ↓ in renal Insuff/elderly **Caution:** [B(PO), C(IV), +] **CI:** Liver Dz, w/ MAOIs, bisulfate allergy **Disp:** Tabs 250, 500 mg; Inj 50 mg/mL **SE:** Discolors urine; initial transient sedation/drowsiness, edema, hemolytic anemia, hepatic disorders, fevers, nightmares **Notes:** tolerance may occur, false (+) Coombs test

Methylergonovine (Methergine)   Uses: *Postpartum bleeding (atony, hemorrhage)* **Action:** Ergotamine derivative, rapid and sustained uterotonic effect **Dose:** 0.2 mg IM after anterior shoulder delivery or puerperium, may repeat in 2–4-h intervals or 0.2–0.4 mg PO q6–12h for 2–7 d **Caution:** [C, ?] w/ Sepsis, obliterative vascular Dz, hepatic/renal impair, w/ CYP3A4 inhibitors (Table 11) **CI:** HTN, PRG, toxemia **Disp:** Inj 0.2 mg/mL; tabs 0.2 mg **SE:** HTN, N/V, CP, ↓ BP, Sz **Notes:** Give IV only if absolutely necessary over >1 min w/ BP monitoring

Methylnaltrexone bromide (Relistor)   Uses: *Opioid-induced constipation in pt w/ advanced illness such as CA* **Action:** Peripheral opioid antagonist **Dose:** *Adults.* Wgt-based *<38 kg/>114 kg:* 0.15 mg/kg SQ; *38–61 kg:* 8 mg SQ; *62–114 kg:* 12 mg SQ, dose q other day PRN, max 1 dose q24h **Caution:** [B, NR] w/ CrCl <30 mL/min ↓ dose 50% **Disp:** Inj 12 mg/0.6 mL **SE:** N/D, Abd pain, dizziness **Notes:** Does not effect opioid analgesic effects or induce withdrawal

Methylphenidate, oral (Concerta, Metadate CD, Methylin Ritalin, Ritalin LA, Ritalin SR, others) [CII]   WARNING: w/ Hx of drug or alcohol dependence, avoid abrupt D/C; chronic use can lead to dependence or psychotic behavior; observe closely during withdrawal of drug **Uses:** *ADHD, narcolepsy,* *depression* **Action:** CNS stimulant, blocks reuptake of norepinephrine and DA **Dose:** *Adults. Narcolepsy:* 10 mg PO 2–3×/d, 60 mg/d max. *Depression:* 2.5 mg q A.M.; ↑ slowly, 20 mg/d max, ÷ bid 7 A.M. & 12 P.M.; use regular release only. *Adults and Peds >6 y: ADHD: IR:* 5–10 mg/d to 60 mg/d, max (2 mg/kg/d); *ER/SR* use total IR dose q day. *CD/LA* 20 mg PO q A.M., ↑ 10–20 mg q wk to 60 mg/d max. *Concerta:* 18 mg PO q A.M. Rx naïve or already on 20 mg/d, 36 mg PO q A.M. if on 40 mg/d or 54 mg PO q A.M. if on 60 mg/d **Caution:** [C, +/–] w/ Hx EtOH/drug abuse, CV Dz, HTN, bipolar Dz, Sz; separate from MAOIs by 14 d **Disp:** Chew tabs 2.5, 5, 10 mg; tabs scored IR (*Ritalin*) 5, 10, 20 mg; Caps ER (*Ritalin LA*) 10, 20, 30, 40 mg. Caps ER (*Metadate CD*) 10, 20, 30, 40, 50, 60 mg (*Methylin ER*) 10, 20 mg. Tabs SR (*Ritalin SR*) 20 mg; ER tabs (*Concerta*) 18, 27, 36, 54 mg. Oral soln 5, 10 mg/5 mL **SE:** CV/CNS stimulation, growth retard, GI upset, pancytopenia, ↑ LFTs **CI:** Marked anxiety, tension, agitation, NAG, motor tics, family Hx or diagnosis of Tourette syndrome, severe HTN, angina, arrhythmias, CHF, recent MI, ↑ thyroid; w/ or w/in 14 d of MAOI **Notes:** See also transdermal form; titrate dose; take 30–45 min ac; do not chew or crush; *Concerta* "ghost tablet" in stool, avoid w/ GI narrowing; Metadate contains sucrose, avoid w/ lactose/galactose problems. Do not use these meds w/ halogenated anesthetics; abuse and diversion concerns; AHA recommends all ADHD peds need Cv assessment and consideration for ECG before Rx

Methylphenidate, transdermal (Daytrana) [CII]   WARNING: w/ Hx of drug or alcohol dependence; chronic use can lead to dependence or psychotic behavior; observe closely during withdrawal of drug **Uses:** *ADHD in children 6–12 y* **Action:** CNS stimulant, blocks reuptake of norepinephrine and DA **Dose:** *Adults & Peds ≥6 y:* Apply to hip in A.M. (2 h before desired effect), remove 9 h later; titrate 1st wk 10 mg/9 h, 2nd wk 15 mg/9 h, 3rd wk 20 mg/9 h, 4th wk 30 mg/9 h **Caution:** [C, +/–] See methylphenidate, oral sensitization may preclude subsequent use of oral forms; abuse and diversion concerns **Disp:** Patches 10, 15, 20, 30 mg **SE:** Local Rxns, N/V, nasopharyngitis, ↓ wgt, ↓ appetite, lability, insomnia, tic **Notes:** Titrate dose weekly; effects last hours after removal; evaluate BP, HR at baseline and periodically; avoid heat exposure to patch, may cause OD, AHA recommends all ADHD peds need CV assessment and consideration for ECG before Rx

Methylprednisolone (Solu-Medrol) [See Steroids page 214 and Table 3]

Metoclopramide (Reglan, Clopra, Octamide) **Uses:** *Diabetic gastroparesis, symptomatic GERD; chemotherapy & post-op N/V, facilitate small-bowel intubation & upper GI radiologic evaluation;* *stimulate gut in prolonged post-op ileus* **Action:** ↑ Upper GI motility; blocks dopamine in chemoreceptor trigger zone, sensitized tissues to ACH **Dose:** *Adults. Gastroparesis:* 10 mg PO 30 min ac & hs for 2–8 wk PRN, or same dose IM/IV for 10 d, then PO. *Reflux:* 10–15 mg PO 30 min ac & hs. *Chemotherapy Antiemetic:* 1–3 mg/kg/dose IV 30 min before chemotherapy, then q2h × 2 doses, then q3h × 3 doses. *Post-op:* 10–20 mg IV/IM q4–6h PRN. *Adults & Peds >14 y: Intestinal intubation:* 10 mg IV × 1 over 1–2 min. *Peds. Reflux:* 0.1 mg/kg/dose PO 30 min ac & hs, max 0.3–0.75 mg/kg/d × 2 wk–6 mo. *Chemotherapy Antiemetic:* 1–2 mg/kg/dose IV as adults. *Post-op:* 0.25 mg/kg IV q6–8h PRN. *Peds intestinal intubation:* **6–14 y:** 2.5–5 mg IV × 1 over 1–2 min; *<6 y:* use 0.1 mg/kg IV × 1 **Caution:** [B, –] Drugs w/ extrapyramidal ADRs, MAOIs, TCAs, sympathomimetics **CI:** EPS meds, GI bleeding, pheochromocytoma, Sz disorders, GI obst **Disp:** Tabs 5, 10 mg; syrup 5 mg/5 mL; Inj 5 mg/mL **SE:** Dystonic Rxns common w/ high doses (Rx w/IV diphenhydramine), fluid retention, restlessness, D, drowsiness

Metolazone (Zaroxolyn) **Uses:** *Mild–mod essential HTN & edema of renal Dz or cardiac failure* **Action:** Thiazide-like diuretic; ↓ distal tubule Na reabsorption **Dose:** *HTN:* 2.5–5 mg PO maint 5–20 mg PO q day *Edema:* 2.5–20 mg/d PO. **Caution:** [D, +] Avoid w/ Li, gout, digitalis, SLE, many interactions **CI:** Anuria, hepatic coma or precoma, sulfa *allergy* **Disp:** Tabs 2.5, 5, 10 mg **SE:** Monitor fluid/lytes; dizziness, ↓ BP, ↓ K⁺, ↑ HR, ↑ uric acid, CP, photosensitivity

Metoprolol Tartrate (Lopressor) Metoprolol Succinate (Toprol XL) **WARNING:** Do not acutely stop therapy as marked worsening of angina can result; taper over 1–2 wk **Uses:** *HTN, angina, AMI, CHF (XL form)* **Action:** β₁-Adrenergic receptor blocker **Dose:** *Adults. Angina:* 50–200 mg PO bid max 400 mg/d; ER form dose q day. *HTN:* 50–200 mg PO bid max 450 mg/d, ER form dose q day. *AMI:* 5 mg IV q2min × 3 doses, then 50 mg PO q6h × 48 h,

then 100 mg PO bid. *CHF: (XL form preferred)* 12.5–25 mg/d PO × 2 wk, ↑ 2-wk intervals, 200 mg/max, use low dose w/ greatest severity; 5 mg slow IV q5min, total 15 mg *(ECC 2005)*. *Peds 1–17 y: HTN* IR form 1–2 mg/kg/d PO, max 6 mg/kg/d (200 mg/d). *≥6 y: HTN* ER form 1 mg/kg/d PO, initial max 50 mg/d, ↑ PRN to 2 mg/kg/d max; ↓ w/ hepatic failure; take w/ meals **Caution:** [C, +] Uncompensated CHF, bradycardia, heart block, hepatic impair, MyG, Raynaud, thyrotoxicosis **CI:** For HTN/angina SSS (unless paced), severe PVD, pheochromocytoma. For MI sinus brady <45 BPM, 1st-degree block (PR >0.24 s), 2nd-, 3rd-degree block, SBP <100 mm Hg, severe CHF, cardiogenic shock **Disp:** Tabs 25, 50, 100 mg; ER tabs 25, 50, 100, 200 mg; Inj 1 mg/mL **SE:** Drowsiness, insomnia, ED, bradycardia, bronchospasm **Notes:** IR:ER 1:1 daily dose but ER/XL is q day. OK to split XL tab but do not crush/chew

Metronidazole (Flagyl, MetroGel)   **WARNING:** Carcinogenic in rats
Uses: *Bone/joint, endocarditis, intra-Abd, meningitis, & skin Infxns; amebiasis and amebic liver abscess; trichomoniasis in pt and partner; bacterial vaginosis; PID; giardiasis; antibiotic associated pseudomembranous colitis (C. difficile), eradicate H. pylori w/ combo therapy, rosacea, prophylactic in post-op colorectal surgery* **Action:** Interferes w/ DNA synth. **Spectrum:** Excellent anaerobic, C. difficile **Dose:** *Adults. Anaerobic Infxns:* 500 mg IV q6–8h. *Amebic dysentery:* 500–750 mg PO q8h × 5–10 d. *Trichomonas:* 250 mg PO tid for 7 d or 2 g PO × 1 (Rx partner). *C. difficile:* 500 mg PO or IV q8h for 7–10 d (PO preferred; IV only if pt NPO), if no response, change to PO vancomycin. *Vaginosis:* 1 applicator intravag q day or bid × 5 d, or 500 mg PO bid × 7 d or 750 mg PO q day × 7 d. *Acne rosacea/skin:* Apply bid. *Giardia:* 500 mg PO bid × 5–7 d. *H. pylori:* 250–500 mg PO w/ meals & hs × 14 d, combine w/ other antibiotic & a proton pump inhibitor or H_2 antagonist. *Peds.* 30 mg/kg PO/IV/d divided q6H, 4 g/d max ÷. *Amebic dysentery:* 35–50 mg/kg/24 h PO in 3 ÷ doses for 5–10 d; Rx 7–10 d for C. difficile. *Trichomonas:* 15–30 mg/kg/d PO ÷ q8h × 7 d. *C. difficile:* 20 mg/kg/d PO ÷ q6h × 10 d, max 2 g/d; ↓ w/ severe hepatic/renal impair **Caution:** [B, +/–] Avoid EtOH, w/ warfarin, CYP3A4 substrates (Table 11), ↑ Li levels **CI:** First tri of PRG **Disp:** Tabs 250, 500 mg; XR tabs 750 mg; caps 375 mg; IV 500 mg/100 mL; lotion 0.75%; gel 0.75, 1%; intravag gel 0.75% (5 g/applicator 37.5 mg in 70-g tube), cream 0.75,1% **SE:** Disulfiram-like Rxn; dizziness, HA, GI upset, anorexia, urine discoloration, flushing, metallic taste **Notes:** For trichomoniasis, Rx pt's partner; no aerobic bacteria activity; use in combo w/ serious mixed Infxns; wait 24 h after 1st dose to breast-feed or 48 h if extended therapy, take ER on empty stomach

Mexiletine (Mexitil)   **WARNING:** Mortality risks noted for flecainide and/or encainide (type 1 antiarrhythmics). Reserve for use in pts with life-threatening ventricular arrhythmias **Uses:** *Suppress symptomatic vent arrhythmias* DN **Action:** Class IB antiarrhythmic (Table 10) **Dose:** *Adults.* 200–300 mg PO q8h. Initial 200 mg q8h, can load w/ 400 mg if needed, ↑ q2–3d, 1200 mg/d max. **Caution:** [C, +] CHF, may worsen severe arrhythmias; interacts w/ hepatic inducers

& suppressors **CI:** Cardiogenic shock or 2nd-/3rd-degree AV block w/o pacemaker **Disp:** Caps 150, 200, 250 mg **SE:** Light-headedness, dizziness, anxiety, incoordination, GI upset, ataxia, hepatic damage, blood dyscrasias, PVCs, N/V, tremor **Notes:** ↓ LFTs, CBC, false (+) ANA

Miconazole (Monistat 1 Combo, Monistat 3, Monistat 7)[OTC] (Monistat-Derm) Uses: *Candidal Infxns, dermatomycoses (tinea pedis/ tinea cruris/tinea corporis/tinea versicolor/Candidiasis)* **Action:** Azole antifungal, alters fungal membrane permeability **Dose:** *Intravag:* 100 mg supp or 2% cream intravag qhs × 7 d or 200 mg supp or 4% cream intravag qhs × 3 d. *Derm:* Apply bid, A.M./P.M.. *Tinea versicolor:* Apply q day. Treat tinea pedis for 1 mo and other Infxns for 2 wk. **Peds ≥12 y:** 100 mg supp or 2% cream intravag qhs × 7 d or 200 mg supp or 4% cream intravag qhs × 3 d **Caution:** [C, ?] Azole sensitivity **Disp:** *Monistat-Derm:* (Rx) cream 2%; *Monistat 1 Combo:* 2% cream w/ 1200 mg supp, *Monistat 3:* Vag cream 4%, supp 200 mg; *Monistat 7:* cream 2%, supp 100 mg; lotion 2%; powder 2%; effervescent tab 2%; oint 2%; spray 2%; Vag supp 100, 200, 1200 mg; Vag cream 2%, 4%; [OTC] **SE:** Vag burning; on skin contact dermatitis, irritation, burning **Notes:** May interfere w/ condom and diaphragm, do not use w/ tampons

Miconazole/zinc oxide/petrolatum (Vusion) Uses: *Candidal diaper rash* **Action:** Combo antifungal **Dose:** *Peds >4 wk:* Apply at each diaper change × 7 d **Caution:** [C, ?] **CI:** None **Disp:** Miconazole/zinc oxide/petrolatum oint 0.25/15/81.35%, 50-, 90- g tube **SE:** None **Notes:** Keep diaper dry, not for prevention

Midazolam (various) [C-IV] **WARNING:** Associated w/ resp depression and resp arrest especially when used for sedation in noncritical care settings. Reports of airway obst, desaturation, hypoxia, and apnea w/ other CNS depressants. Cont monitoring required Uses: *Pre-op sedation, conscious sedation for short procedures & mechanically ventilated pts, induction of general anesthesia* **Action:** Short-acting benzodiazepine **Dose:** *Adults.* 1–5 mg IV or IM or 0.02–0.35 mg/kg based on indication; titrate to effect. *Peds.* Pre-op: *>6 mo:* 0.25–1 mg/kg PO, 20 mg max. *Conscious sedation:* 0.08 mg/kg × 1. *>6 mo:* 0.1–0.15 mg/kg IM × 1 max 10 mg. *General anesthesia:* 0.025–0.1 mg/kg IV q2min for 1–3 doses PRN to induce anesthesia (↓ in elderly, w/ narcotics or CNS depressants) **Caution:** [D, +/–] w/ CYP3A4 substrate (Table 11), multiple drug interactions **CI:** NAG; w/ amprenavir, atazanavir, nelfinavir, ritonavir **Disp:** Inj 1, 5 mg/mL; syrup 2 mg/mL **SE:** Resp depression; ↓ BP w/ conscious sedation, N **Notes:** Reversal w/ flumazenil; monitor for resp depression; not for epidural/intrathecal use

Mifepristone [RU 486] (Mifeprex) **WARNING:** Pt counseling & information required; associated w/ fatal Infxns & bleeding Uses: *Terminate intrauterine pregnancies of <49 d* **Action:** Antiprogestin; ↑ prostaglandins, results in uterine contraction **Dose:** Administered w/ 3 office visits: Day 1: 600 mg PO × 1; day 3, unless abortion confirmed, 400 mcg PO of misoprostol (*Cytotec*); about day 14, verify termination of PRG. Surgical termination if therapy fails. **Caution:** [X, –] w/ Infxn, sepsis **CI:** Ectopic pregnancy, undiagnosed adnexal mass, w/ IUD, adrenal failure, w/ long-term steroid therapy, hemorrhagic Dz, w/ anticoagulants, prostaglandin hypersensitivity. Pts who do not have access to medical facilities or unable to understand treatment or comply. **Disp:** Tabs 200 mg **SE:** Abd pain & 1–2 wk of uterine bleeding, N/V/D, HA **Notes:** Under physician's supervision only, 9–16 d Vag bleed on average after using

Miglitol (Glyset) Uses: *Type 2 DM* Action: α-Glucosidase inhibitor; delays carbohydrate digestion of **Dose:** Initial 25 mg PO tid; maint 50–100 mg tid (w/ 1st bite of each meal), titrate over 4–8 wk **Caution:** [B, –] w/ Digitalis & digestive enzymes **CI:** DKA, obstructive/inflammatory GI disorders; SCr >2 **Disp:** Tabs 25, 50, 100 mg **SE:** Flatulence, D, Abd pain **Notes:** Use alone or w/ sulfonylureas

Milrinone (Primacor) Uses: *CHF acutely decompensated,* calcium antagonist intoxication **Action:** Phosphodiesterase inhibitor, + inotrope & vasodilator; little chronotropic activity **Dose:** 50 mcg/kg, IV over 10 min then 0.375–0.75 mcg/kg/min IV Inf; ↓ w/ renal impair **Caution:** [C, ?] **CI:** Allergy to drug; w/ inamrinone **Disp:** Inj 200 mcg/mL **SE:** Arrhythmias, ↓ BP, HA **Notes:** Monitor fluids, lytes, CBC, Mg^{2+}, BP, HR; not for long-term use

Mineral Oil [OTC] Uses: *Constipation, bowel irrigation, fecal impaction* **Action:** Lubricant laxative **Dose:** *Adults. Constipation:* 15–45 mL PO/d PRN. *Fecal impaction or after barium:* 118 mL rectally × 1. *Peds >6 y: Constipation:* 5–25 mL PO q day. *2–12 y: Fecal impaction:* 118 mL rectally × 1. **Caution:** [C, ?] w/ N/V, difficulty swallowing, bedridden pts; may ↓ absorption of Vit A, D, E, K, warfarin **CI:** Colostomy/ileostomy, appendicitis, diverticulitis, ulcerative colitis **Disp:** All [OTC] liq PO 13.5 mL/15 mL, PO microemulsion 2.5 mL/5 mL, rectal enema 118 mL **SE:** Lipid pneumonia (aspiration of PO), N/V, temporary anal incontinence **Notes:** Take PO upright, do not use PO in peds <6 y

Mineral Oil-Pramoxine HCl-Zinc Oxide (Tucks Ointment, [OTC]) Uses: *Temporary relief of anorectal disorders (itching, etc)* Action: Topical anesthetic **Dose:** *Adults & Peds ≥12 y:* Cleanse, rinse, & dry, apply externally or into anal canal w/ tip 5×/d × 7 d max. **Caution:** [?/?] Do not place into rectum **CI:** None **Disp:** Oint 30-g tube **SE:** Local irritation **Notes:** D/C w/ or if rectal bleeding occurs or if condition worsens or does not improve within 7 d

Minocycline (Dynacin, Minocin, Solodyn) Uses: *Mod–severe nonnodular acne (Solodyn),* anthrax, rickettsiae, gonococcus, skin Infxn, URI, UTI, nongonococcal urethritis, amebic dysentery, asymptomatic meningococcal carrier, *Mycobacterium marinum* Action: Tetracycline, bacteriostatic, ↓ protein synth **Dose:** *Adults & Peds >12 y: Usual:* 200 mg, then 100 mg q12h or 100–200 mg, then 50 mg qid. *Gonococcal urethritis, men:* 100 mg q12h × 5 d. *Syphilis:* usual dose × 10–15 d. *Meningococcal carrier:* 100 mg q12h × 5 d. *M. marinum:* 100 mg q12h × 6–8 wk. *Uncomp urethral, endocervical, or rectal infection:* 100 mg q12h × 7 d minimum. *Adults & Peds> 12 y:* Acne: *(Solodyn)* 1 mg/kg PO q day × 12 wk. *>8 y:* 4 mg/kg initially then 2 mg/kg q12h w/ food to ↓ irritation, hydrate well, ↓ dose or extend interval w/ renal impair. **Caution:** [D, –] Associated w/ pseudomembranous colitis, w/ renal impair, may ↓ OCP, or w/ warfarin may ↑ INR **CI:** Allergy, women of childbearing potential **Dose:** Tabs 50, 75, 100 mg; tabs ER *(Solodyn)* 45, 90, 135 mg, caps *(Minocin)* 50, 100 mg, susp 50 mg/mL **SE:** D, HA, fever, rash, joint pain, fatigue, dizziness, photosensitivity, hyperpigmentation, SLE syndrome, pseudotumor cerebri **Notes:** Do not cut/crush/chew; keep away from children, tooth discoloration in <8 y or w/ use last half of PRG

Minoxidil, oral   **WARNING:** May cause pericardial effusion, occasional tamponade, and angina pectoris may be exacerbated. Only for nonresponders to max doses of 2 other antihypertensives and a diuretic. Administer under supervision with a β-blocker and diuretic. Monitor for ↓ BP in those receiving guanethidine with malignant HTN **Uses:** *Severe HTN* **Action:** Peripheral vasodilator **Dose:** *Adults & Peds >12 y:* 5 mg PO ÷ daily, titrate q3d, 10 mg/d max. *Peds.* 0.2–1 mg/kg/24 h ÷ PO q12–24h, titrate q3d, max 50 mg/d; ↓ w/ elderly, renal insuff **Caution:** [C, +] **CI:** Pheochromocytoma, component allergy, CHF, renal impair **Disp:** Tabs 2.5, 10 mg **SE:** Pericardial effusion & vol overload w/ PO use; hypertrichosis w/ chronic use, edema, ECG changes, wgt gain **Note:** Avoid for 1 mo after MI

Minoxidil, topical (Theroxidil, Rogaine) [OTC]   **Uses:** *Male & female pattern baldness* **Action:** Stimulates vertex hair growth **Dose:** Apply 1 mL bid to area, D/C if no growth in 4 mo. **Caution:** [?, ?] **CI:** Component allergy **Disp:** Soln & aerosol foam 5% **SE:** Changes in hair color/texture **Note:** requires chronic use to maintain hair

Mirtazapine (Remeron, Remeron SolTab)   **WARNING:** ↑ Risk of suicidal thinking and behavior in children, adolescents, and young adults with major depression and other psychological disorders. Not for peds **Uses:** *Depression* **Action:** α₂-Antagonist antidepressant, ↑ norepinephrine & 5-HT **Dose:** 15 mg PO hs, up to 45 mg/d hs **Caution:** [C, ?] Has anticholesterol effects, w/ Sz, clonidine, CNS depressant use, CYP1A2, CYP3A4 inducers/inhibitors **CI:** MAOIs w/in 14 d **Disp:** Tabs 15, 30, 45 mg; rapid dispersion tabs (SolTab) 15, 30, 45 mg **SE:** Somnolence, ↑ cholesterol, constipation, xerostomia, wgt gain, agranulocytosis, ↓ BP, edema, musculoskeletal pain **Notes:** Do not ↑ dose < q1–2wk; handle rapid tabs with dry hands, do not cut or chew

Misoprostol (Cytotec)   **WARNING:** Use in pregnancy can cause abortion, premature birth, or birth defects; do not use to decrease ulcer risk in women of child-bearing age; must comply w/ birth control measures **Uses:** *Prevent NSAID-induced gastric ulcers; medical termination of PRG <49 d w/ mifepristone*; induce labor (cervical ripening); incomplete & therapeutic abortion **Action:** Prostaglandin (PGE-1), antisecretory & mucosal protection; induces uterine contractions **Dose:** *Ulcer prevention:* 200 mcg PO qid w/ meals; in females, start 2nd/3rd d of next nl period. *Induction of labor (term):* 25–50 mcg intravag. *PRG termination:* 400 mcg PO on day 3 of mifepristone; take w/ food **Caution:** [X, –] **CI:** PRG, component allergy **Disp:** Tabs 100, 200 mcg **SE:** Miscarriage w/ severe bleeding; HA, D, Abd pain, constipation. **Note:** Not induction of labor w/ previous C-section or major uterine surgery

Mitomycin (Mutamycin) **WARNING:** Administer only by physician experienced in chemotherapy; myelosuppressive; can induce hemolytic uremic syndrome with irreversible renal failure **Uses:** *Stomach, pancreas,* breast, colon CA; squamous cell carcinoma of the anus; non–small-cell lung, head & neck, cervical; bladder CA (intravesically) **Action:** Alkylating agent; generates oxygen-free radicals w/ DNA strand breaks **Dose:** (Per protocol) 20 mg/m² q6–8wk IV or 10 mg/m² combo w/ other myelosuppressive drugs q6–8wk. *Bladder CA:* 20–40 mg in 40 mL NS via a urethral catheter once/wk × 8 wk, followed by monthly × 12 mo for 1 y; ↓ in renal/hepatic impair **Caution:** [D, –] **CI:** ↓ Plt, ↓ WBC, coagulation disorders, Cr >1.7 mg/dL, ↑ cardiac tox w/ vinca alkaloids/doxorubicin **Disp:** Inj 5, 20, 40 mg **SE:** ↓ BM (persists for 3–8 wk, may be cumulative; minimize w/ lifetime dose <50–60 mg/m²), N/V, anorexia, stomatitis, renal tox, microangiopathic hemolytic anemia w/ renal failure (hemolytic–uremic syndrome), venoocclusive liver Dz, interstitial pneumonia, alopecia, extrav Rxns, contact dermatitis; CHF

Mitoxantrone (Novantrone) **WARNING:** Administer only by physician experienced in chemotherapy; except for acute leukemia, do not use w/ ANC count of <1500 cells/mm³; severe neutropenia can result in Infxn, follow CBC; cardiotoxic (CHF), secondary AML reported **Uses:** *AML (w/ cytarabine), ALL, CML, PCA, MS, Lung CA* breast CA, & NHL **Action:** DNA-intercalating agent; ↓ DNA synth by interacting with topoisomerase II **Dose:** Per protocol; ↓ w/ hepatic impair, leukopenia, thrombocytopenia **Caution:** [D, –] Reports of secondary AML, w/ MS ↑ CV risk, do not treat MS pt w/ low LVEF **CI:** PRG, sig ↓ in LVEF **Disp:** Inj 2 mg/mL **SE:** ↓ BM, N/V, stomatitis, alopecia (infrequent), cardiotox, urine discoloration, secretions & scleras may be blue-green **Notes:** Maintain hydration; baseline CV evaluate w/ ECG & LVEF; cardiac monitoring prior to each dose; not for intrathecal use

Modafinil (Provigil) [C-IV] **Uses:** *Improve wakefulness in pts w/ excess daytime sleepiness (narcolepsy, sleep apnea, shift work sleep disorder)* **Action:** Alters dopamine & norepinephrine release, ↓ GABA-mediated neurotransmission **Dose:** 200 mg PO q A.M.; ↓ dose 50% w/ elderly/hepatic impair **Caution:** [C, ?/–] ↑ effects of warfarin, diazepam, phenytoin; ↓ OCP, cyclosporine, & theophylline effects **CI:** Component allergy **Disp:** Tabs 100, 200 mg **SE:** Serious rash including Stevens-Johnson syndrome, HA, N, D, paresthesias, rhinitis, agitation, psychological Sx **Notes:** cv assessment ok before using

Moexipril (Univasc) **WARNING:** ACE inhibitors can cause fatal injury/death in 2nd/3rd tri; D/C w/ PRG **Uses:** *HTN, post-MI,* DN **Action:** ACE inhibitor **Dose:** 7.5–30 mg in 1–2 ÷ doses 1 h ac ↓ in renal impair **Caution:** [C (1st tri, D 2nd & 3rd tri), ?] **CI:** ACE inhibitor sensitivity **Disp:** Tabs 7.5, 15 mg; **SE:** ↓ BP, edema, angioedema, HA, dizziness, cough, ↑ K⁺

Molindone (Moban) Uses: *Schizophrenia* Action: Piperazine phenothiazine Dose: *Adults.* 50–75 mg/d PO, ↑ to max 225 mg/d q3–4d PRN; Peds 3–5 y: 1–2.5 mg/d PO in 4 ÷ doses. 5–12 y: 0.5–1.0 mg/kg/d in 4 ÷ doses Caution: [C, ?] NAG CI: Drug/EtOH CNS depression, coma Disp: Tabs 5, 10, 25, 50 mg scored; SE: Drowsiness, depression, ↓ BP, tachycardia, arrhythmias, EPS, neuroleptic malignant syndrome, Szs, constipation, xerostomia, blurred vision. Notes: ✓ lipid profile, fasting glucose, HgA1c; may ↑ prolactin

Montelukast (Singulair) Uses: *Prevent/chronic Rx asthma ≥12 mo; seasonal allergic rhinitis ≥2 y; perennial allergic rhinitis ≥6 mo; prevent exercise bronchoconstriction (EIB) ≥15 y; prophylaxis & Rx of chronic asthma, seasonal allergic rhinitis* Action: Leukotriene receptor antagonist Dose: *Asthma: Adults & Peds >15 y:* 10 mg/d PO in P.M.. 6–23 mo: 4-mg pack granules q day. 2–5 y: 4 mg/d PO q P.M.. 6–14 y: 5 mg/d PO q P.M. Caution: [B, M] CI: Component allergy Disp: Tabs 10 mg; chew tabs 4, 5 mg; granules 4 mg/pack SE: HA, dizziness, fatigue, rash, GI upset, Churg-strauss syndrome, flu, cough Notes: Not for acute asthma; do not dose w/in 24 h of previous; recent concern over ↑ suicidal behavior

Morphine (Avinza XR, Astramorph/PF, Duramorph, Infumorph, MS Contin, Kadian SR, Oramorph SR, Roxanol) [C-II] WARNING: Do not crush/chew SR/CR forms Uses: *Rx severe pain* AMI Action: Narcotic analgesic; SR/CR forms for chronic use Dose: *Adults.* Short-term use PO: 5–30 mg q4h PRN; *IV/IM:* 2.5–15 mg q2–6h; *supp:* 10–30 mg q4h. SR formulations 15–60 mg q8–12h (do not chew/crush). *IT/epidural* (Duramorph, Infumorph, Astramorph/PF): Per protocol in Inf device. Peds >6 mo: 0.1–0.2 mg/kg/dose IM/IV q2–4h PRN to 15 mg/dose max; 0.2–0.5 mg/kg PO q4–6h PRN; 0.3–0.6 mg/kg SR taps PO q12h; 2–4 mg IV (over 1–5 min) q5–30 min (ECC 2005) Caution: [C, +/–] Severe resp depression possible, w/ head injury CI: Severe asthma, resp depression, GI obst Disp: IR tabs 15, 30 mg; soln 10, 20, 100 mg/5 mL; supp 5, 10, 15, 20, 30 mg; Inj 2, 4, 5, 8, 10, 15, 25, 50 mg/mL; *MS Contin* CR tabs 15, 30, 60, 100, 200 mg; *Oramorph SR* tabs 15, 30, 60, 100 mg; *Kadian SR caps* 10, 20, 30, 50, 60, 80, 100 mg; *Avinza XR* caps 30, 60, 90, 120 mg; *Duramorph/Astramorph PF* Inj 0.5, 1 mg/mL; *Infumorph* 10, 25 mg/mL, SE: Narcotic SE (resp depression, sedation, constipation, N/V, pruritus, diaphoresis, urinary retention, biliary colic), granulomas w/ IT Notes: May require scheduled dosing to relieve severe chronic pain

Morphine liposomal (DepoDur) Uses: *Long-lasting epidural analgesia* Action: ER morphine analgesia Dose: 10–20 mg lumbar epidural Inj (C-section 10 mg after cord clamped) Caution: [C, +/–] Elderly, biliary Dz (sphincter of Oddi spasm) CI: Ileus, resp depression, asthma, obstructed airway, suspected/known head injury ↑ ICP, allergy to morphine Disp: Inj 10 mg/mL SE: Hypoxia, resp depression, ↓ BP, retention, N/V, constipation, flatulence, pruritus, pyrexia, anemia, HA, dizziness, tachycardia, insomnia, ileus Notes: Effect = 48 h; not for IT/IV/IM

Moxifloxacin (Avelox)   WARNING: Increase risk of tendon rupture and tendonitis. Uses: *Acute sinusitis & bronchitis, skin/soft-tissue/intra-Abd Infxns, conjunctivitis, CAP* Action: 4th-gen quinolone; ↓ DNA synthesis Spectrum: Excellent gram(+) except MRSA & E. faecium; good gram(−) except P. aeruginosa, Stenotrophomonas maltophilia, & Acinetobacter sp; good anaerobic Dose: 400 mg/d PO/IV; avoid cation products, antacids. tid Caution: [C, ?/−] Quinolone sensitivity; interactions w/ Mg⁻, CA⁻, Al⁻, Fe-containing products, & class IA & III antiarrhythmic agents CI: Quinolone/component sensitivity Disp: Tabs 400 mg, ABC Pak 5 tabs, Inj SE: Dizziness, N, QT prolongation, Szs, photosensitivity, tendon rupture

Moxifloxacin ophthalmic (Vigamox ophthalmic)   Uses: *Bacterial conjunctivitis* Action: See Moxifloxacin Dose: 1 gtt tid × 7 d Caution: [C, ?/−] CI: Quinolone/component sensitivity Disp: 4 mL ophthal 0.5% SE: ↓ Visual acuity, ocular pain, itching, tearing, conjunctivitis

Multivitamins, oral [OTC] (Table 13, page 268)

Mupirocin (Bactroban, Bactroban Nasal)   Uses: *Impetigo (oint); skin lesion infect w/ S. aureus or S. pyogenes; eradicate MRSA in nasal carriers* Action: ↓ Bacterial protein synth Dose: Topical: Apply small amount 3×/d × 5–14 d. Nasal: Apply 1/2 single-use tube bid in nostrils × 5 d Caution: [B, ?] CI: Do not use w/ other nasal products Disp: Oint 2%; cream 2%; nasal oint 2% 1-g single-use tubes SE: Local irritation, rash Notes: Pt to contact health-care provider if no improvement in 3–5 d.

Muromonab-CD3 (Orthoclone OKT3)   WARNING: Can cause anaphylaxis; monitor fluid status; cytokine release syndrome Uses: *Acute rejection following organ transplantation* Action: Murine Ab, blocks T-cell Fxn Dose: Per protocol Adults. 5 mg/d IV for 10–14 d. Peds <30 kg: 2.5 mg/d IV for 10–14 d. >30 kg: 5 mg/d IV for 10–14 d Caution: [C, ?/−] w/ Hx of Szs, PRG, uncontrolled HTN CI: Murine sensitivity, fluid overload Disp: Inj 5 mg/5 mL SE: Anaphylaxis, pulm edema, fever/chills w/ 1st dose (premedicate w/ steroid/APAP/antihistamine); cytokine release syndrome (↓ BP, fever, rigors) Notes: Monitor during Inf; use 0.22-micron filter

Mycophenolic Acid (Myfortic)   WARNING: ↑ Risk of Infxns, lymphoma, other CA's, progressive multifocal leukoencephalopathy PML), risk of PRG loss and malformation, female of childbearing potential must use contraception Uses: *Prevent rejection after renal transplant* Action: Cytostatic to lymphocytes Dose: Adults. 720 mg PO bid. Peds. BSA 1.19–1.58 m²: 540 mg bid. BSA >1.8 m²: adult dose; used w/ steroids & cyclosporine ↓ w/ renal Insuff/neutropenia; take on empty stomach Caution: [D, ?/−] CI: Component allergy Disp: Delayed release tabs 180, 360 mg SE: N/V/D, pain, fever, HA, Infxn, HTN, anemia, leukopenia, edema

Mycophenolate Mofetil (CellCept)   WARNING: ↑ Risk of Infxns, lymphoma, other CAs, progressive multifocal leukoencephalopathy (PML); risk of PRG loss and malformation; female of childbearing potential must use contraception **Uses:** *Prevent organ rejection after transplant* **Action:** Cytostatic to lymphocytes **Dose:** *Adults.* 1 g PO bid. *Peds. BSA 1.2–1.5 m²:* 750 mg PO bid. *BSA >1.5 m²:* 1 g PO bid; may taper up to 600 mg/m² PO bid; used w/ steroids & cyclosporine; ↓ in renal Insuff or neutropenia. *IV:* Infuse over >2 h. *PO:* Take on empty stomach, do not open caps **Caution:** [D, ?/–] **CI:** Component allergy; IV use in polysorbate 80 allergy **Disp:** Caps 250, 500 mg; susp 200 mg/mL, Inj 500 mg **SE:** N/V/D, pain, fever, HA, Infxn, HTN, anemia, leukopenia, edema

Nabilone (Cesamet) [CII]   **WARNING:** Psychotomimetic Rxns, may persist for 72 h following D/C; caregivers should be present during initial use or dosage modification; pts should not operate heavy machinery; avoid alcohol, sedatives, hypnotics, other psychoactive substances **Uses:** *Refractory chemotherapy-induced emesis* **Action:** Synthetic cannabinoid **Dose:** *Adults.* 1–2 mg PO bid 1–3 h before chemotherapy, 6 mg/d max; may continue for 48 h beyond final chemotherapy dose **Caution:** [C, ?/–] Elderly, HTN, heart failure, w/ psychological illness, substance abuse; high protein binding w/ 1st-pass metabolism may lead to drug interactions **Disp:** Caps 1 mg **SE:** Drowsiness, vertigo, xerostomia, euphoria, ataxia, HA, difficulty concentrating, tachycardia, ↓ BP **Notes:** May require initial dose evening before chemotherapy; Rx only quantity for single cycle

Nabumetone (Relafen)   **WARNING:** May ↑ risk of cv events & GI bleeding, perforation; CI w/ post-op coronary artery bypass graft **Uses:** *OA and RA,* pain **Action:** NSAID; ↓ prostaglandins **Dose:** 1000–2000 mg/d ÷ daily-bid w/ food **Caution:** [C, –] Severe hepatic Dz **CI:** w/ Peptic ulcer, NSAID sensitivity, after coronary artery bypass graft surgery **Disp:** Tabs 500, 750 mg **SE:** Dizziness, rash, GI upset, edema, peptic ulcer, ↑ BP

Nadolol (Corgard)   **Uses:** *HTN & angina* migraine prophylaxis **Action:** Competitively blocks β-adrenergic receptors (β₁, β₂) **Dose:** 40–80 mg/d; ↑ to 240 mg/d (angina) or 320 mg/d (HTN) at 3–7-d intervals; ↓ in renal Insuff & elderly **Caution:** [C (1st tri; D if 2nd or 3rd tri), +] **CI:** Uncompensated CHF, shock, heart block, asthma **Disp:** Tabs 20, 40, 80, 120, 160 mg **SE:** Nightmares, paresthesias, ↓ BP, bradycardia, fatigue

Nafcillin (Nallpen, Unipen)   **Uses:** *Infxns due to susceptible strains of Staphylococcus & Streptococcus* **Action:** Bactericidal; β-lactamase-resistant PCN; ↓ cell wall synth *Spectrum:* Good gram(+) except MRSA & enterococcus, no gram(–), poor anaerobe **Dose:** *Adults.* 1–2 g IV q4–6h. *Peds.* 50–200 mg/kg/d ÷ q4–6h **Caution:** [B, ?] PCN allergy **CI:** PCN allergy **Disp:** Inj powder 1, 2 g **SE:** Interstitial nephritis, N/D, fever, rash, allergic Rxn **Notes:** No adjustment for renal Fxn

Naftifine (Naftin)   **Uses:** *Tinea pedis, cruris, & corporis* **Action:** Allylamine antifungal, ↓ cell membrane ergosterol synth **Dose:** Apply daily (cream) or bid (gel) **Caution:** [B, ?] **CI:** Component sensitivity **Disp:** 1% cream; gel **SE:** Local irritation

Nalbuphine (Nubain) Uses: *Mod–severe pain; pre-op & obstetric analgesia* Action: Narcotic agonist–antagonist; ↓ ascending pain pathways Dose: *Adults. Pain:* 10 mg/70 kg IV/IM/SQ q3–6h; adjust PRN; 20 mg/dose or 160 mg/d max. *Anesthesia: Induction:* 0.3–3 mg/kg IV over 10–15 min; maint 0.25–0.5 mg/kg IV. *Peds.* 0.2 mg/kg IV or IM, 20 mg max; ↓ w/ renal/in hepatic impair Caution: [B, M] w/ Opiate use CI: Component sensitivity Disp: Inj 10, 20 mg/mL SE: CNS depression, drowsiness; caution, ↓ BP

Naloxone Uses: *Opioid addiction (diagnosis) & OD* Action: Competitive narcotic antagonist Dose: *Adults.* 0.4–2 mg IV, IM, or SQ q2–3 min; total dose 10 mg max. *Peds.* 0.01–0.1 mg/kg/dose IV, IM, or SQ; repeat IV q3min × 3 doses PRN Caution: [B, ?] May precipitate acute withdrawal in addicts Disp: Inj 0.4, 1 mg/mL SE: ↓ BP, tachycardia, irritability, GI upset, pulm edema Notes: If no response after 10 mg, suspect nonnarcotic cause

Naltrexone (Depade, ReVia, Vivitrol) WARNING: Can cause hepatic injury, CI w/ active liver Dz Uses: *EtOH & narcotic addiction* Action: Antagonizes opioid receptors Dose: *EtOH/narcotic addiction:* 50 mg/d PO; must be opioid-free for 7–10 d; *EtOH dependence:* 380 mg IM q4wk (*Vivitrol*) Caution: [C, M] CI: Active hep, liver failure, opioid use Disp: Tabs 50 mg; Inj 380 mg (*Vivitrol*) SE: Hepatotox; insomnia, GI upset, joint pain, HA, fatigue

Naphazoline (Albalon, Naphcon, others), Naphazoline & Pheniramine Acetate (Naphcon A, Visine A) Uses: *Relieve ocular redness & itching caused by allergy* Action: Sympathomimetic (α-adrenergic vasoconstrictor) & antihistamine (pheniramine) Dose: 1–2 gtt up to qid, 3 d max Caution: [C, +] CI: NAG, in children, w/ contact lenses, component allergy SE: CV stimulation, dizziness, local irritation Disp: Ophthal 0.012, 0.025, 0.1%/16 mg; naphazoline & pheniramine 0.025%/0.3% soln

Naproxen (Aleve [OTC], Naprosyn, Anaprox) WARNING: May ↑ risk of cardiovascular events & GI bleeding Uses: *Arthritis & pain* Action: NSAID; ↓ prostaglandins Dose: *Adults & Peds >12 y:* 200–500 mg bid-tid to 1500 mg/d dose. *>2 y:* JRA 5 mg/kg/dose bid; ↓ in hepatic impair Caution: [C, (D 3rd tri), +] CI: NSAID or ASA triad sensitivity, peptic ulcer, post-coronary artery bypass graft pain, 3rd tri PRG Disp: *Tabs:* 220, 250, 375, 500 mg; *DR:* 375 mg, 500 mg; *CR:* 375 mg, 550 mg; susp 125 mL/5 mL. SE: Dizziness, pruritus, GI upset, peptic ulcer, edema Note: Take w/ food to ↓ GI upset

Naratriptan (Amerge) Uses: *Acute migraine* Action: Serotonin 5-HT$_1$ receptor agonist Dose: 1–2.5 mg PO once; repeat PRN in 4 h; 5 mg/24 h max; ↓ in mild renal/hepatic Insuff, take w/ fluids Caution: [C, M] CI: Severe renal/hepatic impair, avoid w/ angina, ischemic heart Dz, uncontrolled HTN, cerebrovascular syndromes, & ergot use Disp: Tabs 1, 2.5 mg SE: Dizziness, sedation, GI upset, paresthesias, ECG changes, coronary vasospasm, arrhythmias

Natalizumab (Tysabri) WARNING: PML reported Uses: *Relapsing MS to delay disability and ↓ recurrences, Crohn Dz* Action: Integrin receptor antagonist **Dose:** *Adults.* 300 mg IV q4wk; 2nd-line Tx only **CI:** PML; immune compromise or w/ immunosuppressant **Caution:** [C, ?/–] Baseline MRI to rule out PML **Disp:** Vial 300 mg **SE:** Infxn, immunosuppression; Inf Rxn precluding subsequent use; HA, fatigue, arthralgia **Notes:** Give slowly to ↓ Rxns; limited distribution (TOUCH Prescribing program); D/C immediately w/ signs of PML (weakness, paralysis, vision loss, impaired speech, cognitive ↓); evaluate at 3 and 6 mo, then q6mo thereafter

Nateglinide (Starlix) **Uses:** *Type 2 DM* **Action:** ↑ Pancreatic insulin release **Dose:** 120 mg PO tid 1–30 min ac; ↓ to 60 mg tid if near target HbA1c **Caution:** [C, –] w/ CYP2C9 metabolized drug (Table 11) **CI:** DKA, type 1 DM **Disp:** Tabs 60, 120 mg **SE:** Hypoglycemia; URI; salicylates, nonselective β-blockers may enhance hypoglycemia

Nebivolol (Bystolic) **Uses:** *HTN* **Action:** β₁-Selective blocker **Dose:** *Adults.* 5 mg PO daily, ↑ q2wk to 40 mg/d max, ↓ w/ CrCl <30 mL/min **Caution:** [D, +/–] w/ Bronchospastic Dz, DM, heart failure, pheochromocytoma, w/ CYP2D6 inhibitors **CI:** Bradycardia, cardiogenic shock, decompensated CHF, severe hepatic impair **Disp:** tabs 5, 10 mg **SE:** HA, fatigue, dizziness

Nefazodone **WARNING:** Fatal hep & liver failure possible, D/C if LFTs >3× ULN, do not retreat; closely monitor for worsening depression or suicidality, particularly in ped pts **Uses:** *Depression* **Action:** ↓ Neuronal uptake of serotonin & norepinephrine **Dose:** Initial 100 mg PO bid; usual 300–600 mg/d in 2 ÷ doses **Caution:** [C, M] **CI:** w/ MAOIs, pimozide, carbamazepine, alprazolam; active liver Dz **Disp:** Tabs 50, 100, 150, 200, 250 mg **SE:** Postural ↓ BP & allergic Rxns; HA, drowsiness, xerostomia, constipation, GI upset, liver failure **Notes:** Monitor LFTs, HR, BP

Nelarabine (Arranon) **WARNING:** Fatal neurotox possible **Uses:** *T-cell ALL or T-cell lymphoblastic lymphoma unresponsive >2 other regimens* **Action:** Nucleoside (deoxyguanosine) analog **Dose:** *Adults.* 1500 mg/m² IV over 2 h days 1, 3, 5 of 21-d cycle. *Peds.* 650 mg/m² IV over 1 h days 1–5 of 21-d cycle **Caution:** [D, ?/–] **Disp:** Vial 250 mg **SE:** Neuropathy, ataxia, Szs, coma, hematologic tox, GI upset, HA, blurred vision **Notes:** Prehydration, urinary alkalinization, allopurinol before dose; monitor CBC

Nelfinavir (Viracept) **Uses:** *HIV Infxn, other agents* **Action:** Protease inhibitor causes immature, noninfectious virion production **Dose:** *Adults.* 750 mg PO tid or 1250 mg PO bid. *Peds.* 25–35 mg/kg PO tid or 45–55 mg/kg bid; take w/ food **Caution:** [B, –] Many drug interactions **CI:** Phenylketonuria, w/ triazolam/midazolam use or drug dependent on CYP3A4 (Table 11) **Disp:** Tabs 250, 625 mg; powder 50 mg/g; **SE:** Food ↑ absorption; interacts w/ St. John's wort; dyslipidemia, lipodystrophy, D, rash **Notes:** pregnancy registry; tabs can be dissolved in water

Neomycin, Bacitracin, & Polymyxin B (Neosporin Ointment) (See Bacitracin, Neomycin, & Polymyxin B Topical, page 51)

Neomycin, Colistin, & Hydrocortisone (Cortisporin-TC Otic Drops); Neomycin, Colistin, Hydrocortisone, & Thonzonium (Cortisporin-TC Otic Susp) Uses: *Otitis externa,* Infxns of mastoid/ fenestration cavities **Action:** Antibiotic w/ anti-inflammatory **Dose:** *Adults.* 5 gtt in ear(s) tid-qid. *Peds.* 3–4 gtt in ear(s) tid-qid **CI:** component allergy; HSV, vaccinia, varicella **Caution:** [B, ?] **Disp:** Otic gtt & susp **SE:** Local irritation, rash **Notes:** Shake well, limit use to 10 d to minimize hearing loss

Neomycin & Dexamethasone (AK-Neo-Dex Ophthalmic, NeoDecadron Ophthalmic) Uses: *Steroid-responsive inflammatory conditions of the cornea, conjunctiva, lid, & anterior segment* **Action:** Antibiotic w/ anti-inflammatory corticosteroid **Dose:** 1–2 gtt in eye(s) q3–4h or thin coat tid-qid until response, then ↓ to daily **Caution:** [C, ?] **Disp:** Cream neomycin 0.5%/dexamethasone 0.1%; oint neomycin 0.35%/dexamethasone 0.05%; soln neomycin 0.35%/dexamethasone 0.1% **SE:** Local irritation **Notes:** Use under ophthalmologist's supervision

Neomycin & Polymyxin B (Neosporin Cream) [OTC] Uses: *Infxn in minor cuts, scrapes, & burns* **Action:** Bactericidal **Dose:** Apply bid-qid **Caution:** [C, ?] **CI:** Component allergy **Disp:** Cream neomycin 3.5 mg/ polymyxin B 10,000 units/g **SE:** Local irritation **Notes:** Different from Neosporin oint

Neomycin, Polymyxin B, & Dexamethasone (Maxitrol) Uses: *Steroid-responsive ocular conditions w/ bacterial Infxn* **Action:** Antibiotic w/ anti-inflammatory corticosteroid **Dose:** 1–2 gtt in eye(s) q3–4h; apply oint in eye(s) tid-qid **CI:** Component allergy; viral, fungal, TB eye Dz **Caution:** [C, ?] **Disp:** Oint neomycin sulfate 3.5 mg/polymyxin B sulfate 10,000 units/dexamethasone 0.1%/g; susp identical/5 mL **SE:** Local irritation **Notes:** Use under supervision of ophthalmologist

Neomycin-Polymyxin Bladder Irrigant [Neosporin GU Irrigant] Uses: *Cont irrigant prevent bacteriuria & gram(–) bacteremia associated w/ indwelling catheter* **Action:** Bactericidal; not for *Serratia* sp or streptococci **Dose:** 1 mL irrigant in 1 L of 0.9% NaCl; cont bladder irrigation w/ 1 L of soln/24 h 10 d max **Caution:** [D] **CI:** Component allergy **Disp:** Soln neomycin sulfate 40 mg & polymyxin B 200,000 units/mL; amp 1, 20 mL **SE:** Rash, neomycin ototox or nephrotox (rare) **Notes:** Potential for bacterial/fungal super-Infxn; not for Inj; use only 3-way catheter for irrigation

Neomycin, Polymyxin, & Hydrocortisone ophthalmic (generic) Uses: *Ocular bacterial Infxns* **Action:** Antibiotic w/ anti-inflammatory **Dose:** Apply a thin layer to the eye(s) or 1 gtt daily-qid **Caution:** [C, ?] **Disp:** Ophthal soln; ophthal oint **SE:** Local irritation

Neomycin, Polymyxin, & Hydrocortisone otic (Cortisporin Otic solution, generic susp) Uses: *Otitis externa and infected mastoidectomy and fenestration cavities* **Action:** Antibiotic & anti-inflammatory

Dose: *Adults.* 3–4 gtt in the ear(s) tid-qid *Peds.* >2 y: 3 gtt in the ear(s) tid-qid **CI:** Viral Infxn, hypersensitivity to components **Caution:** [C, ?] **Disp:** Otic susp (generic); otic soln (Cortisporin) **SE:** Local irritation

Neomycin, Polymyxin B, & Prednisolone (Poly-Pred Ophthalmic) Uses: *Steroid-responsive ocular conditions w/ bacterial Infxn* **Action:** Antibiotic & anti-inflammatory **Dose:** 1–2 gtt in eye(s) q4–6h; apply oint in eye(s) tid-qid **Caution:** [C, ?] **Disp:** Susp neomycin/polymyxin B/prednisolone 0.5%/mL **SE:** Irritation **Notes:** Use under supervision of ophthalmologist

Neomycin Sulfate (Neo-Fradin, generic) WARNING: Systemic absorption of oral route may cause neuro-/oto-/nephrotox; resp paralysis possible with any route of administration **Uses:** *Hepatic coma, bowel preparation* **Action:** Aminoglycoside, poorly absorbed PO; ↓ GI bacterial flora **Dose:** *Adults.* 3–12 g/24 h PO in 3–4 ÷ doses. *Peds.* 50–100 mg/kg/24 h PO in 3–4 ÷ doses **Caution:** [C, ?/–] Renal failure, neuromuscular disorders, hearing impair **CI:** Intestinal obst **Disp:** Tabs 500 mg; PO soln 125 mg/5 mL **SE:** Hearing loss w/ long-term use; rash, N/V **Notes:** Do not use parenterally (↑ tox); part of the Condon bowel preparation; also topical form

Nepafenac (Nevanac) Uses: *Inflammation postcataract surgery* **Action:** NSAID **Dose:** 1 gtt in eye(s) tid 1 d before, and continue 14 d after surgery **CI:** NSAID/aspirin sensitivity **Caution:** [C, ?/–] May ↑ bleeding time, delay healing, cause keratitis **Disp:** Susp 3 mL **SE:** Capsular opacity, visual changes, foreign-body sensation, ↑ IOP **Notes:** Prolonged use ↑ risk of corneal damage; shake well before use; separate from other drops by >5 min

Nesiritide (Natrecor) Uses: *Acutely decompensated CHF* **Action:** Human B-type natriuretic peptide **Dose:** 2 mcg/kg IV bolus, then 0.01 mcg/kg/min IV **Caution:** [C, ?/–] When vasodilators are not appropriate **CI:** SBP <90, cardiogenic shock **Disp:** Vials 1.5 mg **SE:** ↓ BP, HA, GI upset, arrhythmias, ↑ Cr **Notes:** Requires cont BP monitoring; some studies indicate ↑ in mortality

Nevirapine (Viramune) WARNING: Reports of fatal hepatotox even w/ short-term use; severe life-threatening skin Rxns (Stevens–Johnson syndrome, toxic epidermal necrolysis, & allergic Rxns); monitor closely during 1st 8 wk of Rx **Uses:** *HIV Infxn* **Action:** Nonnucleoside RT inhibitor **Dose:** *Adults.* Initial 200 mg/d PO × 14 d, then 200 mg bid. *Peds 2 mo–8 y:* 4 mg/kg/d × 14 d, then 7 mg/kg bid. *>8 y:* 4 mg/kg/d × 14 d, then 4 mg/kg bid max 200 mg/dose for peds (w/o regard to food) **Caution:** [B, –] OCP **Disp:** Tabs 200 mg; susp 50 mg/5 mL **SE:** Life-threatening rash; HA, fever, D, neutropenia, hep **Notes:** HIV resistance when used as monotherapy; use in combo w/ at least 2 additional antiretroviral agents. Not recommended in women if CD4 >250 or men >400 unless benefit > risk of hepatotox

Niacin (Nicotinic acid) (Niaspan, Slo-Niacin, Niacor, Nicolar) [some OTC forms] Uses: *Sig hyperlipidemia/hypercholesteremia, nutritional supl* **Action:** Vit B_3; ↓ lipolysis; ↓ esterification of triglycerides; ↑ lipoprotein lipase **Dose:** *Hypercholesterolemia:* Start 500 mg PO qhs, ↑ 500 mg q4wk, maint 1–2 g/d; 2 g/d max; qhs w/ low fat snack; do not crush/chew; niacin supl 1 ER tab PO q day or 100 mg PO q day; *Pellagra:* Up to 500 mg/d **Caution:** [(C), +] **CI:** Liver Dz, peptic ulcer, arterial hemorrhage **Disp:** ER tabs (*Niaspan*) 500, 750, 1000 mg & (*Slo-Niacin*) 250, 500, 750 mg; tab 500 mg (Niacor); many OTC: tab 50, 100, 250, 500 mg, ER caps 125, 250, 400 mg, ER tab 250, 500, elixir 50 mg/5 mL **SE:** Upper body/facial flushing & warmth; hepatox, HA, paresthesias, liver damage, gout, altered glucose control in DM **Notes:** ASA/NSAID 30–60 min prior to ↓ flushing; ✓ cholesterol, LFTs, if on statins (eg, Lipitor, etc) ✓ CPK and K⁺; *RDA adults:* male 16 mg/d, female 14 mg/d

Niacin & Lovastatin (Advicor)
Uses: *Hypercholesterolemia* **Action:** Combo antilipemic agent, w/ HMG-CoA reductase inhibitor **Dose:** *Adults.* Niacin 500 mg/lovastatin 20 mg, titrate q4wk, max niacin 2000 mg/lovastatin 40 mg **Caution:** [X, –] See individual agents, D/C w/ LFTs >3× ULN **CI:** PRG **Disp:** Niacin/lovastatin: 500/20, 750/20, 1000/20, 1000/40 tabs **SE:** Flushing, myopathy/rhabdomyolysis, nausea, Abd pain, increase LFTs **Notes:** ↓ Flushing by taking ASA or NSAID 30 min before

Niacin & Simvastatin (Simcor)
Uses: *Hypercholesterolemia* **Action:** Combo antilipemic agent w/ HMG-CoA reductase inhibitor **Dose:** *Adults* Niacin 500 mg/simvastatin 20 mg, titrate q4wk to not exceed niacin 2000 mg/simvastatin 40 mg **Caution:** [X, –] See individual agents, discontinue therapy if LFTs >3× nl **CI:** PRG **Disp:** Niacin/simvastatin: 500/20, 750/20, 1000/20 tabs **SE:** Flushing, myopathy/rhabdomyolysis, nausea, Abd pain **Notes:** ↓ Flushing by taking ASA or NSAID 30 min before

Nicardipine (Cardene)
Uses: *Chronic stable angina & HTN*; prophylaxis of migraine **Action:** CCB **Dose:** *Adults.* *PO:* 20–40 mg PO tid. *SR:* 30–60 mg PO bid. *IV:* 5 mg/h IV cont Inf; ↑ by 2.5 mg/h q15min to max 15 mg/h. *Peds.* (Not established) *PO:* 20–30 mg PO q8h. *IV:* 0.5–5 mcg/kg/min; ↓ in renal/hepatic impair **Caution:** [C, ?/–] Heart block, CAD **CI:** Cardiogenic shock, aortic stenosis **Disp:** Caps 20, 30 mg; SR caps 30, 45, 60 mg; Inj 2.5 mg/mL **SE:** Flushing, tachycardia, ↓ BP, edema, HA **Notes:** *PO-to-IV conversion:* 20 mg tid = 0.5 mg/h, 30 mg tid = 1.2 mg/h, 40 mg tid = 2.2 mg/h; take w/ food (not high fat)

Nicotine Gum (Nicorette, others) [OTC]
Uses: *Aid to smoking cessation, relieve nicotine withdrawal* **Action:** Systemic delivery of nicotine **Dose:** Wk 1–6 one piece q1–2h PRN; wk 7–9 one piece q2–4h PRN; wk 10–12 one piece q4–8h PRN; max 24 pieces/d **Caution:** [C, ?] **CI:** Life-threatening arrhythmias, unstable angina **Disp:** 2 mg, 4 mg/piece; mint, orange, original flavors **SE:** Tachycardia, HA, GI upset, hiccups **Notes:** Must stop smoking & perform behavior modification for max effect; use at least 9 pieces first 6 wk; >25 cigarettes/d use 4 mg; <25 cigarettes/d use 2 mg

Nicotine Nasal Spray (Nicotrol NS)
Uses: *Aid to smoking cessation, relieve nicotine withdrawal* **Action:** Systemic delivery of nicotine **Dose:** 0.5 mg/actuation; 1–2 doses/h, 5 doses/h max; 40 doses/d max **Caution:** [D, M] **CI:**

Life-threatening arrhythmias, unstable angina **Disp:** Nasal inhaler 10 mg/mL **SE:** Local irritation, tachycardia, HA, taste perversion **Notes:** Must stop smoking & perform behavior modification for max effect; 1 dose = 1 spray each nostril = 1 mg

Nicotine Transdermal (Habitrol, Nicoderm CQ [OTC], others) **Uses:** *Aid to smoking cessation; relief of nicotine withdrawal* **Action:** Systemic delivery of nicotine **Dose:** Individualized; 1 patch (14–21 mg/d) & taper over 6 wk **Caution:** [D, M] **CI:** Life-threatening arrhythmias, unstable angina **Disp:** *Habitrol & Nicoderm CQ* 7, 14, 21 mg of nicotine/24 h **SE:** Insomnia, pruritus, erythema, local site Rxn, tachycardia, vivid dreams **Notes:** Wear patch 16–24 h; must stop smoking & perform behavior modification for max effect; >10 cigarettes/d start w/ 2-mg patch; <10 cigarettes/d 1-mg patch

Nifedipine (Procardia, Procardia XL, Adalat CC) **Uses:** *Vasospastic or chronic stable angina & HTN*; tocolytic **Action:** CCB **Dose:** *Adults.* SR tabs 30–90 mg/d. *Tocolysis:* per local protocol. *Peds.* 0.25–0.9 mg/kg/24 h ÷ tid-qid **Caution:** [C, +] Heart block, aortic stenosis **CI:** IR preparation for urgent or emergent HTN; acute MI **Disp:** Caps 10, 20 mg; SR tabs 30, 60, 90 mg **SE:** HA common on initial Rx; reflex tachycardia may occur w/ regular-release dosage forms; peripheral edema, ↓ BP, flushing, dizziness **Notes:** Adalat CC & Procardia XL not interchangeable; SL administration not OK

Nilotinib (Tasigna) **WARNING:** May ↑ QT interval; sudden deaths reported, use w/ caution in hepatic failure; administer on empty stomach **Uses:** *Ph+ CML* **Action:** TKI **Dose:** *Adults.* 400 mg bid, on empty stomach 1 h prior or 2 h post meal. **Caution:** [D, ?/–] Avoid w/ CYP3A4 inhibitors/inducers (Table 11), adjust w/ hepatic impair, avoid QT ↑, avoid QT-prolonging agents **CI:** Bilirubin >3× ULN, AST/ALT >5× ULN, resume at 400 mg/d once levels return to normal **Disp:** 200 mg caps **SE:** ↓ WBC, ↓ plt, anemia, N/V/D, rash, edema **Notes:** Use chemotherapy precautions when handling

Nilutamide (Nilandron) **WARNING:** Interstitial pneumonitis possible; most cases in 1st 3 mo; check CXR before and during Rx **Uses:** *Combo w/ surgical castration for metastatic PCa* **Action:** Nonsteroidal antiandrogen **Dose:** 300 mg/d PO in ÷ doses × 30 d, then 150 mg/d **Caution:** [Not used in females] **CI:** Severe hepatic impair, resp Insuff **Disp:** Tabs 150 mg **SE:** Interstitial pneumonitis, hot flashes, ↓ libido, impotence, N/V/D, gynecomastia, hepatic dysfunction **Notes:** May cause Rxn when taken w/ EtOH, follow LFTs

Nimodipine (Nimotop) **WARNING:** Do not give IV or by other parenteral routes can cause death **Uses:** *Prevent vasospasm following subarachnoid hemorrhage* **Action:** CCB **Dose:** 60 mg PO q4h for 21 d; ↓ in hepatic failure **Caution:** [C, ?] **CI:** Component allergy **Disp:** Caps 30 mg **SE:** ↓ BP, HA, constipation **Notes:** Give via NG tube if caps cannot be swallowed whole

Nisoldipine (Sular) **Uses:** *HTN* **Action:** CCB **Dose:** 8.5–34 mg/d PO; take on empty stomach; ↓ start doses w/ elderly or hepatic impair **Caution:** [C, –] **Disp:** ER tabs 8.5, 17, 25.5, 34 mg **SE:** Edema, HA, flushing, ↓ BP

Nitazoxanide (Alinia) Uses: **Cryptosporidium or Giardia lamblia-*induced D* Action: Antiprotozoal interferes w/ pyruvate ferredoxin oxidoreductase. *Spectrum: Cryptosporidium, Giardia* Dose: *Adults.* 500 mg PO q12h × 3 d. *Peds 1–3 y:* 100 mg PO q12h × 3 d. *4–11 y:* 200 mg PO q12h × 3 d. *>12 y:* 500 mg q12h × 3 d; take w/ food Caution: [B, ?] Not effective in HIV or immunocompromised D* Disp: 100 mg/5 mL PO susp, 500 tab SE: Abd pain Notes: Susp contains sucrose, interacts w/ highly protein-bound drugs

Nitrofurantoin (Furadantin, Macrodantin, Macrobid) WARNING: Pulm fibrosis possible Uses: **Prophylaxis & Rx UTI** Action: Bacteriocidal; interferes w/ carbohydrate metabolism. *Spectrum:* Some gram(+) & (–) bacteria; *Pseudomonas, Serratia,* & most *Proteus* resistant Dose: *Adults.* Prophylaxis: 50–100 mg/d PO. *Rx:* 50–100 mg PO qid × 7 d; *Macrobid* 100 mg PO bid × 7 d. *Peds.* Prophylaxis: 1–2 mg/kg/d ÷ 1–2 doses, max 100 mg/d. *Rx:* 5–7 mg/kg/24 h in 4 ÷ doses (w/ food/milk/antacid) Caution: [B, +/not OK if child <1 mo] Avoid w/ CrCl <60 mL/min CI: Renal failure, infants <1 mo, pregnancy at term Disp: Caps 25, 50, 100 mg; susp 25 mg/5 mL SE: GI effects, dyspnea, various acute/chronic pulm Rxns, peripheral neuropathy, hemolytic anemia w/ G6PD deficiency, rare aplastic anemia Notes: Macrocrystals (Macrodantin) < N than other forms; not for comp UTI; may turn urine brown

Nitroglycerin (Nitrostat, Nitrolingual, Nitro-Bid Ointment, Nitro-Bid IV, Nitrodisc, Transderm-Nitro, NitroMist, others) Uses: **Angina pectoris, acute & prophylactic therapy, CHF, BP control** Action: Relaxes vascular smooth muscle, dilates coronary arteries Dose: *Adults. SL:* 1 tab q5min SL PRN for 3 doses. *Translingual:* 1–2 metered-doses sprayed onto PO mucosa q3–5min, max 3 doses. *PO:* 2.5–9 mg tid. *IV:* 5–20 mcg/min, titrated to effect. *Topical:* Apply 1/2 inch of oint to chest wall tid, wipe off at night. *Transdermal:* 0.2–0.4 mg/h/patch daily; aerosol 1 spray at 5-min intervals, max 3 doses (*ECC 2005*). *Peds.* 0.25–0.5 mcg/kg/min IV, titrated Caution: [B, ?] Restrictive cardiomyopathy CI: w/ Sildenafil, tadalafil, vardenafil, head trauma, NAG, pericardial tamponade, constrictive pericarditis. Disp: SL tabs 0.3, 0.4, 0.6 mg; translingual spray 0.4 mg/dose; SR caps 2.5, 6.5, 9 mg; Inj 0.1, 0.2, 0.4 mg/mL (premixed); 5 mg/mL Inj soln; oint 2%; transdermal patches 0.1, 0.2, 0.4, 0.6 mg/h; aerosol (*NitroMist*) 0.4 mg/spray SE: HA, ↓ BP, light-headedness, GI upset Notes: Nitrate tolerance w/ chronic use after 1–2 wk; minimize by providing 10–12 h nitrate-free period daily, using shorter-acting nitrates tid, & removing LA patches & oint before sleep to ↓ tolerance

Nitroprusside (Nipride, Nitropress) Uses: **Hypertensive crisis,* CHF, controlled ↓ BP perioperation (↓ bleeding),* aortic dissection, pulm edema Action: ↓ Systemic vascular resistance Dose: *Adults & Peds.* 0.5–10 mcg/kg/min IV Inf, titrate; usual dose 3 mcg/kg/min Caution: [C, ?] ↓ Cerebral perfusion CI: High output failure, compensatory HTN Disp: Inj 25 mg/mL SE: Excessive hypotensive effects, palpitations, HA Notes: Thiocyanate (metabolite w/ renal excretion) w/ tox at 5–10 mg/dL, more likely if used for >2–3 d; w/ aortic dissection use w/ β-blocker

Nizatidine (Axid, Axid AR [OTC]) Uses: *Duodenal ulcers, GERD, heartburn* Action: H$_2$-receptor antagonist Dose: *Adults.* Active ulcer: 150 mg PO bid or 300 mg PO hs; maint 150 mg PO hs. GERD: 150 mg PO bid. Heartburn: 75 mg PO bid. *Peds. GERD:* 10 mg/kg PO bid in ÷ doses, 150 mg bid max; ↓ in renal impair Caution: [B, ?] CI: H$_2$-receptor antagonist sensitivity Disp: Tab 75 mg [OTC]; caps 150, 300 mg; soln 15 mg/mL SE: Dizziness, HA, constipation, D

Norepinephrine (Levophed) Uses: *Acute ↓ BP, cardiac arrest (adjunct)* Action: Peripheral vasoconstrictor of arterial/venous beds Dose: *Adults.* 8–30 mcg/min IV, titrate. *Peds.* 0.05–0.1 mcg/kg/min IV, titrate Caution: [C, ?] CI: ↓ BP due to hypovolemia, vascular thrombosis, ↓ in renal or w/ cyclopropane/ halothane anesthetics Disp: Inj 1 mg/mL SE: Bradycardia, arrhythmia Notes: Correct vol depletion as much as possible before vasopressors; interaction w/ TCAs leads to severe HTN; use large vein to avoid extrav; phentolamine 5–10 mg/10 mL NS injected locally for extrav

Norethindrone acetate/ethinyl estradiol tablets (Femhrt) (See estradiol/norethindrone acetate)

Norfloxacin (Noroxin, Chibroxin ophthal) WARNING: Use associated with tendon rupture and tendonitis (pending) Uses: *Comp & uncomp UTI due to gram(–) bacteria, prostatitis, gonorrhea,* infectious D, conjunctivitis Action: Quinolone, ↓ DNA gyrase, bactericidal *Spectrum:* Broad gram(+) and (–) E. faecalis, E. coli, K. pneumoniae, P. mirabilis, P. aeruginosa, S. epidermidis, S. saprophyticus Dose: Uncomp UTI (E. coli, K. pneumoniae, P. mirabilis): 400 mg PO bid × 3 d; other uncomp UTI Rx × 7–10 d. Comp UTI: 400 mg q12h for 10–21 d PO bid. Gonorrhea: 800 mg × 1 dose. Prostatitis: 400 mg PO bid × 28 d. Gastroenteritis, traveler's D: 400 mg PO × 1–3 d; take 1 h ac or 2 h pc. Adults & Peds >1 y: Ophthal: 1 gtt each eye qid for 7 d; QCrl <30 mL/min use 400 mg q day Caution: [C, –] Quinolone sensitivity, w/ some antiarrhythmics CI: Hx allergy or tendon problems Disp: Tabs 400 mg; ophthal 3 mg/mL SE: Photosensitivity, HA, dizziness, asthenia, GI upset, pseudomembranous colitis; ocular burning w/ ophthal Notes: Interactions w/ antacids, theophylline, caffeine; good conc in the kidney & urine, poor blood levels; not for urosepsis; CDC suggests do not use for GC

Nortriptyline (Pamelor) WARNING: ↑ Suicide risk in pts <24 y w/ major depressive/other behavioral disorders especially during 1st month of Tx; risk ↓ pts >65 y; observe all pts for clinical Sxs; not for ped use Uses: *Endogenous depression* Action: TCA; ↑ synaptic CNS levels of serotonin &/or norepinephrine Dose: *Adults.* 25 mg PO tid-qid; >150 mg/d not OK. *Elderly:* 10–25 mg hs. *Peds 6–7 y:* 10 mg/d. *8–11 y:* 10–20 mg/d. *>11 y:* 25–35 mg/d, ↓ w/ hepatic Insuff Caution: [D, –] NAG, CV Dz CI: TCA allergy, use w/ MAOI Disp: Caps 10, 25, 50, 75 mg; soln 10 mg/5 mL SE: Anticholinergic (blurred vision, retention, xerostomia, sedation) Notes: Max effect may take >2–3 wk

Nystatin (Mycostatin) Uses: *Mucocutaneous *Candida* Infxns (oral, skin, vaginal)* Action: Alters membrane permeability. *Spectrum:* Susceptible *Candida* sp Dose: *Adults & Peds. PO:* 400,000–600,000 units PO "swish & swallow" qid. *Vaginal:* 1 tab vaginally hs × 2 wk. *Topical:* Apply bid-tid to area. *Peds Infants:* 200,000 units PO q6h. Caution: [B (C PO), +] Disp: PO susp 100,000 units/mL; PO tabs 500,000 units; troches 200,000 units; Vag tabs 100,000 units; topical cream/oint 100,000 units/g; powder 100,000 units/g SE: GI upset, Stevens-Johnson syndrome Notes: Not absorbed PO; not for systemic Infxns

Octreotide (Sandostatin, Sandostatin LAR) Uses: *↓ Severe D associated w/ carcinoid & neuroendocrine GI tumors (eg, vasoactive intestinal peptide-secreting tumor (VIPoma), ZE syndrome), acromegaly*; bleeding esophageal varices Action: LA peptide; mimics natural somatostatin Dose: *Adults.* 100–600 mcg/d SQ/IV in 2–4 ÷ doses; start 50 mcg daily-bid. *Sandostatin LAR (depot):* 10–30 mg IM q4wk. *Peds.* 1–10 mcg/kg/24 h SQ in 2–4 ÷ doses Caution: [B, +] Hepatic/renal impair Disp: Inj 0.05, 0.1, 0.2, 0.5, 1 mg/mL; 10, 20, 30 mg/5 mL LAR depot SE: N/V, Abd discomfort, flushing, edema, fatigue, cholelithiasis, hyper-/hypoglycemia, hep, hypothyroidism Notes: Stabilize for at least 2 wk before changing to LAR form

Ofloxacin (Floxin) WARNING: Use associated with tendon rupture and tendonitis (pending) Uses: *Lower resp tract, skin & skin structure, & UTI, prostatitis, uncomp gonorrhea, & *Chlamydia* Infxns* Action: Bactericidal; ↓ DNA gyrase. *Broad spectrum gram(+) & (–): S. pneumoniae, S. aureus, S. pyogenes, H. influenzae, P. mirabilis, N. gonorrhoeae, C. trachomatis, E. coli* Dose: *Adults.* 200–400 mg PO or IV q12h. *Adults & Peds >1 y: Ophthal:* 1–2 gtt in eye(s) q2–4h for 2 d, then qid × 5 more d. *Adults & Peds >12 y: Otic:* 10 gtt in ear(s) bid for 10 d. *Peds 1–12 y: Otic:* 5 gtt in ear(s) for 10 d; ↓ in renal impair, take on empty stomach Caution: [C, –] ↓ Absorption w/ antacids, sucralfate, Al⁻, Ca⁻, Mg⁻, Fe⁻, Zn-containing drugs CI: Quinolone allergy Disp: Tabs 200, 300, 400 mg; Inj 20, 40 mg/mL; ophthal & otic 0.3% SE: N/V/D, photosensitivity, insomnia, HA, local irritation Notes: Ophthal form OK in ears

Ofloxacin, ophthalmic (Ocuflox Ophthalmic) Uses: *Bacterial conjunctivitis, corneal ulcer* Action: See Ofloxacin Dose: *Adults & Peds >1 y:* 1–2 gtt in eye(s) q2–4h × 2 d, then qid × 5 more d Caution: [C, +/–] CI: Quinolone allergy Disp: Ophthal 0.3% soln SE: Burning, hyperemia, bitter taste, chemosis, photophobia

Ofloxacin, otic (generic) Uses: *Otitis externa; chronic suppurative otitis media w/ perf drums; otitis media in peds w/ tubes* Action: See Ofloxacin Dose: *Adults & Peds >13 y: Otitis externa:* 10 gtt in ear(s) × 7–14 d. *Peds 1–12 y: Otitis media* 5 gtt in ear(s) bid × 10 d Caution: [C, –] CI: Quinolone allergy Disp: Otic 0.3% soln SE: Local irritation Notes: OK with tubes/perforated drums; 10 gtt = 0.5 mL

Olanzapine (Zyprexa, Zyprexa Zydis)   WARNING: ↑ Mortality in elderly w/ dementia-related psychosis Uses: *Bipolar mania, schizophrenia,* psychotic disorders, acute agitation in schizophrenia Action: Dopamine & serotonin antagonist. Dose: *Bipolar/schizophrenia:* 5–10 mg PO, weekly PRN, 20 mg/d max. *Agitation:* 5–10 mg IM q2–4h PRN, 30 mg d/max Caution: [C, –] Disp: Tabs 2.5, 5, 7.5, 10, 15, 20 mg; PO disintegrating tabs (*Zyprexa Zydis*) 5, 10, 15, 20 mg; Inj 10 mg SE: HA, somnolence, orthostatic ↓ BP, tachycardia, dystonia, xerostomia, constipation, hyperglycemia Notes: Takes wk to titrate dose; smoking ↓ levels; may be confused w/ Zyrtec

Olopatadine, nasal (Patanase)   Uses: *Seasonal allergic rhinitis* Action: H_1-receptor antagonist Dose: 2 sprays each nostril bid Caution: [C, ?] Disp: 0.6% 240-Spray bottle SE: Epistaxis, bitter taste somnolence, HA, rhinitis

Olopatadine ophthalmic (Patanol, Pataday)   Uses: *Allergic conjunctivitis* Action: H_1-receptor antagonist Dose: *Patanol:* 1–2 gtt in eye(s) bid; *Pataday:* 1 gtt in eye(s) q day Caution: [C, ?] Disp: *Patanol:* Soln 0.1% 5 mL *Pataday:* 0.2% 2.5 mL SE: Local irritation, HA, rhinitis Notes: Wait 10 min after to insert contacts

Olsalazine (Dipentum) Uses: *Maintain remission in UC* Action: Topical anti-inflammatory Dose: 500 mg PO bid (w/ food) Caution: [C, –] CI: Salicylate sensitivity Disp: Caps 250 mg SE: D, HA, blood dyscrasias, hep

Omalizumab (Xolair)   WARNING: Reports of anaphylaxis 2–24 h after administration, even in previously treated pts Uses: *Mod–severe asthma in ≥12 y w/ reactivity to an allergen & when Sxs inadequately controlled w/ inhaled steroids* Action: Anti-IgE Ab Dose: 150–375 mg SQ q2–4wk (dose/frequency based on serum IgE level & body wgt; see package insert) Caution: [B, ?/–] CI: Component allergy, acute bronchospasm Disp: 150-mg single-use 5-mL vial SE: Site Rxn, sinusitis, HA, anaphylaxis reported in 3 pts Notes: Continue other asthma meds as indicated

Omega-3 fatty acid [fish oil] (Lovaza)   Uses: *Rx hypertriglyceridemia* Action: Omega-3 acid ethyl esters, ↓ thrombus inflammation & triglycerides Dose: *Hypertriglyceridemia:* 4 g/d ÷ in 1–2 doses Caution: Fish hypersensitivity; PRG risk factor [C, –], w/ anticoagulant use, w/ bleeding risk CI: Hypersensitivity to components Disp: 1000-mg gel caps SE: Dyspepsia, N, GI pain, rash, flu-like syndrome Notes: Only FDA-approved fish oil supl; not for exogenous hypertriglyceridemia (type 1 hyperchylomicronemia); many OTC products (page 242). D/C after 2 mo if triglyceride levels do not ↓; previously called "Omacor"

Omeprazole (Prilosec, Prilosec OTC, Zegerid)   Uses: *Duodenal/ gastric ulcers, prevent NSAID ulcers, esophagitis, ZE syndrome, GERD,* H. pylori Infxns Action: Proton pump inhibitor; *Zegerid* w/ sodium bicarb Dose: Adults. 20–40 mg PO daily-bid × 4–8 wk; H. pylori 20 mg PO bid × 10 d w/ amoxicillin & clarithromycin; 80 mg/d max. *Peds 2–16 y <20 kg:* 10 mg PO q day. *>20 kg:* 20 mg PO q day; 40 mg/d max Caution: [C, –/+] Disp: OTC DR tabs 20 mg; DR caps 20, 40 mg;

Zegerid (omeprazole mg/sodium bicarb mg) caps 20/1100, 40/1100; powder packet for oral susp 20/1680, 40/1680 **SE:** HA, D **Notes:** Combo w/ antibiotic Rx for *H. pylori*, take Zegerid 1 h ac; Zegerid powder mix in small cup w/ 2 tbsp H_2O (not food or other liq) refill and drink; do not open Zegerid caps

Ondansetron (Zofran, Zofran ODT) Uses: *Prevent chemotherapy-associated & post-op N/V* **Action:** Serotonin receptor (5-HT_3) antagonist **Dose: Adults & Peds.** *Chemotherapy:* 0.15 mg/kg/dose IV prior to chemotherapy, then 4 & 8 h after 1st dose or 4–8 mg PO tid; 1st dose 30 min prior to chemotherapy & give on schedule, not PRN. **Adults.** *Postoperation:* 4 mg IV immediately preanesthesia or postoperation. **Peds.** *Postoperation:* *<40 kg:* 0.1 mg/kg. *>40 kg:* 4 mg IV; ↓ w/ hepatic impair **Caution:** [B, +/–] **Disp:** Tabs 4, 8, 24 mg, soln 4 mg/5 mL, Inj 2 mg/mL, 32 mg/50 mL; Zofran ODT tabs 4, 8 mg **SE:** D, HA, constipation, dizziness

Oprelvekin (Neumega) WARNING: Allergic Rxn w/ anaphylaxis reported; D/C w/ any allergic Rxn **Uses:** *Prevent ↓ plt w/ chemotherapy* **Action:** ↑ Proliferation & maturation of megakaryocytes (IL-11) **Dose: Adults.** 50 mcg/kg/d SQ for 10–21 d. **Peds >12 y:** 75–100 mcg/kg/d SQ for 10–21 d. **<12 y:** Use only in clinical trials; ↓ w/ CrCt <30 mL/min 25 mcg/kg. **Caution:** [C, ?/–] **Disp:** 5 mg powder for Inj **SE:** Tachycardia, palpitations, arrhythmias, edema, HA, dizziness, visual disturbances, papilledema, insomnia, fatigue, fever, N, anemia, dyspnea, allergic Rxns including anaphylaxis

Oral Contraceptives, Biphasic, Monophasic, Triphasic, Progestin Only (Table 6) WARNING: Cigarette smoking ↑ risk of serious CV side effects; ↑ risk w/ >15 cigarettes/d, >35 y; strongly advise women on OCP to not smoke. Patients should be counseled that these products do not protect against HIV and other STD **Uses:** *Birth control; regulation of anovulatory bleeding; dysmenorrhea; endometriosis; polycystic ovaries; acne** (Note: FDA approvals vary widely, see insert) **Action:** *Birth control:* Suppresses LH surge, prevents ovulation; progestins thicken cervical mucus; ↓ fallopian tubule cilia, ↓ endometrial thickness to ↓ chances of fertilization. *Anovulatory bleeding:* Cyclic hormones mimic body's natural cycle & regulate endometrial lining, results in regular bleeding q28d; may ↓ uterine bleeding & dysmenorrhea **Dose:** Start day 1 menstrual cycle or 1st Sunday after onset of menses; 28-d cycle pills take daily; 21-d cycle pills take daily, no pills during last 7 d of cycle (during menses); some available as transdermal patch **Caution:** [X, +] Migraine, HTN, DM, sickle cell Dz, gallbladder Dz; monitor for breast Dz, ✓ K^+ if taking drugs with ↑ K^+ risk **CI:** AUB, PRG, estrogen-dependent malignancy, ↑ hypercoagulation/liver Dz, hemiplegic migraine, smokers >35 y **Disp:** 28-d cycle pills (21 active pills + 7 placebo or Fe supl) 21-d cycle pills (21 active pills) **SE:** Intramenstrual bleeding, oligomenorrhea, amenorrhea, ↑ appetite/wgt gain, ↓ libido, fatigue, depression, mood swings, mastalgia, HA, melasma, ↑ Vag discharge, acne/greasy skin, corneal edema, N **Notes:** Taken correctly, 99.9% effective for contraception;

no STDs prevention, use additional barrier contraceptive; long-term, can ↓ risk of ectopic PRG, benign breast Dz, ovarian & uterine CA.

* *Rx menstrual cycle control:* Start w/ monophasic × 3 mo before switching to another brand; w/ continued bleeding change to pill w/ ↑ estrogen
* *Rx birth control:* Choose pill w/ lowest SE profile for particular pt; SEs numerous; due to estrogenic excess or progesterone deficiency; each pill's SE profile can be unique (see insert); newer extended-cycle combos have shorter/fewer hormone-free intervals, ? ↓ PRG risk; OCP troubleshooting SE w/ suggested OCP.

  * *Absent menstrual flow:* ↑ Estrogen, ↓ progestin: Brevicon, Necon 1/35, Norinyl 1/35, Modicon, Necon 1/50, Norinyl 1/50, Ortho-Cyclen, Ortho-Novum 1/35, Ortho-Novum 1/35, Ovcon 35
  * *Acne:* Use ↑ estrogen, ↓ androgenic: Brevicon, Ortho-Cyclen, Demulen 1/50, Ortho Tri-Cyclen, Mircette, Modicon, Necon, Ortho Evra, Yasmin, Yaz
  * *Break-through bleed:* ↑ Estrogen, ↑ progestin, ↓ androgenic: Demulen 1/50, Desogen, Estrostep, Loestrin 1/20, Ortho-Cept, Ovcon 50, Yasmin, Zovia 1/50E
  * *Breast tenderness or ↑ wgt:* ↓ Estrogen, ↓ progestin: Use ↓ estrogen pill rather than current; Alesse, Levlite, Loestrin 1/20 Fe, Ortho Evra, Yasmin, Yaz
  * *Depression:* ↓ Progestin: Alesse, Brevicon, Levlite, Modicon, Necon, Ortho Evra, Ovcon 35, Ortho-Cyclen, Ortho Tri-Cyclen Tri-Levlen, Triphasil, Trivora
  * *Endometriosis:* ↓ Estrogen, ↑ progestin: Demulen 1/35, Loestrin 1.5/30, Loestrin 1/20 Fe, Lo Ovral, Levlen, Levora, Nordette, Zovia 1/35; cont w/o placebo pills or w/ 4 d of placebo pills
  * *HA:* ↓ Estrogen, ↓ progestin: Alesse, Levlite, Ortho Evra
  * *Moodiness &/or irritability:* ↓ Progestin: Alesse, Brevicon, Levlite, Modicon, Necon 1/35, Ortho Evra, Ortho-Cyclen, Ortho Tri-Cyclen, Ovcon 35, Tri-Levlen, Triphasil, Trivora
  * *Severe menstrual cramping:* ↑ Progestin: Demulen 1/50, Desogen, Loestrin 1.5/30, Mircette, Ortho-Cept, Yasmin, Yaz, Zovia 1/50E, Zovia 1/35E

Orlistat (Xenical, Alli [OTC]).
Uses: *Manage obesity w/ body mass index ≥30 kg/m² or ≥27 kg/m² w/ other risk factors; type 2 DM, dyslipidemia* **Action:** Reversible inhibitor of gastric & pancreatic lipases. **Dose:** 120 mg PO tid w/ a fat-containing meal; Alli (OTC) 60 mg PO tid w/ fat-containing meals **Caution:** [B, ?] May ↓ cyclosporine & warfarin dose requirements **CI:** Cholestasis, malabsorption, organ transplant **Disp:** Capsules 120 mg; Alli OTC 60 mg caps **SE:** Abd pain/discomfort, fatty stools, fecal urgency **Notes:** Do not use if meal contains no fat; GI effects ↑ w/ higher-fat meals; supl w/ fat-soluble vits

Orphenadrine (Norflex)
Uses: *Discomfort associated w/ painful musculoskeletal conditions* **Action:** Central atropine-like effect; indirect skeletal muscle relaxation, euphoria, analgesia **Dose:** 100 mg PO bid, 60 mg IM/IV q12h **Caution:** [C, +/−] **CI:** NAG, GI or bladder obst, cardiospasm, MyG **Disp:** SR tabs 100 mg; Inj 30 mg/mL **SE:** Drowsiness, dizziness, blurred vision, flushing, tachycardia, constipation

Oseltamivir (Tamiflu)   **Uses:** *Prevention & Rx influenza A & B* **Action:** ↓ Viral neuraminidase **Dose: *Adults. Tx:*** 75 mg PO bid for 5 d; *Prophylaxis:* 75 mg PO daily × 10 D. ***Peds. Tx:*** PO bid; dosing: *<15 kg:* 30 mg. *15–23 kg:* 45 mg. *23–40 kg:* 60 mg. *>40 kg:* adult dose. *Prophylaxis:* same dosing but q day; ↓ w/ renal impair **Caution:** [C, ?/–] **CI:** Component allergy **Disp:** Caps 75 mg, powder 12 mg/mL **SE:** N/V, insomnia, reports of neuropsychological events in children (self-injury, confusion, delirium) **Notes:** Initiate w/in 48 h of Sx onset or exposure

Oxacillin (Prostaphlin)   **Uses:** *Infxns due to susceptible S. aureus & Streptococcus* **Action:** Bactericidal; ↓ cell wall synth. *Spectrum:* Excellent gram(+), poor gram(–) **Dose: *Adults.*** 250–500 mg (2 g severe) IM/IV q4–6h. ***Peds.*** 150–200 mg/kg/d IV ÷ q4–6h **Caution:** [B, M] **CI:** PCN sensitivity **Disp:** Powder for Inj 500 mg, 1, 2, 10 g **SE:** GI upset, interstitial nephritis, blood dyscrasias

Oxaliplatin (Eloxatin)   **WARNING:** Administer w/ supervision of physician experienced in chemotherapy. Appropriate management is possible only w/ adequate diagnostic & Rx facilities. Anaphylactic-like Rxns reported **Uses:** *Adjuvant Rx stage-III colon CA (primary resected) & metastatic colon CA w/ 5-FU* **Action:** Metabolized to platinum derivatives, crosslinks DNA **Dose:** Per protocol; see insert. *Premedicate:* Antiemetic w/ or w/o dexamethasone **Caution:** [D, –] See Warning **CI:** Allergy to components or platinum **Disp:** Inj 50, 100 mg **SE:** Anaphylaxis, granulocytopenia, paresthesia, N/V/D, stomatitis, fatigue, neuropathy, hepatotox, pulm tox **Notes:** 5-FU & leucovorin are given in combo; epi, corticosteroids, & antihistamines alleviate severe Rxns

Oxaprozin (Daypro, Daypro ALTA)   **WARNING:** May ↑ risk of cardiovascular events & GI bleeding **Uses:** *Arthritis & pain* **Action:** NSAID; ↓ prostaglandin synth **Dose: *Adults.*** 600–1200 mg/daily (÷ dose helps GI tolerance); ↓ w/ renal/hepatic impair ***Peds. JRA (Daypro):* 22–31 kg:** 600 mg/d. *32–54 kg:* 900 mg/d **Caution:** [C (D in 3rd tri), ?] Peptic ulcer, bleeding disorders **CI:** ASA/NSAID sensitivity perioperative pain w/ coronary artery bypass graft **Disp:** *Daypro ALTA* tab 600 mg; caplets 600 mg **SE:** CNS inhibition, sleep disturbance, rash, GI upset, peptic ulcer, edema, renal failure, anaphylactoid Rxn w/ ASA triad (asthmatic w/ rhinitis, nasal polyps and bronchospasm w/ NSAID use)

Oxazepam [C-IV]   **Uses:** *Anxiety, acute EtOH withdrawal,* anxiety w/ depressive Sxs **Action:** Benzodiazepine; diazepam metabolite **Dose: *Adults.*** 10–15 mg PO tid-qid; severe anxiety & EtOH withdrawal may require up to 30 mg qid. ***Peds.*** 1 mg/kg/d ÷ doses **Caution:** [D, ?/–] **CI:** Component allergy, NAG **Disp:** Caps 10, 15, 30 mg; tabs 15 mg **SE:** Sedation, ataxia, dizziness, rash, blood dyscrasias, dependence **Notes:** Avoid abrupt D/C

Oxcarbazepine (Trileptal)   **Uses:** *Partial Szs,* bipolar disorders **Action:** Blocks voltage-sensitive Na^+ channels, stabilization of hyperexcited neural membranes **Dose: *Adults.*** 300 mg PO bid, ↑ weekly to target maint 1200–2400 mg/d.

Peds. 8–10 mg/kg bid, 600 mg/d max, ↑ weekly to target maint dose; ↓ w/ renal Insuff **Caution:** [C, –] Carbamazepine sensitivity; **CI:** Components sensitivity **Disp:** Tabs 150, 300, 600 mg; susp 300 mg/5 mL **SE:** ↓ Na⁺, HA, dizziness, fatigue, somnolence, GI upset, diplopia, concentration difficulties, fatal skin/multi-organ hypersensitivity Rxns **Notes:** Do not abruptly D/C, ✓ Na⁺ if fatigued; advise about Stevens–Johnson syndrome and topic epidermal necrolysis

Oxiconazole (Oxistat)   **Uses:** *Tinea cruris, tinea corporis, tinea pedis, tinea versicolor* **Action:** ? ↓ Ergosterols in fungal cell membrane. *Spectrum:* Most *Epidermophyton floccosum, Trichophyton mentagrophytes, Trichophyton rubrum, Malassezia furfur* **Dose:** Apply thin layer daily-bid **Caution:** [B, M] **CI:** Component allergy **Disp:** Cream, lotion 1% **SE:** Local irritation

Oxybutynin (Ditropan, Ditropan XL)   **Uses:** *Symptomatic relief of urgency, nocturia, incontinence w/ neurogenic or reflex neurogenic bladder* **Action:** Anticholinergic, relaxes bladder smooth muscle, ↑ bladder capacity **Dose:** *Adults.* 5 mg bid-tid, 5 mg qid max. XL 5–10 mg/d, 30 mg/d max. *Peds >5 y:* 5 mg PO bid-tid; 15 mg/d max. *Peds 1–5 y:* 0.2 mg/kg/dose bid-qid (syrup 5 mg/5 mL); 15 mg/d max; in elderly; periodic drug holidays OK **Caution:** [B, ?] **CI:** NAG, MyG, GI/GU obst, ulcerative colitis, megacolon **Disp:** Tabs 5 mg; XL tabs 5, 10, 15 mg; syrup 5 mg/5 mL **SE:** Anticholinergic (drowsiness, xerostomia, constipation, tachycardia), ER form shell expelled in stool

Oxybutynin Transdermal System (Oxytrol)   **Uses:** *Rx OAB* **Action:** Anticholinergic, relaxes bladder smooth muscle, ↑ bladder capacity **Dose:** One 3.9 mg/d system apply 2×/wk (q3–4d) to abdomen, hip, or buttock **Caution:** [B, ?/–] GI/GU obst, NAG **Disp:** 3.9 mg/d transdermal patch **SE:** Anticholinergic, itching/redness at site **Notes:** Do not apply to same site w/in 7 d

Oxycodone [Dihydro hydroxycodeinone] (OxyContin, OxyIR, Roxicodone) [C-II]   **WARNING:** High-abuse potential; controlled release only for extended chronic pain, not for PRN use; 60-, 80-, 160-mg tab for opioid-tolerant pts **Uses:** *Mod–severe pain, usually in combo w/ nonnarcotic analgesics* **Action:** Narcotic analgesic **Dose:** *Adults.* 5 mg PO q6h PRN (IR). *Mod–severe chronic pain:* 10–160 mg PO q12h (ER). *Peds 6–12 y:* 1.25 mg PO q6h PRN. *>12 y:* 2.5 mg q6h PRN; ↓ w/ severe liver/renal Dz, elderly; w/ food **Caution:** [B (D if prolonged use/near term)] **CI:** Allergy, resp depression, acute asthma, ileus w/ microsomal morphine **Disp:** IR caps (OxyIR) 5 mg; CR Roxicodone tabs 15, 30 mg; ER (OxyContin) 10, 15, 20, 30, 40, 60, 80 mg; liq 5 mg/5 mL; soln conc 20 mg/mL **SE:** ↓ BP, sedation, resp depression, dizziness, GI upset, constipation, risk of abuse **Notes:** OxyContin for chronic CA pain; do not crush/chew/cut ER product; sought after as drug of abuse

Oxycodone & Acetaminophen (Percocet, Tylox) [C-II]   **Uses:** *Mod–severe pain* **Action:** Narcotic analgesic **Dose:** *Adults.* 1–2 tabs/caps PO q4–6h PRN (acetaminophen max dose 4 g/d). *Peds.* Oxycodone 0.05–0.15 mg/ kg/dose q 4–6h PRN, 5 mg/dose max **Caution:** [C (D prolonged use or near term), M] **CI:** Allergy, paralytic ileus, resp depression **Disp:** Percocet tabs, mg oxycodone/mg APAP: 2.5/325, 5/325, 7.5/325, 10/325, 7.5/500, 10/650; Tylox caps 5 mg oxycodone, 500 mg APAP; soln 5 mg oxycodone & 325 mg APAP/5 mL **SE:** ↓ BP, sedation, dizziness, GI upset, constipation

Oxycodone & Aspirin (Percodan) [C-II]   **Uses:** *Mod–severe pain* **Action:** Narcotic analgesic w/ NSAID **Dose:** *Adults.* 1–2 tabs/caps PO q4–6h PRN. *Peds.* Oxycodone 0.05–0.15 mg/kg/dose q 4–6h PRN, up to 5 mg/dose; ↓ in severe hepatic failure **Caution:** [D, –] Peptic ulcer **CI:** Component allergy, children (<16 y) with viral Infxn, resp depression, ileus **Disp:** *Generics:* 4.83 mg oxycodone hydrochloride, 0.38 mg oxycodone terephthalate, 325 mg ASA; *Percodan* 4.83 mg oxycodone hydrochloride, 325 mg ASA **SE:** Sedation, dizziness, GI upset/ulcer, constipation, allergy

Oxycodone/Ibuprofen (Combunox) [C-II]   **WARNING:** May ↑ risk of serious CV events; CI in perioperative coronary artery bypass graft pain; ↑ risk of GI events such as bleeding **Uses:** *Short-term (not >7 d) management of acute mod–severe pain* **Action:** Narcotic w/ NSAID **Dose:** 1 tab q6h PRN 4 tab max/24 h; 7 d max **Caution:** [C, –] w/ Impaired renal/hepatic Fxn; COPD, CNS depression, avoid in PRG **CI:** Paralytic ileus, 3rd tri PRG, allergy to ASA or NSAIDs, where opioids are CI **Disp:** Tabs 5 mg oxycodone/400 mg ibuprofen **SE:** N/V, somnolence, dizziness, sweating, flatulence, ↑ LFTs **Notes:** ✓ renal Fxn; abuse potential w/ oxycodone

Oxymorphone (Opana, Opana ER) [C-II]   **WARNING:** (Opana ER) Abuse potential, controlled release only for chronic pain; do not consume EtOH-containing beverages, may cause fatal OD **Uses:** *Mod/severe pain, sedative* **Action:** Narcotic analgesic **Dose:** 10–20 mg PO q4–6h PRN if opioid-naïve or 1–1.5 mg SQ/IM q4–6h PRN or 0.5 mg IV q4–6h PRN; start 20 mg/dose max PO; *Chronic pain:* ER 5 mg PO q12h; if opioid-naïve ↑ PRN 5–10 mg PO q12h q3–7d; take 1 h pc or 2 h ac; ↓ dose w/ elderly, renal/hepatic impair **Caution:** [B, ?] **CI:** ↑ ICP, severe resp depression, w/ EtOH or liposomal morphine, severe hepatic impair **Disp:** Tabs 5, 10 mg; ER 5, 10, 20, 40 mg **SE:** ↓ BP, sedation, GI upset, constipation, histamine release **Notes:** Related to hydromorphone

Oxytocin (Pitocin)   **Uses:** *Induce labor, control postpartum hemorrhage* **Action:** Stimulate muscular contractions of the uterus **Dose:** 0.0005–0.001 units/min IV Inf; titrate 0.001–0.002 units/min q30–60min **Caution:** [Uncategorized, +/–] **CI:** Where Vag delivery not favorable, fetal distress **Disp:** Inj 10 units/mL **SE:** Uterine rupture, fetal death; arrhythmias, anaphylaxis, H_2O intoxication **Notes:** Monitor vital signs; nasal form for breast-feeding only

Paclitaxel (Taxol, Abraxane)   **WARNING:** Administration only by physician experienced in chemotherapy; fatal anaphylaxis and hypersensitivity possible; severe myelosuppression possible **Uses:** *Ovarian & breast CA, PCa,* Kaposi sarcoma, NSCLC **Action:** Mitotic spindle poison; promotes microtubule assembly & stabilization against depolarization **Dose:** Per protocols; use glass

or polyolefin containers (eg, nitroglycerin tubing set); PVC sets leach plasticizer; ↓ in hepatic failure **Caution:** [D, –] **CI:** Neutropenia <1500 WBC/mm³; solid tumors, component allergy **Disp:** Inj 6 mg/mL, 5 mg/mL albumin bound (Abraxane) **SE:** ↓ BM, peripheral neuropathy, transient ileus, myalgia, bradycardia, ↓ BP, mucositis, N/V/D, fever, rash, HA, diarrhea; hematologic tox schedule-dependent; leukopenia dose-limiting by 24-h Inf; neurotox limited w/ short (1–3 h) Inf; allergic Rxns (dyspnea, ↓ BP, urticaria, rash) **Notes:** Maintain hydration; allergic Rxn usually w/in 10 min of Inf; minimize w/ corticosteroid, antihistamine pretreatment

Palivizumab (Synagis)   **Uses:** *Prevent RSV Infxn* **Action:** MoAb **Dose:** *Peds.* 15 mg/kg IM monthly, typically Nov–Apr **Caution:** [C, ?] Renal/hepatic dysfunction **CI:** Component allergy **Disp:** Vials 50, 100 mg **SE:** hypersensitivity Rxn, URI, rhinitis, cough, ↑ LFTs, local irritation

Palifermin (Kepivance)   **Uses:** *Oral mucositis w/ BMT* **Action:** Synthetic keratinocyte GF **Dose:** *Phase 1:* 60 mcg/kg IV daily × 3, 3rd dose 24–48 h before chemotherapy. *Phase 2:* 60 mcg/kg IV daily × 3, immediately after stem cell Inf **Caution:** [C, ?/–] **CI:** N/A **Disp:** Inj 6.25 mg **SE:** Unusual mouth sensations, tongue thickening, rash, ↑ amylase & lipase **Notes:** *E. coli* derived; separate phases by 4 d; safety unknown w/ nonhematologic malignancies

Paliperidone (Invega)   **WARNING:** Not for dementia-related psychosis **Uses:** *Schizophrenia* **Action:** Risperidone metabolite, antagonizes dopamine, and serotonin receptors **Dose:** 6 mg PO q A.M., 12 mg/d max; $CrCl$ 50–79: 6 mg/d max; $CrCl$ 10–49: 3 mg/d max **Caution:** [C; ?/–] w/ Bradycardia, ↓ K⁺/Mg²⁺, renal/hepatic impair **CI:** Risperidone hypersensitivity, w/ phenothiazines, ranolazine, ziprasidone, prolonged QT, Hx arrhythmia **Disp:** ER tabs 3, 6, 9 mg **SE:** Impaired temperature regulation, ↑ QT & HR, HA, anxiety, dizziness, N, dry mouth, fatigue, EPS **Notes:** Do not chew/cut/crush pill

Palonosetron (Aloxi)   **WARNING:** May ↑ QTc interval **Uses:** *Prevention acute & delayed N/V w/ emetogenic chemotherapy; prevent postoperative N/V* **Action:** 5-HT₃-receptor antagonist **Dose:** *Chemotherapy:* 0.25 mg IV 30 min prior to chemotherapy. *Postoperative N/V:* 0.75 mg immediately before induction **Caution:** [B, ?] **CI:** Component allergy **Disp:** 0.25 mg/5 mL vial **SE:** HA, constipation, dizziness, Abd pain, anxiety

Pamidronate (Aredia)   **Uses:** *Hypercalcemia of malignancy, Paget Dz, palliate symptomatic bone metastases* **Action:** Bisphosphonate; ↓ nl & abnormal bone resorption **Dose:** *Hypercalcemia:* 60–90 mg IV over 2–24 h or 90 mg IV over 24 h if severe; may repeat in 7 d. *Paget Dz:* 30 mg/d IV slow Inf over 4 h × 3 d. *Osteolytic bone mets in myeloma:* 90 mg IV over 4 h q mo. *Osteolytic bone mets breast CA:* 90 mg IV over 2 h q3–4wk; 90 mg/max single dose. **Caution:** [D, ?/–] Avoid invasive dental procedures w/ use **CI:** PRG, bisphosphonate sensitivity **Disp:** Inj 30, 60, 90 mg **SE:** Fever, malaise, convulsions, Inj site Rxn, uveitis, fluid overload, HTN, Abd pain, N/V, constipation, UTI, bone pain, ↓ K⁺, ↓ Ca²⁺, ↓ Mg²⁺, hypophosphatemia; jaw osteonecrosis, renal tox **Notes:** Perform dental exam pretherapy; follow Cr, hold dose if Cr ↑ by 0.5 mg/dL w/ nl baseline or by 1 mg/dL w/ abnormal baseline; restart when Cr returns w/in 10% of baseline

Pancrelipase (Pancrease, Cotazym, Creon, Ultrase) Uses: *Exocrine pancreatic secretion deficiency (eg, CF, chronic pancreatitis, pancreatic Insuff), steatorrhea of malabsorption* Action: Pancreatic enzyme supl Dose: 1–3 caps (tabs) w/ meals & snacks; ↑ to 8 caps (tabs); do not crush or chew EC products; dose dependent on digestive requirements of pt; avoid antacids Caution: [C, ?/–] CI: Pork product allergy, acute pancreatitis Disp: Caps, tabs SE: N/V, Abd cramps Notes: Individualize therapy

Pancuronium (Pavulon) WARNING: Should only be administered by adequately trained individuals Uses: *Paralysis w/ mechanical ventilation* Action: Nondepolarizing neuromuscular blocker Dose: Adults & Peds >1 mo: Initial 0.06–0.1 mg/kg; maint 0.01 mg/kg 60–100 min after, then 0.01 mg/kg q25–60min PRN; ↓ w/ renal/hepatic impair; intubate pt & keep on controlled ventilation; use adequate sedation or analgesia Caution: [C, ?/–] CI: Component or bromide sensitivity Disp: Inj 1, 2 mg/mL SE: Tachycardia, HTN, pruritus, other histamine Rxns

Panitumumab (Vectibix) WARNING: Derm tox common (89%) and severe in 12%; can be associated w/ Infxn (sepsis, abscesses requiring I&D; w/ severe derm tox, hold or D/C and monitor for Infxn; severe Inf Rxns (anaphylactic Rxn, bronchospasm, fever, chills, hypotension) in 1%; w/ severe Rxns, immediately D/C Inf and possibly permanent discontinuation Uses: *Rx EGFR-expressing metastatic colon CA* Action: Anti-EGFR MoAB Dose: 6 mg/kg IV Inf over 60 min q14d; doses >1000 mg over 90 min ↓ Inf rate by 50% w/ grade 1–2 Inf Rxn, D/C permanently w/ grade 3–4 Rxn. For derm tox, hold until <grade 2 tox. If improves <1 mo, restart 50% original dose. If tox recurs or resolution >1 mo permanently D/C. If ↓ dose tolerated, ↑ dose by 25% Caution: [C; –] D/C nursing during, 2 mo after Disp: Vial 20 mg/mL SE: Rash, acneiform dermatitis, pruritus, paronychia, ↓ Mg^{2+}, Abd pain, N/V/D, constipation, fatigue, dehydration, photosensitivity, conjunctivitis, ocular hyperemia, ↑ lacrimation, stomatitis, mucositis, pulm fibrosis, severe derm tox, Inf Rxns Notes: May impair female fertility; ✓ lytes; wear sunscreen/hats, limit sun exposure

Pantoprazole (Protonix) Uses: *GERD, erosive gastritis,* ZE syndrome, PUD Action: Proton pump inhibitor Dose: 40 mg/d PO; do not crush/ chew tabs; 40 mg IV/d (not >3 mg/min, use Protonix filter) Caution: [B, ?/–] Disp: Tabs, DR 20, 40 mg; 40 mg powder for oral susp (mix in applesauce or juice, give immediately) Inj 40 mg SE: Chest pain, anxiety, GI upset, ↑ LFTs

Paregoric [Camphorated Tincture of Opium] [C-III] Uses: *D,* pain & neonatal opiate withdrawal syndrome Action: Narcotic Dose: Adults. 5–10 mL PO daily–qid PRN. Peds. 0.25–0.5 mL/kg daily–qid. Neonatal withdrawal: 3–6 gtt PO q3–6h PRN to relieve Sxs × 3–5 d, then taper over 2–4 wk Caution: [B (D w/ prolonged use/high dose near term, +] CI: Toxic D; convulsive disorder, morphine sensitivity **Disp:** Liq 2 mg morphine = 20 mg opium/5 mL **SE:** ↓ BP, sedation, constipation **Notes:** Contains anhydrous morphine from opium; short-term use only

Paroxetine (Paxil, Paxil CR, Pexeva)   WARNING: Closely monitor for worsening depression or emergence of suicidality, particularly in children, adolescents, and young adults; not for use in peds **Uses:** *Depression, obsessive-compulsive disorder, panic disorder, social anxiety disorder,* PMDD **Action:** SSRI **Dose:** 10–60 mg PO single daily dose in A.M.; CR 25 mg/d PO; ↑ 12.5 mg/d (max range 26–62.5 mg/d) **Caution:** [D, ?/] ↑ Bleeding risk **CI:** w/ MAOI, thioridazine, pimozide **Disp:** Tabs 10, 20, 30, 40 mg; susp 10 mg/5 mL; CR 12.5, 25, 37.5 mg **SE:** HA, somnolence, dizziness, GI upset, N/D, ↓ appetite, sweating, xerostomia, tachycardia, ↓ libido

Pegfilgrastim (Neulasta)   Uses: *↓ Frequency of Infxn in pts w/ non-myeloid malignancies receiving myelosuppressive anti-CA drugs that cause febrile neutropenia* **Action:** Granulocyte- and macrophage-stimulating factor **Dose:** *Adults.* 6 mg SQ × 1/chemotherapy cycle. **Caution:** [C, M] w/ Sickle cell **CI:** Allergy to *E. coli*-derived proteins or filgrastim **Disp:** *Syringes:* 6 mg/0.6 mL **SE:** Splenic rupture, HA, fever, weakness, fatigue, dizziness, insomnia, edema, N/V/D, stomatitis, anorexia, constipation, taste perversion, dyspepsia, Abd pain, granulocytopenia, neutropenic fever, ↑ LFTs & uric acid, arthralgia, myalgia, bone pain, ARDS, alopecia, worsen sickle cell Dz **Notes:** Never give between 14 d before & 24 h after dose of cytotoxic chemotherapy

Peginterferon Alfa-2a (Pegasys)   WARNING: Can cause or aggravate fatal or life-threatening neuropsychological, autoimmune, ischemic, and infectious disorders. Monitor pts closely **Uses:** *Chronic hep C w/ compensated liver Dz* **Action:** Immune modulator **Dose:** 180 mcg (1 mL) SQ q wk × 48 wk; ↓ in renal impair **Caution:** [C, /?−] **CI:** Autoimmune hep, decompensated liver Dz **Disp:** 180 mcg/mL Inj **SE:** Depression, insomnia, suicidal behavior, GI upset, ↓ WBC and plt, alopecia, pruritus

Peginterferon Alfa-2b (PEG-Intron)   WARNING: Can cause or aggravate fatal or life-threatening neuropsychological, autoimmune, ischemic, and infectious disorders; monitor pts closely **Uses:** *Rx hep C* **Action:** Immune modulator **Dose:** 1 mcg/kg/wk SQ; 1.5 mcg/kg/wk combo w/ ribavirin; w/ depression **Caution:** [C, ?/−] w/ Psychological disorder Hx **CI:** Autoimmune hep, decompensated liver Dz, hemoglobinopathy **Disp:** Vials 50, 80, 120, 150 mcg/0.5 mL; Redipen 50, 80, 120, 150 mcg/5 mL; reconstitute w/ 0.7 mL w/ sterile water **SE:** Depression, insomnia, suicidal behavior, GI upset, neutropenia, thrombocytopenia, alopecia, pruritus **Notes:** Give hs or w/ APAP to ↓ flu-like Sxs; monitor CBC/platelets; use immediately or store in refrigerator × 24 h; do not freeze

Pemetrexed (Alimta)   Uses: *w/ Cisplatin in nonresectable mesothelioma,* NSCLC **Action:** Antifolate antineoplastic **Dose:** 500 mg/m^2 IV over 10 min q3wk; hold if CrCl <45 mL/min; give w/ vit B$_{12}$ (1000 mcg IM q9wk) & folic acid

(350–1000 mcg PO daily); start 1 wk before; dexamethasone 4 mg PO bid × 3, start 1 d before each Rx **Caution:** [D, –] w/ Renal/hepatic/BM impair **CI:** Component sensitivity **Disp:** 500-mg vial **SE:** Neutropenia, thrombocytopenia, N/V/D, anorexia, stomatitis, renal failure, neuropathy, fever, fatigue, mood changes, dyspnea, anaphylactic Rxns **Notes:** Avoid NSAIDs, follow CBC/platelets; ↓ dose w/ grade 3–4 mucositis

Pemirolast (Alamast) **Uses:** *Allergic conjunctivitis* **Action:** Mast cell stabilizer **Dose:** 1–2 gtt in each eye qid **Caution:** [C, ?/–] **Disp:** 0.1% (1 mg/mL) in 10-mL bottles **SE:** HA, rhinitis, cold/flu Sxs, local irritation **Notes:** Wait 10 min before inserting contacts

Penbutolol (Levatol) **Uses:** *HTN* **Action:** β-Adrenergic receptor blocker, β₁, β₂ **Dose:** 20–40 mg/d; ↓ in hepatic Insuff **Caution:** [C 1st tri; D if 2nd/3rd tri] **CI:** Asthma, cardiogenic shock, cardiac failure, heart block, bradycardia, COPD, pulm edema **Disp:** Tabs 20 mg **SE:** Flushing, ↓ BP, fatigue, hyperglycemia, GI upset, sexual dysfunction, bronchospasm

Penciclovir (Denavir) **Uses:** *Herpes simplex (herpes labialis/cold sores)* **Action:** Competitive inhibitor of DNA polymerase **Dose:** Apply at 1st sign of lesions, then q2h while awake × 4 d **Caution:** [B, ?/–] **CI:** Allergy, previous Rxn to famciclovir **Disp:** Cream 1% **SE:** Erythema, HA **Notes:** Do not apply to mucous membranes

Penicillin G, Aqueous (Potassium or Sodium) (Pfizerpen, Pentids) **Uses:** *Bacteremia, endocarditis, pericarditis, resp tract Infxns, meningitis, neurosyphilis, skin/skin structure Infxns* **Action:** Bactericidal; ↓ cell wall synth. *Spectrum:* Most gram(+) (not staphylococci), streptococci, *N. meningitidis*, syphilis, clostridia, & anaerobes (not *Bacteroides*) **Dose:** *Adults.* Based on indication range 0.6–24 million units/d in ÷ doses q4h. *Peds Newborns <1 wk:* 25,000–50,000 units/kg/dose IV q12h. *Infants 1 wk–<1 mo:* 25,000–50,000 units/kg/dose IV q8h. *Children:* 100,000–300,000 units/kg/24h IV ÷ q4h; ↓ in renal impair **Caution:** [B, M] **CI:** Allergy **Disp:** Powder for Inj **SE:** Allergic Rxns; interstitial nephritis, D, Szs **Contains** 1.7 mEq of K⁺/million units

Penicillin G Benzathine (Bicillin) **Uses:** *Single-dose regimen for streptococcal pharyngitis, rheumatic fever, glomerulonephritis prophylaxis, & syphilis* **Action:** Bactericidal; ↓ cell wall synth. *Spectrum:* See Penicillin G **Dose:** *Adults.* 1.2–2.4 million units deep IM Inj q2–4wk. *Peds.* 50,000 units/kg/dose, 2.4 million units/dose max; deep IM Inj q2–4 wk **Caution:** [B, M] **CI:** Allergy **Disp:** Inj 300,000, 600,000 units/mL; Bicillin L-A benzathine salt only; Bicillin C-R combo of benzathine & procaine (300,000 units procaine w/ 300,000 units benzathine/mL or 900,000 units benzathine w/ 300,000 units procaine/2 mL) **SE:** Inj site pain, acute interstitial nephritis, anaphylaxis **Notes:** IM use only; sustained action, w/ levels up to 4 wk; drug of choice for noncongenital syphilis

Penicillin G Procaine (Wycillin, others) **Uses:** *Infxns of resp tract, skin/soft tissue, scarlet fever, syphilis* **Action:** Bactericidal; ↓ cell wall synth. *Spectrum:* PCN G-sensitive organisms that respond to low, persistent serum levels **Dose:** *Adults.* 0.6–4.8 million units/d in ÷ doses q12–24h; give probenecid at least 30 min prior to PCN to prolong action. *Peds.* 25,000–50,000 units/kg/d IM ÷ daily-bid **Caution:** [B, M] **CI:** Allergy **Disp:** Inj 300,000, 500,000, 600,000 units/mL **SE:** Pain at Inj site, interstitial nephritis, anaphylaxis **Notes:** LA parenteral PCN; levels up to 15 h

Penicillin V (Pen-Vee K, Veetids, others)
Uses: Susceptible streptococcal Infxns, otitis media, URIs, skin/soft-tissue Infxns (PCN-sensitive staphylococci) **Action:** Bactericidal; ↓ cell wall synth. *Spectrum:* Most gram(+), including streptococci **Dose:** *Adults.* 250–500 mg PO q6h, q8h, q12h. *Peds.* 25–50 mg/kg/25h PO in 4 doses; ↓ in renal impair; take on empty stomach **Caution:** [B, M] **CI:** Allergy **Disp:** Tabs 125, 250, 500 mg; susp 125, 250 mg/5 mL **SE:** GI upset, interstitial nephritis, anaphylaxis, convulsions **Notes:** Well-tolerated PO PCN; 250 mg = 400,000 units of PCN G

Pentamidine (Pentam 300, NebuPent)
Uses: *Rx & prevention of PCP* **Action:** ↓ DNA, RNA, phospholipid, & protein synth **Dose:** *Rx: Adults & Peds.* 4 mg/kg/24 h IV daily × 14–21 d. *Prevention: Adults & Peds >5 y:* 300 mg once q4wk, give via Respigard II nebulizer; ↓ IV w/ renal impair **Caution:** [C, ?] **CI:** Component allergy, use w/ didanosine **Disp:** Inj 300 mg/vial; aerosol 300 mg **SE:** Pancreatic cell necrosis w/ hyperglycemia; pancreatitis, CP, fatigue, dizziness, rash, GI upset, renal impair, blood dyscrasias (leukopenia, thrombocytopenia) **Notes:** Follow CBC, glucose, pancreatic Fxn monthly for 1st 3 mo; monitor for ↓ BP following IV dose; prolonged use may ↑ Infxn risk

Pentazocine (Talwin, Talwin Compound, Talwin NX) [C-IV]
WARNING: Oral use only; severe and potentially lethal Rxns from misuse by Inj **Uses:** *Mod–severe pain* **Action:** Partial narcotic agonist–antagonist **Dose:** *Adults.* 30 mg IM or IV; 50–100 mg PO q3–4h PRN. *Peds 5–8 y:* 15 mg IM q4h PRN. *8–14 y:* 30 mg IM q4h PRN; ↓ in renal/hepatic impair **CI:** Allergy, ↑ ICP (unless ventilated) **Disp:** *Talwin Compound* tab 12.5 mg + 325 mg ASA; *Talwin NX* 50 mg + 0.5 mg naloxone; Inj 30 mg/mL **SE:** Considerable dysphoria; drowsiness, GI upset, xerostomia, Szs **Notes:** 30–60 mg IM = 10 mg of morphine IM; Talwin NX has naloxone to curb abuse by nonoral route

Pentobarbital (Nembutal, others) [C-II]
Uses: *Insomnia (short-term), convulsions,* induce coma w/ severe head injury **Action:** Barbiturate **Dose:** *Adults. Sedative:* 150–200 mg IM × 1100 mg IV, repeat PRN to 500 mg/max. *Hypnotic:* 100–200 mg PO or PR hs PRN. *Induced coma:* Load 5–10 mg/kg IV, w/ maint 1–3 mg/kg/h IV. *Peds. Induced coma:* As adult **Caution:** [D, +/–] Severe hepatic impair **CI:** Allergy **Disp:** Caps 50, 100 mg; elixir 18.2 mg/5 mL (= 20 mg pentobarbital); supp 30, 60, 120, 200 mg; Inj 50 mg/mL **SE:** Resp depression, ↓ BP w/ aggressive IV use for cerebral edema; bradycardia, ↓ BP, sedation, lethargy, resp ↓, hangover, rash, Stevens-Johnson syndrome, blood dyscrasias **Notes:** Tolerance to sedative–hypnotic effect w/in 1–2 wk

Pentosan Polysulfate Sodium (Elmiron)   Uses: *Relieve pain/discomfort w/ interstitial cystitis* Action: Bladder wall buffer Dose: 100 mg PO tid; on empty stomach w/ H_2O 1 h ac or 2 h pc Caution: [B, ?/–] CI: Allergy Disp: Caps 100 mg SE: Alopecia, N/D, HA, ↑ LFTs, anticoagulant effects, ↓ plts, rectal bleeding Notes: Reassess after 3 mo

Pentoxifylline (Trental)   Uses: *Rx Sxs of peripheral vascular Dz* Action: ↓ Blood cell viscosity, restores RBC flexibility Dose: *Adults.* 400 mg PO tid pc; Rx min 8 wk for effect; ↓ to bid w/ GI/CNS SEs Caution: [C, +/–] CI: Cerebral/retinal hemorrhage, methylxanthine (caffeine) intolerance Disp: Tabs CR 400 mg; Tabs ER 400 mg SE: Dizziness, HA, GI upset

Perindopril Erbumine (Aceon)   WARNING: ACE inhibitors can cause death to developing fetus; D/C immediately w/ pregnancy Uses: *HTN,* CHF, DN, post-MI Action: ACE inhibitor Dose: 4–8 mg/d ÷ dose; 16 mg/d max; avoid w/ food; ↓ w/ elderly/renal impair Caution: [C (1st tri), D 2nd & 3rd tri), ?/–] ACE inhibitor-induced angioedema CI: Bilateral RAS, primary hyperaldosteronism Disp: Tabs 2, 4, 8 mg SE: Weakness, HA, ↓ BP, dizziness, GI upset, cough Notes: OK w/ diuretics

Permethrin (Nix, Elimite) [OTC]   Uses: *Rx lice/scabies* Action: Pediculicide Dose: *Adults & Peds. Lice:* Saturate hair & scalp; allow 10 min before rinsing. *Scabies:* Apply cream head to toe; leave for 8–14 h, wash w/H_2O Caution: [B, ?/–] CI: Allergy Disp: Topical lotion 1%; cream 5% SE: Local irritation Notes: Sprays available (Rid, A200, Nix) to disinfect clothing, bedding, combs, & brushes; lotion not OK in peds <2 y; may repeat after 7 d

Perphenazine (Trilafon)   Uses: *Psychotic disorders, severe N,* intractable hiccups Action: Phenothiazine, blocks brain dopaminergic receptors Dose: *Adults. Antipsychotic:* 4–16 mg PO tid; max 64 mg/d. *Hiccups:* 5 mg IM q6h PRN or 1 mg IV at intervals not <1–2 mg/min, 5 mg max. *Peds 1–6 y:* 4–6 mg/d PO in ÷ doses. *6–12 y:* 6 mg/d PO in ÷ doses. *>12 y:* 4–16 mg PO bid-qid; ↓ in hepatic Insuff Caution: [C, ?/–] NAG, severe ↑/↓ BP CI: Phenothiazine sensitivity, BM depression, severe liver or cardiac Dz Disp: Tabs 2, 4, 8, 16 mg; PO conc 16 mg/5 mL; Inj 5 mg/mL SE: ↓ BP, tachycardia, bradycardia, EPS, drowsiness, Szs, photosensitivity, skin discoloration, blood dyscrasias, constipation

Phenazopyridine (Pyridium, Azo-Standard, Urogesic, many others)   Uses: *Lower urinary tract irritation* Action: Anesthetic on urinary tract mucosa Dose: *Adults.* 100–200 mg PO tid; 2 d max w/ antibiotics for UTI; ↓ w/ renal Insuff Caution: [B, ?] Hepatic Dz CI: Renal failure Disp: Tabs 100, 200 mg SE: GI disturbances, red-orange urine color (can stain clothing, contacts), HA, dizziness, acute renal failure, methemoglobinemia, tinting of sclera/skin Notes: Take w/ food

Phenelzine (Nardil)   WARNING: Antidepressants increase the risk of suicidal thinking and behavior in children and adolescents w/ major depressive disorder and other psychological disorders; not for peds use Uses: *Depression,* bulimia **Action:** MAOI **Dose:** *Adults.* 15 mg PO tid, ↑ to 60–90 mg/d ÷ doses. *Elderly:* 15–60 mg/d ÷ doses **Caution:** [C, –] Interacts w/ SSRI, ergots, triptans **CI:** CHF, Hx liver Dz, pheochromocytoma **Disp:** Tabs 15 mg **SE:** Postural ↓ BP; edema, dizziness, sedation, rash, sexual dysfunction, xerostomia, constipation, urinary retention **Notes:** 2–4 wk for effect; avoid tyramine-containing foods (eg, cheeses)

Phenobarbital [C-IV] **Uses:** *Sz disorders,* insomnia, anxiety **Action:** Barbiturate **Dose:** *Adults. Sedative–hypnotic:* 30–120 mg/d PO or IM PRN. *Anticonvulsant:* Load 10–12 mg/kg in 3 ÷ doses, then 1–3 mg/kg/24 h PO, IM, or IV. *Peds. Sedative–hypnotic:* 2–3 mg/kg/24 h PO or IM hs PRN. *Anticonvulsant:* Load 15–20 mg/kg ÷ in 2 equal doses 4 h apart, then 3–5 mg/kg/24h PO ÷ in 2–3 doses; ↓ w/ CrCl <10 **Caution:** [D, M] **CI:** Porphyria, hepatic impair, dyspnea, airway obst **Disp:** Tabs 15, 16, 30, 32, 60, 65, 100 mg; elixir 15, 20 mg/5 mL; Inj 30, 60, 65, 130 mg/mL **SE:** Bradycardia, ↓ BP, hangover, Stevens-Johnson syndrome, blood dyscrasias, resp depression **Notes:** Tolerance develops to sedation; paradoxic hyperactivity seen in ped pts; long half-life allows single daily dosing. *Levels: Trough:* Just before next dose. *Therapeutic: Trough:* 15–40 mcg/mL; *Toxic Trough:* >40 mcg/mL. *Half-life:* 40–120 h

Phenylephrine, nasal (Neo-Synephrine Nasal) (OTC) **WARNING:** Not for use in Peds <2 y **Uses:** *Nasal congestion* **Action:** α-Adrenergic agonist **Dose:** *Adults.* 1–2 sprays/nostril q4h (usual 0.25%) PRN. *Peds 2–6 y:* 0.125% 1 drop/nostril q2–4h. *6–12 y:* 1–2 sprays/nostril q4h 0.25% 2–3 drops **Caution:** [C, +/–] HTN, acute pancreatitis, hep, coronary Dz, NAG, hyperthyroidism **CI:** Bradycardia, arrhythmias **Disp:** Nasal soln 0.125, 0.25, 0.5, 1%; liq 7.5 mg/5 mL; drops 2.5 mg/mL **SE:** Arrhythmias, HTN, nasal irritation, dryness, sneezing, rebound congestion w/ prolonged use, HA **Notes:** Do not use >3 d

Phenylephrine, ophthalmic (Neo-Synephrine Ophthalmic, AK-Dilate, Zincfrin [OTC]) **Uses:** *Mydriasis, ocular redness [OTC],* perioperative mydriasis, posterior synechiae, uveitis w/ posterior synechiae* **Action:** α-Adrenergic agonist **Dose:** *Adults. Redness:* 1 gtt 0.12% q3–4h PRN. *Exam mydriasis:* 1 gtt 2.5% (15 min–1 h for effect). *Pre-op:* 1 gtt 2.5–10% 30–60 min pre-op. *Ocular disorders:* 1 gtt 2.5–10% daily-tid *Peds.* As adult, only use 2.5% for exam, pre-op, and ocular conditions **Caution:** [C, May cause late-term fetal anoxia/bradycardia, +/–] HTN, w/ elderly w/ CAD **CI:** NAG **Disp:** Ophthal soln 0.12% (Zincfrin OTC), 2.5, 10% **SE:** Tearing, HA, irritation, eye pain, photophobia, arrhythmia, tremor

Phenylephrine, oral (Sudafed PE, SudoGest PE, Nasop, Lusonal, AH-chew D, Sudafed PE quick dissolve) (OTC) **WARNING:** Not for use in peds <2 y **Uses:** *Nasal congestion* **Action:** α-Adrenergic agonist **Dose:** *Adults.* 10–20 mg PO q4h PRN, max 60 mg/d **Peds.** 5 mg PO q4h PRN, max 60 mg/d **Caution:** [C, +/–] HTN, acute pancreatitis, hep, coronary Dz, NAG, hyperthyroidism **CI:** MAOI w/in 14 d, NAG, severe ↑ BP or

CAD, urinary retention **Disp:** Liq 7.5 mg/5 mL; drops 2.5 mg/mL; tabs 5, 10 mg; chew tabs 10 mg; tabs once daily 10 mg; strips 10 mg. **SE:** Arrhythmias, HTN, HA, agitation, anxiety, tremor, palpitations

Phenylephrine, systemic (Neo-Synephrine) **WARNING:** Prescribers should be aware of full prescribing information before use **Uses:** *Vascular failure in shock, allergy, or drug-induced ↓ BP* **Action:** α-Adrenergic agonist **Dose:** *Adults. Mild–mod ↓ BP:* 2–5 mg IM or SQ ↑ BP for 2 h; 0.1–0.5 mg IV elevates BP for 15 min. *Severe ↓ BP/shock:* Cont Inf at 100–180 mcg/min; after BP stable, maint 40–60 mcg/min. *Peds. ↓ BP:* 5–20 mcg/kg/dose IV q10–15min or 0.1–0.5 mcg/kg/min IV Inf, titrate to effect **Caution:** [C, +/–] HTN, acute pancreatitis, hep, coronary Dz, NAG, hyperthyroidism **CI:** Bradycardia, arrhythmias **Disp:** Inj 10 mg/mL **SE:** Arrhythmias, HTN, peripheral vasoconstriction ↑ w/ oxytocin, MAOIs, & TCAs; HA, weakness, necrosis, ↓ renal perfusion **Notes:** Restore blood vol if loss has occurred; use large veins to avoid extrav; phentolamine 10 mg in 10–15 mL of NS for local Inj to Rx extrav

Phenytoin (Dilantin) **Uses:** *Sz disorders* **Action:** ↓ Sz spread in the motor cortex **Dose:** *Adults & Peds. Load:* 15–20 mg/kg IV, 50 mg/min max or PO in 400-mg doses at 4-h intervals; *Adults. Maint:* Initial 200 mg PO or IV bid or 300 mg hs then follow levels. →; alternatively 5–7 mg/kg/d based on ideal body weight ÷ daily-tid, *Peds. Maint:* 4–7 mg/kg/24h PO or IV ÷ daily-bid; avoid PO susp (erratic absorption) **Caution:** [D, +] **CI:** Heart block, sinus bradycardia **Disp:** *Dilantin Infatab:* chew 50 mg. *Dilantin/Phenytek:* caps 100 mg; caps, ER 30, 100, 200, 300 mg; susp 125 mg/5 mL; Inj 50 mg/mL **SE:** Nystagmus/ataxia early signs of tox; gum hyperplasia w/ long-term use. *IV:* ↓ BP, bradycardia, arrhythmias, phlebitis; peripheral neuropathy, rash, blood dyscrasias, Stevens-Johnson syndrome **Notes:** Levels: *Trough:* just before next dose. *Therapeutic:* 10–20 mcg/mL. *Toxic:* >20 mcg/mL. Phenytoin albumin bound, levels = bound & free phenytoin; w/ ↓ albumin & azotemia, low levels may be therapeutic (nl free levels); do not change dosage at intervals <7–10 d; hold tube feeds 1 h before and after dose if using oral susp; avoid large dose ↑

Physostigmine (Antilirium) **Uses:** *Antidote for TCA, atropine, & scopolamine OD; glaucoma* **Action:** Reversible cholinesterase inhibitor **Dose:** *Adults.* 0.5–2 mg IV or IM q20min *Peds.* 0.01–0.03 mg/kg/dose IV q5–10min up to 2 mg total PRN **Caution:** [C, ?] **CI:** GI/GU obst, CV Dz, asthma **Disp:** Inj 1 mg/mL **SE:** Rapid IV administration associated w/ Szs; cholinergic SEs; sweating, salivation, lacrimation, GI upset, asystole, changes in HR **Notes:** Excessive readministration can result in cholinergic crisis; crisis reversed w/ atropine

Phytonadione [Vitamin K] (AquaMEPHYTON, others) **Uses:** *Coagulation disorders due to faulty formation of factors II, VII, IX, X*; hyperalimentation **Action:** Cofactor for production of factors II, VII, IX, & X **Dose:** *Adults & Peds. Anticoagulant-induced prothrombin deficiency:* 1–10 mg PO or IV slowly. *Hyperalimentation:* 10 mg IM or IV q wk. *Infants.* 0.5–1 mg/dose IM, SQ, or PO

Caution: [C, +] **CI:** Allergy **Disp:** Tabs 5 mg; Inj 2, 10 mg/mL **SE:** Anaphylaxis from IV dosage; give IV slowly; GI upset (PO), Inj site Rxns **Notes:** w/ Parenteral Rx, 1st change in PT/INR usually seen in 12–24 h; use makes rewarfarinization more difficult

Pimecrolimus (Elidel)   WARNING: Associated with rare skin malignancies and lymphoma, limit to area, not for age <2 y Uses: *Atopic dermatitis* refractory, severe perianal itching **Action:** Inhibits T-lymphocytes **Dose:** *Adults & Peds >2 y:* Apply bid; use at least 1 wk following resolution **Caution:** [C, ?/–] w/ Local Infxn, lymphadenopathy; avoid in pts <2 y **CI:** Allergy component, <2 y **Disp:** Cream 1% **SE:** Phototox, local irritation/burning, flu-like Sxs, may ↑ malignancy **Notes:** Use on dry skin only; wash hands after; 2nd-line/short-term use only

Pindolol (Visken)   Uses: *HTN* **Action:** β-Adrenergic receptor blocker, β₁, β₂, ISA **Dose:** 5–10 mg bid, 60 mg/d max; ↓ in hepatic/renal failure **Caution:** [B (1st tri; D if 2nd or 3rd tri), +/–] **CI:** Uncompensated CHF, cardiogenic shock, bradycardia, heart block, asthma, COPD **Disp:** Tabs 5, 10 mg **SE:** Insomnia, dizziness, fatigue, edema, GI upset, dyspnea; fluid retention may exacerbate CHF

Pioglitazone (Actos)   WARNING: May cause or worsen CHF Uses: *Type 2 DM* **Action:** ↑ Insulin sensitivity **Dose:** 15–45 mg/d PO **Caution:** [C, –] **CI:** CHF, hepatic impair **Disp:** Tabs 15, 30, 45 mg **SE:** Wgt gain, myalgia, URI, HA, hypoglycemia, edema, ↑ fracture risk in women

Pioglitazone/Metformin (ACTOplus Met)   WARNING: Metformin can cause lactic acidosis, fatal in 50% of cases; pioglitazone may cause or worsen CHF **Uses:** *Type 2 DM as adjunct to diet and exercise* **Action:** Combined ↑ insulin sensitivity w/ ↓ hepatic glucose release **Dose:** Initial 1 tab PO daily or bid, titrate; max daily pioglitazone 45 mg & metformin 2550 mg; give w/ meals **Caution:** [C, –] Stop w/ radiologic contrast agents **CI:** CHF, renal impair, acidosis **Disp:** Tabs pioglitazone mg/metformin mg: 15/500, 15/850 **SE:** Lactic acidosis, CHF, ↓ glucose, edema, wgt gain, myalgia, URI, HA, GI upset, liver damage **Notes:** Follow LFTs; ↑ fracture risk in women receiving pioglitazone

Piperacillin (Pipracil)   Uses: *Infxns of skin, bone, resp, & urinary tract, abdomen, sepsis* **Action:** 4th-Gen PCN; bactericidal; ↓ cell wall synth. **Spectrum:** Primarily gram(+), better *Enterococcus, H. influenzae*, not staphylococci; gram(–) *E. coli, Proteus, Shigella, Pseudomonas*, not β-lactamase producing **Dose:** *Adults.* 2–4 g IV q4–6h. *Peds.* 200–300 mg/kg/d IV ÷ q4–6h; ↓ in renal failure **Caution:** [B, M] **CI:** PCN/β-lactam sensitivity **Disp:** *Powder for Inj:* 2, 3, 4, 40 g **SE:** ↓ Plt aggregation, interstitial nephritis, renal Insuff, anaphylaxis, hemolytic anemia **Notes:** Often used w/ aminoglycoside

Piperacillin–Tazobactam (Zosyn)   Uses: *Infxns of skin, bone, resp & urinary tract, abdomen, sepsis* **Action:** 4th-Gen PCN plus β-lactamase inhibitor; bactericidal; ↓ cell wall synth. **Spectrum:** Good gram(+), excellent gram(–); anaerobes & β-lactamase producers **Dose:** *Adults.* 3.375–4.5 g IV q6h; ↓ in renal Insuff **Caution:** [B, M] **CI:** PCN or β-lactam sensitivity **Disp:** *Powder for*

Inj: Frozen, premix Inj 3.25, 3.375, 4.5 g **SE:** D, HA, insomnia, GI upset, serum sickness-like Rxn, pseudomembranous colitis **Notes:** Often used in combo w/ aminoglycoside

Pirbuterol (Maxair) **Uses:** *Prevention & Rx reversible bronchospasm* **Action:** β_2-Adrenergic agonist **Dose:** 2 Inh q4–6h; max 12 Inh/d **Caution:** [C, ?/–] **Disp:** Aerosol 0.2 mg/actuation **SE:** Nervousness, restlessness, trembling, HA, taste changes, tachycardia **Note:** Teach patient proper inhaler technique

Piroxicam (Feldene) **WARNING:** May ↑ risk of cardiovascular events & GI bleeding **Uses:** *Arthritis & pain* **Action:** NSAID; ↓ prostaglandins **Dose:** 10–20 mg/d **Caution:** [B (1st tri; D if 3rd tri or near term), +] GI bleeding **CI:** ASA/NSAID sensitivity **Disp:** Caps 10, 20 mg **SE:** Dizziness, rash, GI upset, edema, acute renal failure, peptic ulcer

Plasma Protein Fraction (Plasmanate, others) **Uses:** *Shock & ↓ BP* **Action:** Plasma vol expander **Dose:** *Adults. Initial:* 250–500 mL IV (not >10 mL/min); subsequent Inf based on response. *Peds.* 10–15 mL/kg/dose IV; subsequent Inf based on response **Caution:** [C, +] **CI:** Renal Insuff, CHF, cardiopulmonary bypass **Disp:** Inj 5% **SE:** ↓ BP w/ rapid Inf; hypocoagulability, metabolic acidosis, PE **Notes:** 130–160 mEq Na/L; not substitute for blood

Pneumococcal 7-Valent Conjugate Vaccine (Prevnar) **Uses:** *Immunization against pneumococcal Infxns in infants & children* **Action:** Active immunization **Dose:** 0.5 mL IM/dose; series of 3 doses; 1st dose age 2 mo; then doses q2mo, 4th dose at age 12–15 mo **Caution:** [C, +] Thrombocytopenia **CI:** Diphtheria toxoid sensitivity, febrile illness **Disp:** Inj **SE:** Local Rxns, arthralgia, fever, myalgia

Pneumococcal Vaccine, Polyvalent (Pneumovax-23) **Uses:** *Immunization against pneumococcal Infxns in pts at high risk (eg, all pts ≥ 65 y)* **Action:** Active immunization **Dose:** 0.5 mL IM. **Caution:** [C, ?] **CI:** *Do not* vaccinate during immunosuppressive therapy **Disp:** Inj 0.5 mL **SE:** Fever, Inj site Rxn, hemolytic anemia, thrombocytopenia, anaphylaxis

Podophyllin (Podocon-25, Condylox Gel 0.5%, Condylox) **Uses:** *Topical therapy of benign growths (genital & perianal warts [condylomata acuminata],* papillomas, fibromas) **Action:** Direct antimitotic effect; exact mechanism unknown **Dose:** *Condylox gel & Condylox:* Apply bid for 3 consecutive d/wk for 4 wk; 0.5 mL/d max; *Podocon-25:* Use sparingly on the lesion, leave on for 1–4 h, thoroughly wash off **Caution:** [X, ?] Immunosuppression **CI:** DM, bleeding lesions **Disp:** Podocon-25 (w/ benzoin) 15-mL bottles; Condylox gel 0.5% 35-g clear gel; Condylox soln 0.5% 35-g clear **SE:** Local Rxns, sig absorption; anemias, tachycardia, paresthesias, GI upset, renal/hepatic damage **Notes:** Podocon-25 applied by the clinician; do not dispense directly to patient

Polyethylene Glycol [PEG]-Electrolyte Soln (GoLYTELY, CoLyte) **Uses:** *Bowel preparation prior to examination or surgery* **Action:** Osmotic cathartic **Dose:** *Adults.* Following 3–4-h fast, drink 240 mL of soln q10min until 4 L consumed or until BMs are clear. **Peds.** 25–40 mL/kg/h for 4–10 h **Caution:** [C, ?] **CI:** GI obst, bowel perforation, megacolon, ulcerative colitis **Disp:** Powder for recons to 4 L **SE:** Cramping or N, bloating **Notes:** 1st BM should occur in approximately 1 h; chilled soln more palatable

Polyethylene Glycol [PEG] 3350 (MiraLAX) **Uses:** *Occasional constipation* **Action:** Osmotic laxative **Dose:** 17-g powder (1 heaping Tbsp) in 8 oz (1 cup) of H_2O & drink; max 14 d **Caution:** [C, ?] Rule out bowel obst before use **CI:** GI obst, allergy to PEG **Disp:** Powder for reconstitution; bottle cap holds 17 g **SE:** Upset stomach, bloating, cramping, gas, severe D, hives **Notes:** Can add to H_2O, juice, soda, coffee, or tea

Polymyxin B & Hydrocortisone (Otobiotic Otic) **Uses:** *Superficial bacterial Infxns of external ear canal* **Action:** Antibiotic/anti-inflammatory combo **Dose:** 4 gtt in ear(s) tid-qid **Caution:** [B, ?] **Disp:** Soln polymyxin B 10,000 units/hydrocortisone 0.5%/mL **SE:** Local irritation **Notes:** Useful in neomycin allergy

Posaconazole (Noxafil) **Uses:** *Prevent Aspergillus* and *Candida* Infxns in severely immunocompromised; Rx oropharyngeal candida* **Action:** ↓ Cell membrane ergosterol synth **Dose:** *Adults. Invasive fungal prophylaxis:* 200 mg PO tid. *Oropharyngeal candidiasis:* 100 mg PO daily × 13 d, if refractory 40 mg PO bid **Peds >13 y:** 200 mg PO tid; take w/ meal **Caution:** [C; ?] Multiple drug interactions; ↑ QT, cardiac Dzs, severe renal/liver impair **CI:** Component hypersensitivity; w/ many drugs including alfuzosin, astemizole, alprazolam, phenothiazines, terfenadine, triazolam, others **Disp:** Soln 40 mg/mL **SE:** ↑ QT, ↑ LFTs, hepatic failure, fever, N/V/D, HA, Abd pain, anemia, ↓ plt, ↓ K^+ rash, dyspnea, cough, anorexia, fatigue **Notes:** Monitor LFTs, CBC, lytes

Potassium Citrate (Urocit-K) **Uses:** *Alkalinize urine, prevention of urinary stones (uric acid, calcium stones if hypocitraturic)* **Action:** Urinary alkalinizer **Dose:** 1 packet dissolved in H_2O or 15–30 mL pc & hs 10–20 mEq PO tid w/ meals, max 100 mEq/d **Caution:** [A, +] **CI:** Severe renal impair, dehydration, ↑ K^+, peptic ulcer; w/ K^+-sparing diuretics, salt substitutes **Disp:** 540, 1080 mg tabs **SE:** GI upset, ↓ Ca^{2+}, ↑ K^+, metabolic alkalosis **Notes:** Tabs 540 mg = 5 mEq, 1080 mg = 10 mEq

Potassium Citrate & Citric Acid (Polycitra-K) **Uses:** *Alkalinize urine, prevent urinary stones (uric acid, CA stones if hypocitraturic)* **Action:** Urinary alkalinizer **Dose:** 10–20 mEq PO tid w/ meals, max 100 mEq/d **Caution:** [A, +] **CI:** Severe renal impair, dehydration, ↑ K^+, peptic ulcer; w/ use of K^+-sparing diuretics or salt substitutes **Disp:** Soln 10 mEq/5 mL; powder 30 mEq/packet **SE:** GI upset, ↓ Ca^{2+}, ↑ K^+, metabolic alkalosis

Potassium Iodide [Lugol Soln] (SSKI, Thyro-Block, ThyroSafe, ThyroShield) **Uses:** *Thyroid storm,* ↓ vascularity before thyroid surgery, block thyroid uptake of radioactive iodine, thin bronchial secretions **Action:** Iodine supl **Dose:** *Adults & Peds >2 y: Pre-op thyroidectomy:* 50–250 mg PO tid (2–6 gtt strong iodine soln); give 10 d pre-op. *Protection:* 130 mg/d. **Peds.** *Protection: <1 y:*

16.25 mg q day. *1 mo–3y:* 32.5 mg q day. *3–12 y:* 1/2 adult dose **Caution:** [D, +] ↑ K⁺, TB, PE, bronchitis, renal impair **CI:** Iodine sensitivity **Disp:** Tabs 65, 130 mg; soln (saturated soln of potassium iodide (SSKI)) 1 g/mL; Lugol soln, strong iodine 100 mg/mL; syrup 325 mg/5 mL **SE:** Fever, HA, urticaria, angioedema, goiter, GI upset, eosinophilia **Notes:** w/ Nuclear radiation emergency; give until radiation exposure no longer exists

Potassium Supplements (Kaon, Kaochlor, K-Lor, Slow-K, Micro-K, Klorvess, others) Uses: *Prevention or Rx of ↓ K⁺* (eg, diuretic use) **Action:** K⁺ supl **Dose:** *Adults.* 20–100 mEq/d PO ÷ daily-bid; IV 10–20 mEq/h, max 40 mEq/h & 150 mEq/d (monitor K⁺ levels frequently and in presence of continuous ECG monitoring w/ high-dose IV). *Peds.* Calculate K⁺ deficit; 1–3 mEq/kg/d PO ÷ daily–qid; IV max dose 0.5–1 mEq/kg/h **Caution:** [A, +] Renal Insuff, use w/ NSAIDs & ACE inhibitors **CI:** ↑ K⁺ **Disp:** PO forms (Table 7); Inj **SE:** GI irritation; bradycardia, ↑ K⁺, heart block **Notes:** Mix powder & liq w/ beverage (unsalted tomato juice, etc); follow K⁺; Cl⁻ salt OK w/ alkalosis; w/ acidosis use acetate, bicarbonate, citrate, or gluconate salt

Pramipexole (Mirapex) Uses: *Parkinson Dz, restless leg syndrome* **Action:** Dopamine agonist **Dose:** 1.5–4.5 mg/d PO ÷ 3 doses; titrate slowly **Caution:** [C, ?/–] ↓ Renal impair **CI:** Component allergy **Disp:** Tabs 0.125, 0.25, 0.5, 1, 1.5 mg **SE:** Postural ↓ BP, asthenia, somnolence, abnormal dreams, GI upset, EPS, hallucinations (elderly)

Pramoxine (Anusol Ointment, ProctoFoam-NS, others) Uses: *Relief of pain & itching from hemorrhoids, anorectal surgery*; topical for burns & dermatosis **Action:** Topical anesthetic **Dose:** Apply freely to anal area q3h **Caution:** [C, ?] **Disp:** [OTC] All 1%; foam (ProctoFoam-NS), cream, oint, lotion, gel, pads, spray **SE:** Contact dermatitis, mucosal thinning w/ chronic use

Pramoxine + Hydrocortisone (Enzone, ProctoFoam-HC) Uses: *Relief of pain & itching from hemorrhoids* **Action:** Topical anesthetic, anti-inflammatory **Dose:** Apply freely to anal area tid-qid **Caution:** [C, ?/–] **Disp:** *Cream* pramoxine 1% acetate 0.5/1%; *foam* pramoxine 1% hydrocortisone 1%; *lotion* pramoxine 1% hydrocortisone 0.25/1/2.5%, pramoxine 2.5% & hydrocortisone 1% **SE:** Contact dermatitis, mucosal thinning with chronic use

Pravastatin (Pravachol) Uses: *↓ Cholesterol* **Action:** HMG-CoA reductase inhibitor **Dose:** 10–80 mg PO hs; ↓ in sig renal/hepatic impair **Caution:** [X, –] w/ Gemfibrozil **CI:** Liver Dz or persistent LFTs ↑ **Disp:** Tabs 10, 20, 40, 80 mg **SE:** Use caution w/ concurrent gemfibrozil; HA, GI upset, hep, myopathy, renal failure

Prazosin (Minipress) Uses: *HTN* **Action:** Peripherally acting α-adrenergic blocker **Dose:** *Adults.* 1 mg PO tid; can ↑ to 20 mg/d max PRN. *Peds.* 0.05–0.1 mg/kg/d in 3 ÷ doses; max 0.5 mg/kg/d **Caution:** [C, ?] **CI:** Component allergy, concurrent use of PDE5 inhibitors **Disp:** Caps 1, 2, 5 mg; tabs ER 2.5,

5 mg **SE:** Dizziness, edema, palpitations, fatigue, GI upset **Notes:** Can cause orthostatic ↓ BP, take the 1st dose hs; tolerance develops to this effect; tachyphylaxis may result

Prednisolone [See Steroids page 214 and Table 3, page 251]

Prednisone [See Steroids page 214 and Table 3, page 251]

Pregabalin (Lyrica)   WARNING: Increased risk of suicidal behavior ideation **Uses:** *DM peripheral neuropathy pain; postherpetic neuralgia; fibromyalgia; adjunct w/ adult partial onset Szs* **Action:** Nerve transmission modulator, antinociceptive, antiseizure effect; mechanism?; related to gabapentin **Dose:** *Neuropathic pain:* 50 mg PO tid, ↑ to 300 mg/d w/in 1 wk based on response, 300 mg/d max. *Postherpetic neuralgia:* 75–150 mg bid, or 50–100 mg tid; start 75 mg bid or 50 mg tid; ↑ to 300 mg/d w/in 1 wk PRN; if pain persists after 2–4 wk, ↑ to 600 mg/d. *Epilepsy:* Start 150 mg/d (75 mg bid or 50 mg tid) may ↑ to max 600 mg/d; ↓ w/ renal Insuff; w/ or w/o food **Caution:** [C, –] w/ Sig renal impair (see insert), w/ elderly & severe CHF avoid abrupt D/C w/ PRG **Disp:** Caps 25, 50, 75, 100, 150, 200, 225, 300 mg **SE:** Dizziness, drowsiness, xerostomia, edema, blurred vision, wgt gain, difficulty concentrating **Notes:** w/ D/C, taper over at least 1 wk

Probenecid (Benemid, others)   **Uses:** *Prevent gout & hyperuricemia; prolongs levels of PCNs & cephalosporins* **Action:** Uricosuric, renal tubular blocker of organic anions **Dose:** *Adults. Gout:* 250 mg bid × 1 wk, then 0.5 g PO bid; can ↑ by 500 mg/mo up to 2–3 g/d. *Antibiotic effect:* 1–2 g PO 30 min before dose. *Peds >2 y:* 25 mg/kg, then 40 mg/kg/d PO ÷ qid **Caution:** [B, ?] **CI:** High-dose ASA, mod–severe renal impair, age <2 y **Disp:** Tabs 500 mg **SE:** HA, GI upset, rash, pruritus, dizziness, blood dyscrasias **Notes:** Do not use during acute gout attack

Procainamide (Pronestyl, Pronestyl SR, Procanbid) **WARNING:** Positive antinuclear antibody titer or SLE w/ prolonged use; only use in life-treating arrhythmias; hematologic tox can be severe, follow CBC **Uses:** *Supraventricular/ventricular arrhythmias* **Action:** Class 1A antiarrhythmic (Table 10) **Dose:** *Adults.* Recurrent VF/VT: 20 mg/min IV (total 17 mg/kg max). *Maint:* 1–4 mg/min. *Stable wide-complex tachycardia of unknown origin, AF w/ rapid rate in WPW:* 20 mg/min IV until arrhythmia suppression, ↓ BP, or QRS widens >50%, then 1–4 mg/min. *Chronic dosing:* 50 mg/kg/d PO in ÷ doses q4–6h. *Recurrent VF/VT:* 20–50 mg/min IV; max total 17 mg/kg. *Others:* 20 mg/min IV until one these: arrhythmia stopped, hypotension, QRS widens >50%, total 17 mg/kg; then 1–4 mg/min *(ECC 2005).* **Peds.** *Chronic maint:* 15–50 mg/kg/24 h PO ÷ q3–6h; ↓ in renal/hepatic impair **Caution:** [C, +] **CI:** Complete heart block, 2nd- or 3rd-degree heart block w/o pacemaker, torsade de pointes, SLE **Disp:** Tabs & caps 250, 500 mg; SR tabs 500, 750, 1000 mg; Inj 100, 500 mg/mL **SE:** ↓ BP, lupus-like syndrome, GI upset, taste perversion, arrhythmias, tachycardia, heart block, angioneurotic edema, blood dyscrasias **Notes:** Levels: *Trough:*

Just before next dose. *Therapeutic:* 4–10 mcg/mL; *N*-acetyl procainamide (NAPA) + procaine 5–30 mcg/mL; *Toxic:* >10 mcg/mL; NAPA + procaine >30 mcg/mL. *Half-life:* procaine 3–5 h, NAPA 6–10 h

Procarbazine (Matulane) **WARNING:** Highly toxic; handle w/ care
Uses: *Hodgkin Dz,* *NHL, brain & lung tumors **Action:** Alkylating agent; ↓ DNA & RNA synth **Dose:** Per protocol **Caution:** [D, ?] w/ EtOH ingestion **CI:** Inadequate BM reserve **Disp:** Caps 50 mg **SE:** ↓ BM, hemolytic Rxns (w/ G6PD deficiency), N/V/D; disulfiram-like Rxn; cutaneous & constitutional Sxs, myalgia, arthralgia, CNS effects, azoospermia, cessation of menses

Prochlorperazine (Compazine) **Uses:** *N/V, agitation, & psychotic disorders* **Action:** Phenothiazine; blocks postsynaptic dopaminergic CNS receptors **Dose:** *Adults.* *Antiemetic:* 5–10 mg PO tid-qid or 25 mg PR bid or 5–10 mg deep IM q4–6h. *Antipsychotic:* 10–20 mg IM acutely or 5–10 mg PO tid-qid for maint; ↑ doses may be required for antipsychotic effect. *Peds.* 0.1–0.15 mg/kg/dose IM q4–6h or 0.4 mg/kg/24 h PO ÷ tid-qid **Caution:** [C, +/–] Narrow, severe liver/cardiac Dz **CI:** Phenothiazine sensitivity, BM suppression; age <2 y or wgt <9 kg **Disp:** Tabs 5, 10, 25 mg; SR caps 10, 15 mg; syrup 5 mg/5 mL; supp 2.5, 5, 25 mg; Inj 5 mg/mL **SE:** EPS common; Rx w/ diphenhydramine & benztropine

Promethazine (Phenergan) **Uses:** *N/V, motion sickness* **Action:** Phenothiazine; blocks CNS postsynaptic mesolimbic dopaminergic receptors **Dose:** *Adults.* 12.5–50 mg PO, PR, or IM bid-qid PRN. *Peds.* 0.1–0.5 mg/kg/dose PO or IM q2–6h PRN **Caution:** [C, +/–] Use w/ agents w/ resp depressant effects **CI:** Component allergy, NAG, age <2 y **Disp:** Tabs 12.5, 25, 50 mg; syrup 6.25 mg/5 mL, 25 mg/5 mL; supp 12.5, 25, 50 mg; Inj 25, 50 mg/mL **SE:** Drowsiness, tardive dyskinesia, EPS, lowered Sz threshold, ↓ BP, blood dyscrasias, photosensitivity, resp depression in children

Propafenone (Rythmol) **WARNING:** Excess mortality or nonfatal cardiac arrest possible; avoid use in asymptomatic and symptomatic non–life-threatening ventricular arrhythmias **Uses:** *Life-threatening ventricular arrhythmias, AF* **Action:** Class IC antiarrhythmic (Table 10) **Dose:** *Adults.* 150–300 mg PO q8h. *Peds.* 8–10 mg/kg/d ÷ in 3–4 doses; may ↑ 2 mg/kg/d, 20 mg/kg/d max **Caution:** [C, ?] w/ Amprenavir, ritonavir, MI w/in 2 y, w/ liver/renal impair **CI:** Uncontrolled CHF, bronchospasm, cardiogenic shock, AV block w/o pacer **Disp:** Tabs 150, 225, 300 mg; ER caps 225, 325, 425 mg **SE:** Dizziness, unusual taste, 1st-degree heart block, arrhythmias, prolongs QRS & QT intervals; fatigue, GI upset, blood dyscrasias

Propantheline (Pro-Banthine) **Uses:** *PUD,* symptomatic Rx of small intestine hypermotility, spastic colon, ureteral spasm, bladder spasm, pylorospasm **Action:** Antimuscarinic **Dose:** *Adults.* 15 mg PO ac & 30 mg PO hs; ↓ in elderly. *Peds.* 2–3 mg/kg/24 h PO ÷ tid-qid **Caution:** [C, ?] **CI:** NAG, ulcerative colitis, toxic megacolon, GI/GU obst **Disp:** Tabs 7.5, 15 mg **SE:** Anticholinergic (eg, xerostomia, blurred vision)

Propofol (Diprivan) Uses: *Induction & maint of anesthesia; sedation in intubated pts* Action: Sedative–hypnotic; mechanism unknown; acts in 40 s Dose: *Adults. Anesthesia:* 2–2.5 mg/kg (also *ECC 2005*), then 0.1–0.2 mg/kg/min Inf. *ICU sedation:* 5 mcg/kg/min IV × 5 min, ↑ PRN 5–10 mcg/kg/min q5–10min, 5–50 mcg/kg/min cont Inf. *Peds. Anesthesia:* 2.5–3.5 mg/kg induction; then 125–300 mcg/kg/min; ↓ in elderly, debilitated, ASA II/IV pts **Caution:** [B, +] CI: If general anesthesia CI, sensitivity to egg, egg products, soybeans, soybean products Disp: Inj 10 mg/mL SE: May ↑ triglycerides w/ extended dosing; ↓ BP, pain at site, apnea, anaphylaxis Notes: 1 mL has 0.1 g fat

Propoxyphene (Darvon); Propoxyphene & Acetaminophen (Darvocet); Propoxyphene & Aspirin (Darvon Compound-65, Darvon-N + Aspirin) [C-IV] WARNING: Excessive doses alone or in combo w/ other CNS depressants can be cause of suicidal death; use w/ caution in depressed or suicidal pts Uses: *Mild–mod pain* Action: Narcotic analgesic Dose: 1–2 PO q4h PRN; ↓ in hepatic impair, elderly **Caution:** [C (D if prolonged use), M] Hepatic impair (APAP), peptic ulcer (ASA); severe renal impair, Hx EtOH abuse CI: Allergy, suicide risk, Hx drug abuse Disp: *Darvon:* Propoxyphene HCl caps 65 mg. *Darvon-N:* Propoxyphene napsylate 100-mg tabs. *Darvocet-N:* Propoxyphene napsylate 50 mg/APAP 325 mg. *Darvocet-N 100:* Propoxyphene napsylate 100 mg/APAP 650 mg. *Darvon Compound-65:* Propoxyphene HCl caps 65-mg/ASA 389 mg/caffeine 32 mg. *Darvon-N w/ ASA:* Propoxyphene napsylate 100 mg/ASA 325 mg SE: OD can be lethal; ↓ BP, dizziness, sedation, GI upset, ↑ LFTs

Propranolol (Inderal) Uses: *HTN, angina, MI, hyperthyroidism, essential tremor, hypertrophic subaortic stenosis, pheochromocytoma; prevents migraines & atrial arrhythmias* Action: β-Adrenergic receptor blocker, β₁, β₂; only β-blocker to block conversion of T_4 to T_3 Dose: *Adults. Angina:* 80–320 mg/d PO ÷ bid-qid or 80–160 mg/d SR. *Arrhythmia:* 10–80 mg PO tid-qid or 1 mg IV slowly, repeat q5min, 5 mg max. *HTN:* 40 mg PO bid or 60–80 mg/d SR, ↑ weekly to max 640 mg/d. *Hypertrophic subaortic stenosis:* 20–40 mg PO tid-qid. *MI:* 180–240 mg PO ÷ tid-qid. *Migraine prophylaxis:* 80 mg/d ÷ qid-tid, ↑ weekly 160–240 mg/d ÷ tid-qid max; wean if no response in 6 wk. *Pheochromocytoma:* 30–60 mg/d ÷ tid-qid. *Thyrotoxicosis:* 1–3 mg IV × 1; 10–40 mg PO q6h. *Tremor:* 40 mg PO bid, ↑ PRN 320 mg/d max; 0.1 mg/kg slow IV push, divided 3 equal doses q2–3min, max 1 mg/min; repeat in 2 min PRN *(ECC 2005). Peds. Arrhythmia:* 0.5–1.0 mg/kg/d ÷ tid-qid, ↑ PRN q3–7d to 60 mg/d max; 0.01–0.1 mg/kg IV over 10 min, 1 mg max. *HTN:* 0.5–1.0 mg/kg ÷ bid-qid, ↑ PRN q3–7d to 2 mg/kg/d max; ↓ in renal impair **Caution:** [C (1st tri, D if 2nd or 3rd tri), +] CI: Uncompensated CHF, cardiogenic shock, bradycardia, heart block, PE, severe resp Dz Disp: Tabs 10, 20, 40, 80 mg; SR caps 60, 80, 120, 160 mg; oral soln 4, 8, mg/mL; Inj 1 mg/mL SE: Bradycardia, ↓ BP, fatigue, GI upset, ED

Propylthiouracil [PTU] Uses: *Hyperthyroidism* Action: ↓ Production of T_3 & T_4 & conversion of T_4 to T_3 Dose: *Adults.* Initial: 100 mg PO q8h (may need up to 1200 mg/d); after pt euthyroid (6–8 wk), taper dose by 1/2 q4–6wk to maint, 50–150 mg/24 h; can usually D/C in 2–3 y; ↓ in elderly. *Peds.* Initial: 5–7 mg/kg/24 h PO ÷ q8h. Maint: 1/3–2/3 of initial dose Caution: [D, –] CI: Allergy Disp: Tabs 50 mg SE: Fever, rash, leukopenia, dizziness, GI upset, taste perversion, SLE-like syndrome Notes: Monitor pt clinically, ✓ TFT

Protamine (generic) Uses: *Reverse heparin effect* Action: Neutralize heparin by forming a stable complex Dose: Based on degree of heparin reversal; give IV slowly; 1 mg reverses ~ 100 units of heparin given in the preceding 3–4 h, 50 mg max Caution: [C, ?] CI: Allergy Disp: Inj 10 mg/mL SE: Follow coagulants; anticoagulant effect if given w/o heparin; ↓ BP, bradycardia, dyspnea, hemorrhage Notes: ✓ aPTT ~ 15 min after use to assess response

Pseudoephedrine (Sudafed, Novafed, Afrinol, others) [OTC] WARNING: Not for use in peds <2 y Uses: *Decongestant* Action: Stimulates α-adrenergic receptors w/ vasoconstriction Dose: *Adults.* 30–60 mg PO q6–8h. *Peds 2–5 y:* 15 mg q 4–6h, 60 mg/24h max. *6–12 y:* 30 mg q4–6h, 120 mg/24 h max; ↓ w/ renal Insuff Caution: [C, +] CI: Poorly controlled HTN or CAD, w/ MAOIs Disp: Tabs 30, 60 mg; caps 60 mg; SR tabs 120, 240 mg; liq 7.5 mg/0.8 mL, 15, 30 mg/5 mL SE: HTN, insomnia, tachycardia, arrhythmias, nervousness, tremor Notes: Found in many OTC cough/cold preparations; OTC restricted distribution

Psyllium (Metamucil, Serutan, Effer-Syllium) Uses: *Constipation & colonic diverticular Dz* Action: Bulk laxative Dose: 1 tsp (7 g) in glass of H_2O PO daily–tid Caution: [B, ?] Effer-Syllium (effervescent psyllium) usually contains K^+, caution w/ renal failure; phenylketonuria (in products w/ aspartame) CI: Suspected bowel obst Disp: Granules 4, 25 g/tsp; powder 3.5 g/packet, caps 0.52g (3 g/6 caps), wafers 3.4 g/dose SE: D, Abd cramps, bowel obst, constipation, bronchospasm

Pyrazinamide (generic) Uses: *Active TB in combo w/ other agents* Action: Bacteriostatic; unknown mechanism Dose: *Adults.* 15–30 mg/kg/24 h PO ÷ tid-qid; max 2 g/d; dosing based on lean body wgt; ↓ dose in renal/hepatic impair. *Peds.* 15–30 mg/kg/d PO ÷ daily-bid; ↓ w/ renal/hepatic impair Caution: [C, +/–] CI: Severe hepatic damage, acute gout Disp: Tabs 500 mg SE: Hepatotox, malaise, GI upset, arthralgia, myalgia, gout, photosensitivity Notes: Use in combo w/ other anti-TB drugs; consult *MMWR* for latest TB recommendations; dosage regimen differs for "directly observed" therapy

Pyridoxine [Vitamin B₆] Uses: *Rx & prevention of vit B_6 deficiency* Action: Vit B_6 supl Dose: *Adults.* Deficiency: 10–20 mg/d PO. *Drug-induced neuritis:* 100–200 mg/d; 25–100 mg/d prophylaxis. *Peds.* 5–25 mg/d × 3 wk Caution: [A (C if doses exceed RDA), +] CI: Component allergy Disp: Tabs 25, 50, 100 mg; Inj 100 mg/mL SE: Allergic Rxns, HA, N

Quetiapine (Seroquel, Seroquel XR) **WARNING:** Closely monitor pts for worsening depression or emergence of suicidality, particularly in ped pts; not for use in peds; ↑ mortality in elderly with dementia-related psychosis **Uses:** *Acute exacerbations of schizophrenia* **Action:** Serotonin & dopamine antagonism **Dose:** 150–750 mg/d; initiate at 25–100 mg bid-tid; slowly ↑ dose; XR: 400–800 mg PO q P.M.; start 300 mg/d, ↑ 300 mg d max ↓ 800 mg d max ↓ mortality w/ hepatic & geriatric pts **Caution:** [C, –] **CI:** Component allergy **Disp:** Tabs 25, 50, 100, 200, 300, 400 mg; 200, 300, 400 XR **SE:** Confusion w/ nefazodone; HA, somnolence, ↑ wgt, ↓ BP, dizziness, cataracts, neuroleptic malignant syndrome, tardive dyskinesia, ↑ QT internal

Quinapril (Accupril) **WARNING:** ACE inhibitors used during PRG can cause fetal injury & death **Uses:** *HTN, CHF, DN, post-MI* **Action:** ACE inhibitor **Dose:** 10–80 mg PO daily; ↓ in renal impair **Caution:** [D, +] w/ RAS, vol depletion **CI:** ACE inhibitor sensitivity, angioedema, PRG **Disp:** Tabs 5, 10, 20, 40 mg **SE:** Dizziness, HA, ↓ BP, impaired renal Fxn, angioedema, taste perversion, cough

Quinidine (Quinidex, Quinaglute) **WARNING:** Mortality rates increased when used to treat non-life threatening arrhythmias **Uses:** *Prevention of tachydysrhythmias, malaria* **Action:** Class 1A antiarrhythmic **Dose:** *Adults.* *AF/flutter conversion:* After digitalization, 200 mg q2–3h × 8 doses; ↑ daily to 3–4 g max or nl rhythm. *Peds.* 15–60 mg/kg/24 h PO in 4–5 ÷ doses; ↓ in renal impair **Caution:** [C, +] w/ Ritonavir **CI:** Digitalis tox & AV block; conduction disorders **Disp:** *Sulfate:* Tabs 200, 300 mg; SR tabs 300 mg. *Gluconate:* SR tabs 324 mg; Inj 80 mg/mL **SE:** Extreme ↓ BP w/ IV use; syncope, QT prolongation, GI upset, arrhythmias, fatigue, cinchonism (tinnitus, hearing loss, delirium, visual changes), fever, hemolytic anemia, thrombocytopenia, rash **Notes:** Levels: *Trough:* just before next dose. *Therapeutic:* 2–5 mcg/mL. *Toxic:* >10 mcg/mL. *Half-life:* 6–8h; sulfate salt 83% quinidine; gluconate salt 62% quinidine; use w/ drug that slows AV conduction (eg, digoxin, diltiazem, β-blocker)

Quinupristin–Dalfopristin (Synercid) **Uses:** *Vancomycin-resistant Infxns due to E. faecium & other gram(+) Infxns* **Action:** ↓ Ribosomal protein synth. *Spectrum:* Vancomycin-resistant *E. faecium*, methicillin-susceptible *S. aureus*, *S. pyogenes*; not against *E. faecalis* **Dose:** *Adults & Peds.* 7.5 mg/kg IV q8–12h (central line preferred); incompatible w/ NS or heparin; flush IV w/ dextrose; ↓ w/ hepatic failure **Caution:** [B, M] Multiple drug interactions w/ drugs metabolized by CYP3A4 (eg, cyclosporine) **CI:** Component allergy **Disp:** Inj 500 mg (150 mg quinupristin/350 mg dalfopristin) 600 mg (180 quinupristin/420 mg dalfopristin) **SE:** Hyperbilirubinemia, Inf site Rxns & pain, arthralgia, myalgia

Rabeprazole (AcipHex) **Uses:** *PUD, GERD, ZE* *H. pylori* **Action:** Proton pump inhibitor **Dose:** 20 mg/d; may ↑ to 60 mg/d; *H. pylori* 20 mg PO bid × 7 d (w/ amoxicillin and clarithromycin); do not crush/chew tabs **Caution:** [B, ?/–] **Disp:** Tabs 20 mg ER **SE:** HA, fatigue, GI upset

Raloxifene (Evista) **WARNING:** Increased risk of venous thromboembolism and death from stroke **Uses:** *Prevent osteoporosis, breast CA prevention*

Action: Partial antagonist of estrogen, behaves like estrogen **Dose:** 60 mg/d **Caution:** [X, –] **CI:** Thromboembolism, PRG **Disp:** Tabs 60 mg **SE:** Chest pain, insomnia, rash, hot flashes, GI upset, hepatic dysfunction, leg cramps

Raltegravir (Isentress)   **Uses:** *HIV in combo w/ other agents* **Action:** HIV-integrase strand transfer inhibitor **Dose:** 100 mg PO bid **Caution:** [C, –] **CI:** None **Disp:** tabs 400 mg **SE:** N/D, HA, fever

Ramipril (Altace)   **WARNING:** ACE inhibitors used during PRG can cause fetal injury & death **Uses:** *HTN, CHF, DN, post-MI* **Action:** ACE inhibitor **Dose:** 2.5–20 mg/d PO ÷ daily-bid; ↓ in renal failure **Caution:** [D, +] **CI:** ACE inhibitor-induced angioedema **Disp:** Caps 1.25, 2.5, 5, 10 mg **SE:** Cough, HA, dizziness, ↓ BP, renal impair, angioedema **Notes:** OK in combo w/ diuretics

Ranibizumab (Lucentis)   **Uses:** *Neovascular "wet" macular degeneration* **Action:** Vascular endothelial growth factor inhibitor **Dose:** 0.5 mg intravitreal Inj q mo **Caution:** [C; ?] Hx thromboembolism **CI:** periocular Infxn **Disp:** Inj **SE:** Endophthalmitis, retinal detachment/hemorrhage, cataract, intraocular inflammation, conjunctival hemorrhage, eye pain, floaters

Ranitidine Hydrochloride (Zantac)   **Uses:** *Duodenal ulcer, active benign ulcers, hypersecretory conditions, & GERD* **Action:** H_2-receptor antagonist **Dose:** *Adults. Ulcer:* 150 mg PO bid, 300 mg PO hs, or 50 mg IV q6–8h; or 400 mg IV/d cont Inf, then maint of 150 mg PO hs. *Hypersecretion:* 150 mg PO bid, up to 600 mg/d. *GERD:* 300 mg PO bid; maint 300 mg PO hs. *Dyspepsia:* 75 mg PO daily-bid. *Peds.* 0.75–1.5 mg/kg/dose IV q6–8h or 1.25–2.5 mg/kg/dose PO q12h; ↓ in renal Insuff/failure **Caution:** [B, +] **CI:** Component allergy **Disp:** Tabs 75 [OTC], 150, 300 mg; caps 150, 300 mg; effervescent tabs 150 mg; syrup 15 mg/mL; Inj 25 mg/mL **SE:** Dizziness, sedation, rash, GI upset **Notes:** PO & parenteral doses differ

Ranolazine (Ranexa)   **Uses:** *Chronic angina* **Action:** ↓ Ischemia-related Na^+ entry into myocardium **Dose:** *Adults.* 500bid-1000 mg PO bid **CI:** w/ Hepatic impair, CYP3A inhibitors (Table 11); w/ agents that ↑ QT interval; ↓ K^+ **Caution:** [C, ?/–] HTN may develop w/ renal impair **Disp:** SR tabs 500 mg **SE:** Dizziness, HA, constipation, arrhythmias **Notes:** Not first line; use w/ amlodipine, nitrates, β-blockers

Rasagiline mesylate (Azilect)   **Uses:** *Early Parkinson Dz monotherapy; levodopa adjunct w/ advanced Dz* **Action:** MAO B inhibitor **Dose:** *Adults. Early Dz:* 1 mg PO daily, start 0.5 mg PO daily w/ levodopa; ↓ w/ CYP1A2 inhibitors or hepatic impair **CI:** MAOIs, sympathomimetic amines, meperidine, methadone, tramadol, propoxyphene, dextromethorphan, mirtazapine, cyclobenzaprine, St. John's wort, sympathomimetic vasoconstrictors, general anesthetics, SSRIs **Caution:** [C, ?] Avoid tyramine-containing foods; mod/severe hepatic impair **Disp:** Tabs 0.5, 1 mg **SE:** Arthralgia, indigestion, dyskinesia, hallucinations, ↓ wgt, postural ↓ BP, N, V, constipation, xerostomia, rash, sedation, CV conduction disturbances **Notes:** Rare melanoma reported; do periodic skin exams; D/C 14 d prior to elective surgery; initial ↓ levodopa dose ok

Rasburicase (Elitek) Uses: *Reduce ↑ uric acid due to tumor lysis (peds)* Action: Catalyzes uric acid Dose: *Peds.* 0.15 or 0.20 mg/kg IV over 30 min, daily × 5 Caution: [C, ?/–] Falsely ↑ uric acid values CI: Anaphylaxis, screen for G6PD deficiency to avoid hemolysis, methemoglobinemia Disp: 1.5 mg Inj SE: Fever, neutropenia, GI upset, HA, rash Note: Place blood test tube for uric acid level on ice to stop enzymatic Rxn; removed by dialysis

Repaglinide (Prandin) Uses: *Type 2 DM* Action: ↑ Pancreatic insulin release Dose: 0.5–4 mg ac, PO start 1–2 mg, ↑ to 16 mg/d max; take pc Caution: [C, ?/–] DKA, type 1 DM Disp: Tabs 0.5, 1, 2 mg SE: HA, hyper-/hypoglycemia, GI upset

Retapamulin (Altabax) Uses: *Topical Rx impetigo in pts >9 mo* Action: Pleuromutilin antibiotic, bacteriostatic, ↓ bacteria protein synth; *Spectrum: S. aureus (not MRSA), S. pyogenes* Dose: Apply bid × 5 d Caution: [B; ?] Disp: 10 mg/1 g SE: Local irritation

Reteplase (Retavase) Uses: *Post-AMI* Action: Thrombolytic Dose: 10 units IV over 2 min, 2nd dose in 30 min, 10 units IV over 2 min; 10 units IV bolus over 2 min; 30 min later, 10 units IV bolus over 2 min NS flush before and after each dose (*ECC 2005*) Caution: [C, ?/–] CI: Internal bleeding, spinal surgery/trauma, Hx AVM/CVA, bleeding diathesis, severe uncontrolled ↑ BP, sensitivity to thrombolytics Disp: Inj 10.8 units/2 mL SE: Bleeding including CNS, allergic Rxns

Ribavirin (Virazole, Copegus) WARNING: Monotherapy for chronic hep C ineffective; hemolytic anemia possible, teratogenic and embryocidal; use 2 forms of birth control for up to 6 mo after D/C drug; decrease in resp fxn when used in infants as Inh Uses: *RSV Infxn in infants [Virazole]; hep C (in combo w/ interferon alfa-2b [Copegus]* Action: Unknown *RSV:* 6 g in 300 mL sterile H_2O, inhale over 12–18 h. *hep C:* 600 mg PO bid in combo w/ interferon alfa-2b (see Rebetron) Caution: [X, ?] May accumulate on soft contact lenses CI: PRG, autoimmune hep, CrCl <50 mL/min Disp: Powder for aerosol 6 g; tabs 200, 400, 600 mg, caps 200 mg, soln 40 mg/mL SE: Fatigue, HA, GI upset, anemia, myalgia, alopecia, bronchospasm, ↓ HCT Notes: Virazole aerosolized by a SPAG, monitor resp Fxn closely; ✓ Hgb/Hct; PRG test monthly; hep C viral genotyping may modify dose

Rifabutin (Mycobutin) Uses: *Prevent MAC Infxn in AIDS pts w/ CD4 count <100* Action: ↓ DNA-dependent RNA polymerase activity Dose: Adults. 150–300 mg/d PO. *Peds 1 y:* 15–25 mg/kg/d PO. *2–10 y:* 4.4–18.8 mg/kg/d PO. *14–16 y:* 2.8–5.4 mg/kg/d PO Caution: [B; ?/–] WBC <1000/mm³ or platelets <50,000/mm³; ritonavir CI: Allergy Disp: Caps 150 mg SE: Discolored urine, rash, neutropenia, leukopenia, myalgia, ↑ LFTs Notes: SE/interactions similar to rifampin

Rifampin (Rifadin) Uses: *TB & Rx & prophylaxis of N. meningitidis, H. influenzae, or S. aureus carriers*; adjunct w/ severe S. aureus Action:

↓ DNA-dependent RNA polymerase **Dose:** *Adults. N. meningitidis & H. influenzae carrier:* 600 mg/d PO for 4 d. *TB:* 600 mg PO or IV daily or 2×/wk w/ combo regimen. *Peds.* 10–20 mg/kg/dose PO or IV daily-bid; ↓ in hepatic failure **Caution:** [C, +] Amprenavir, multiple drug interactions **CI:** Allergy, active *N. meningitidis* Infxn, w/ saquinavir/ritonavir **Disp:** Caps 150, 300 mg; Inj 600 mg **SE:** Red-orange–colored bodily fluids, ↓ LFTs, flushing, HA **Notes:** Never use as single agent w/ active TB

Rifapentine (Priftin)   **Uses:** *Pulm TB* **Action:** ↓ DNA-dependent RNA polymerase. *Spectrum: Mycobacterium tuberculosis* **Dose:** *Intensive phase:* 600 mg PO 2×/wk for 2 mo; separate doses by >3 d. *Continuation phase:* 600 mg/wk for 4 mo; part of 3–4 drug regimen **Caution:** [C, red-orange breast milk] Strong CYP3A4 inducer, ↓ protease inhibitor efficacy, antiepileptics, β-blockers, CCBs **CI:** Rifamycins allergy **Disp:** 150-mg tabs **SE:** Neutropenia, hyperuricemia, HTN, HA, dizziness, rash, GI upset, blood dyscrasias, ↑ LFTs, hematuria, discolored secretions **Notes:** Monitor LFTs

Rifaximin (Xifaxan)   **Uses:** *Traveler's D (noninvasive strains of E. coli) in pts >12 y* **Action:** Not absorbed, derivative of rifamycin. *Spectrum: E. coli* **Dose:** 1 tab PO daily × 3 d **Caution:** [C, ?/–] Hx allergy; pseudomembranous colitis **CI:** Allergy to rifamycins **Disp:** Tabs 200 mg **SE:** Flatulence, HA, Abd pain, GI distress, fever **Notes:** D/C if Sx worsen or persist >24–48 h, or w/ fever or blood in stool

Rimantadine (Flumadine)   **Uses:** *Prophylaxis & Rx of influenza A viral Infxns* **Action:** Antiviral **Dose:** *Adults & Peds >9 y:* 100 mg PO bid. *Peds 1–9 y:* 5 mg/kg/d PO, 150 mg/d max; daily w/ severe renal/hepatic impair & elderly; initiate w/in 48 h of Sx onset **Caution:** [C, –] w/ Cimetidine; avoid w/ PRG, breast-feeding **CI:** Component & amantadine allergy **Disp:** Tabs 100 mg; syrup 50 mg/5 mL **SE:** Orthostatic ↓ BP, edema, dizziness, GI upset, ↓ Sz threshold **Note:** See CDC *(MMWR)* for current Influenza A guidelines

Rimexolone (Vexol Ophthalmic)   **Uses:** *Post-op inflammation & uveitis* **Action:** Steroid **Dose:** *Adults & Peds >2 y: Uveitis:* 1–2 gtt/h daytime & q2h at night, taper to 1 gtt q4h. *Post-op:* 1–2 gtt qid = 2 wk **Caution:** [C, ?/–] Ocular Infxns **Disp:** Susp 1% **SE:** Blurred vision, local irritation **Notes:** Taper dose

Risedronate (Actonel, Actonel w/ calcium)   **Uses:** *Paget Dz; Rx/prevention glucocorticoid-induced/postmenopausal osteoporosis; ↑ bone mass in osteoporotic men; w/ calcium only FDA approved for female osteoporosis* **Action:** Bisphosphonate; ↓ osteoclast-mediated bone resorption **Dose:** *Paget Dz:* 30 mg/d PO for 2 mo. *Osteoporosis Rx/prevention:* 5 mg daily or 35 mg q wk; 30 min before 1st food/drink of the d; stay upright for at least 30 min after taking **Caution:** [C, ?/–] CA supls & antacids ↓ absorption **CI:** Component allergy, ↓ Ca^{2+}, esophageal abnormalities, unable to stand/sit for 30 min, CrCl <30 mL/min **Disp:** Tabs 5, 30, 35, 75 mg; Risedronate 35 mg (4 tabs)/calcium carbonate 1250 mg (24 tabs) **SE:** HA, D, Abd pain, arthralgia; flu-like Sxs, rash, esophagitis, bone pain **Notes:** Monitor LFTs, Ca^{2+}, PO^{3+}, K^+; severe bone, joint muscle pain may have black box warning

Risperidone, oral (Risperdal, Risperdal M-Tab) **WARNING:** ↑ Mortality in elderly with dementia-related psychosis **Uses:** *Psychotic disorders (schizophrenia),* dementia of the elderly, bipolar disorder, mania, Tourette disorder, autism **Action:** Benzisoxazole antipsychotic **Dose:** *Adults.* 0.5–6 mg PO bid; *M-Tab:* 1–6 mg/d start 1–2 mg/d, titrate q3–7d. *Peds.* 0.25 mg PO bid, ↑ q5–7d; ↓ start dose w/ elderly, renal/hepatic impair **Caution:** [C, –], ↑ BP w/ antihypertensives, clozapine **CI:** Component allergy **Disp:** Tabs 0.25, 0.5, 1, 2, 3, 4 mg; soln 1 mg/mL, M-Tab (orally disintegrating) tabs 0.5, 1, 2, 3, 4 mg **SE:** Orthostatic ↓ BP, EPS w/ high dose, tachycardia, arrhythmias, sedation, dystonias, neuroleptic malignant syndrome, sexual dysfunction, constipation, xerostomia, blood dyscrasias, cholestatic jaundice **Notes:** Several wk for effect

Risperidone, parenteral (Risperdal Consta) **WARNING:** Not approved for dementia-related psychosis; ↑ mortality risk in elderly dementia pts on atypical antipsychotics; most deaths due to CV or infectious events **Uses:** Schizophrenia **Action:** Benzisoxazole antipsychotic **Dose:** 25 mg q2wk IM may ↑ to max 50 mg q2wk; w/ renal/hepatic impair start PO Risperdal 0.5 mg PO bid × 1 wk titrate weekly **Caution:** [C, –], ↑ BP w/ antihypertensives, clozapine **CI:** Component allergy **Disp:** Inj 25, 37.5, 50 mg/vial **SE:** See risperidone oral **Note:** Long-acting Inj

Ritonavir (Norvir) **WARNING:** Life-threatening adverse events when used with certain nonsedating antihistamines, sedative hypnotics, antiarrhythmics, or ergot alkaloids due to inhibited drug metabolism **Uses:** *HIV* **Actions:** Protease inhibitor; ↓ maturation of immature noninfectious virions to mature infectious virus **Dose:** *Adults.* Initial 300 mg PO bid, titrate over 1 wk to 600 mg PO bid (titration will ↓ GI SE). *Peds >1 mo:* 250 mg/m^2 titrate to 400 mg bid (adjust w/ amprenavir, indinavir, nelfinavir, & saquinavir); take w/ food **Caution:** [B, +] w/ Ergotamine, amiodarone, bepridil, flecainide, propafenone, quinidine, pimozide, midazolam, triazolam **CI:** Component allergy **Disp:** Caps 100 mg; soln 80 mg/mL **SE:** ↑ Triglycerides, ↑ LFTs, N/V/D, Abd pain, taste perversion, anemia, weakness, HA, fever, malaise, rash, paresthesias **Notes:** Refrigerate

Rivastigmine (Exelon) **Uses:** *Mild–mod dementia in Alzheimer Dz* **Action:** Enhances cholinergic activity **Dose:** 1.5 mg bid; ↑ to 6 mg bid, w/ ↑ at 2-wk intervals (take w/ food) **Caution:** [B, ?] w/ β-Blockers, CCBs, smoking, neuromuscular blockade, digoxin **CI:** Rivastigmine or carbamate allergy **Disp:** Caps 1.5, 3, 4.5, 6 mg; soln 2 mg/mL **SE:** Dose-related GI upset, N/V/D, dizziness, insomnia, fatigue, tremor, diaphoresis, HA, wgt loss (in 18–26%) **Notes:** Swallow caps whole, do not break/chew/crush; avoid EtOH

Rivastigmine transdermal (Exelon Patch) **Uses:** *Mild/mod Alzheimer and Parkinson Dz dementia* **Action:** Acetylcholinesterase inhibitor **Dose:** *Initial:* 4.6-mg patch/d applied to back, chest, upper arm, ↑ 9.5 mg after

4 wk if tolerated **Caution:** [?; ?] Sick sinus syndrome, conduction defects, asthma, COPD, urinary obst, Szs **CI:** Hypersensitivity to rivastigmine, other carbamates **Disp:** Transdermal patch 5 cm² (4.6 mg/24 h), 10 cm² (9.5 mg/24 h) **SE:** N/V/D

Rizatriptan (Maxalt, Maxalt MLT)
Uses: *Rx acute migraine* **Action:** Vascular serotonin receptor agonist **Dose:** 5–10 mg PO, repeat in 2 h, PRN, 30 mg/d max **Caution:** [C, M] **CI:** Angina, ischemic heart Dz, ischemic bowel Dz, hemiplegic/basilar migraine, uncontrolled HTN, ergot or serotonin 5-HT_1 agonist use w/in 24 h, MAOI use w/in 14 d **Disp:** Tab 5, 10 mg; *Maxalt MLT:* OD tabs 5, 10 mg. **SE:** Chest pain, palpitations, nausea, vomiting, asthenia, dizziness, somnolence, fatigue

Rocuronium (Zemuron)
Uses: *Skeletal muscle relaxation during rapid-sequence intubation, surgery, or mechanical ventilation* **Action:** Nondepolarizing neuromuscular blocker **Dose:** *Rapid sequence intubation:* 0.6–1.2 mg/kg IV. *Continuous Inf:* 5–12.5 mcg/kg/min IV; adjust/titrate based on monitoring; ↓ in hepatic impair **Caution:** [C, ?] Aminoglycosides, vancomycin, tetracycline, polymyxins enhance blockade **CI:** Component or pancuronium allergy **Disp:** Inj preservative-free 10 mg/mL **SE:** BP changes, tachycardia

Ropinirole (Requip)
Uses: *Rx of Parkinson Dz, restless leg syndrome* **Action:** Dopamine agonist **Dose:** Initial 0.25 mg PO tid, weekly ↑ 0.25 mg/dose, to 3 mg max, max 4 mg for restless leg syndrome **Caution:** [C, ?/–] Severe CV, renal, or hepatic impair **CI:** Component allergy **Disp:** Tabs 0.25, 0.5, 1, 2, 3, 4, 5 mg **SE:** Syncope, postural ↓ BP, N/V, HA, somnolence, dosed-related hallucinations, dyskinesias, dizziness **Notes:** D/C w/ 7-d taper

Rosiglitazone (Avandia)
WARNING: May cause or worsen CHF; may increase myocardial ischemia **Uses:** *Type 2 DM* **Action:** Thiazolidinedione; ↑ insulin sensitivity **Dose:** 4–8 mg/d PO or in 2 ÷ doses (w/o regard to meals) **Caution:** [C, –] w/ ESRD, CHF, edema, **CI:** DKA, severe CHF (NYHA class III), ALT >2.5 ULN **Disp:** Tabs 2, 4, 8 mg **SE:** May ↑ CV, CHF & ? CA risk; wgt gain, hyperlipidemia, HA, edema, fluid retention, worsen CHF, hyper-/hypoglycemia, hepatic damage w/ ↑ LFTs **Notes:** Not ok in class III, IV heart Dz

Rosuvastatin (Crestor)
Uses: *Rx primary hypercholesterolemia & mixed dyslipidemia* **Action:** HMG-CoA reductase inhibitor **Dose:** 5–40 mg PO daily; max 5 mg/d w/ cyclosporine, 10 mg/d w/ gemfibrozil or CrCl <30 mL/min (avoid Al-/Mg-based antacids for 2 h after) **Caution:** [X, ?/–] **CI:** Active liver Dz, unexplained ↑ LFTs **Disp:** Tabs 5, 10, 20, 40 mg **SE:** Myalgia, constipation, asthenia, Abd pain, N, myopathy, rarely rhabdomyolysis **Notes:** May ↑ warfarin effect; monitor LFTs at baseline, 12 wk, then q6mo; ↓ dose in Asian pts

Rotavirus vaccine, live, oral, attenuated (Rotarix)
Uses: *Prevent rotavirus gastroenteritis in peds* **Action:** Vaccine w/ live attenuated rotavirus **Dose:** *Peds 6–24 wk:* 1st dose PO at 6 wk of age, wait at least 4 wk then a second dose by 24 wk of age. **Caution:** [C, ?] **CI:** Uncorrected congenital GI

malformation **Disp:** single dose vial **SE:** Fussiness/irritability, cough, runny nose, fever, ↓ appetite, V

Rotavirus vaccine, live, oral, pentavalent (RotaTeq) Uses: *Prevent rotavirus gastroenteritis* **Action:** Active immunization **Dose:** *Peds.* Single dose PO at 2, 4, and 6 mo **Caution:** [?, ?] **Disp:** Oral susp 2-mL single-use tubes **SE:** D, V **Notes:** Begin series by age 12 wk and conclude by age 32 wk

Salmeterol (Serevent Diskus) **WARNING:** Long-acting β₂-agonists, such as salmeterol, may ↑ the risk of asthma-related death. Should not be used alone, only as additional therapy for pts not controlled on other asthma meds **Uses:** *Asthma, exercise-induced asthma, COPD* **Action:** Sympathomimetic bronchodilator, β₂-agonist **Dose:** *Adults & Peds >12 y:* 1 Diskus-dose inhaled bid **Caution:** [C, ?/–] **CI:** Acute asthma; w/in 14 d of MAOI **Disp:** 50 mcg/dose, dry powder discus, metered-dose inhaler, 21 mcg/activation **SE:** HA, pharyngitis, tachycardia, arrhythmias, nervousness, GI upset, tremors **Notes:** Not for acute attacks; also prescribe short-acting β-agonist

Saquinavir (Fortovase, Invirase) **WARNING:** Invirase and Fortovase not bioequivalent/interchangeable; must use Invirase in combo w/ ritonavir, which provides saquinavir plasma levels = to those w/ Fortovase **Uses:** *HIV Infxn* **Action:** HIV protease inhibitor **Dose:** 1200 mg PO tid w/in 2 h pc (dose adjust w/ ritonavir, delavirdine, lopinavir, & nelfinavir) **Caution:** [B, +] w/ Ketoconazole, statins, sildenafil **CI:** w/ Rifampin, severe hepatic impair, allergy, sun exposure w/o sunscreen/clothing, triazolam, midazolam, ergots, **Disp:** Caps 200, tabs 500 mg **SE:** Dyslipidemia, lipodystrophy, rash, hyperglycemia, GI upset, weakness **Notes:** Take 2 h after meal, avoid direct sunlight

Sargramostim [GM-CSF] (Leukine) **Uses:** *Myeloid recovery following BMT or chemotherapy* **Action:** Recombinant GF, activates mature granulocytes & macrophages **Dose:** *Adults & Peds.* 250 mcg/m²/d IV for 21 d (BMT) **Caution:** [C, ?/–] Lithium, corticosteroids **CI:** >10% blasts, allergy to yeast, concurrent chemotherapy/RT **Disp:** Inj 250, 500 mcg **SE:** Bone pain, fever, ↓ BP, tachycardia, flushing, GI upset, myalgia **Notes:** Rotate Inj sites; use APAP PRN for pain

Scopolamine, Scopolamine transdermal & ophthalmic (Scopace, Transderm-Scop) **Uses:** *Prevent N/V associated w/ motion sickness, anesthesia, opiates; mydriatic,* cycloplegic, Rx uveitis & iridocyclitis **Action:** Anticholinergic, inhibits iris & ciliary bodies, antiemetic **Dose:** 1 mg/72 h, 1 patch behind ear q3d; apply >4 h before exposure; cycloplegic 1–2 gtt 1 h preprocedure, uveitis 1–2 gtt up to qid max; ↓ in elderly **Caution:** [C, +] w/APAP, levodopa, ketoconazole, digitalis, KCl **CI:** NAG, GI or GU obst, thyrotoxicosis, paralytic ileus **Disp:** Patch 1.5 mg, (releases 1 mg over 72 h), ophthal 0.25% **SE:** Xerostomia, drowsiness, blurred vision, tachycardia, constipation **Notes:** Do not blink excessively after dose, wait 5 min before dosing other eye; antiemetic activity w/ patch requires several hours

Secobarbital (Seconal) [C-II]   Uses: *Insomnia, short-term use,* pre-anesthetic agent **Action:** Rapid-acting barbiturate **Dose:** *Adults.* 100–200 mg hs, 100–300 mg pre-op. *Peds.* 2–6 mg/kg/dose, 100 mg/max, ↓ in elderly **Caution:** [D, +] CYP2C9, 3A3/4, 3A5/7 inducer (Table 11); ↑ tox w/ other CNS depressants **CI:** Porphyria, w/ voriconazole, PRG **Disp:** Caps 50, 100 mg **SE:** Tolerance in 1–2 wk; resp depression, CNS depression, porphyria, photosensitivity

Selegiline, oral (Eldepryl, Zelapar)   WARNING: Closely monitor pts for worsening depression or emergence of suicidality, particularly in ped pts **Uses:** *Parkinson Dz* **Action:** MAOI **Dose:** 5 mg PO bid; 1.25–2.5 once daily tabs PO q A.M. (before breakfast w/o liq) 2.5 mg/d max; ↓ in elderly **Caution:** [C, ?] w/ Drugs that induce CYP3A4 (Table 11) (eg, phenytoin, carbamazepine, nafcillin, phenobarbital, & rifampin); avoid w/ antidepressants **CI:** w/ Meperidine, MAOI, dextromethorphan, general anesthesia w/in 10 d, pheochromocytoma **Disp:** Tabs/caps 5 mg; once-daily tabs 1.25 mg **SE:** N, dizziness, orthostatic ↓ BP, arrhythmias, tachycardia, edema, confusion, xerostomia **Notes:** ↓ Carbidopa/levodopa if used in combo; see transdermal form

Selegiline, transdermal (Emsam)   WARNING: May ↑ risk of suicidal thinking and behavior in children and adolescents with major depression disorder **Uses:** *Depression* **Action:** MAOI **Dose:** *Adults.* Apply patch daily to upper torso, upper thigh, or outer upper arm **CI:** Tyramine-containing foods w/ 9- or 12-mg doses; serotonin-sparing agents **Caution:** [C, –] ↑ Carbamazepine and oxcarbazepine levels **Disp:** ER Patches 6, 9, 12 mg **SE:** Local Rxns requiring topical steroids; HA, insomnia, orthostatic, ↓ BP, serotonin syndrome, suicide risk **Notes:** Rotate site; see oral form

Selenium Sulfide (Exsel Shampoo, Selsun Blue Shampoo, Selsun Shampoo)   Uses: *Scalp seborrheic dermatitis,* scalp itching & flaking due to *dandruff;* tinea versicolor **Action:** Antiseborrheic **Dose:** *Dandruff, seborrhea:* Massage 5–10 mL into wet scalp, leave on 2–3 min, rinse, repeat; use 2× wk, then once q1–4wk PRN. *Tinea versicolor:* Apply 2.5% daily on area & lather w/ small amounts of water; leave on 10 min, then rinse **Caution:** [C, ?] **CI:** Open wounds **Disp:** Shampoo [OTC]; 2.5% lotion **SE:** Dry or oily scalp, lethargy, hair discoloration, local irritation **Notes:** Do not use more than 2×/wk

Sertaconazole (Ertaczo)   Uses: *Topical Rx interdigital tinea pedis* **Action:** Imidazole antifungal. *Spectrum: Trichophyton rubrum, Trichophyton mentagrophytes, Epidermophyton floccosum* **Dose:** *Adults & Peds >12:* Apply between toes & immediate surrounding healthy skin bid × 4 wk **Caution:** [C, ?] **CI:** Component allergy **Disp:** 2% Cream **SE:** Contact dermatitis, dry/burning skin, tenderness **Notes:** Use in immunocompetent pts; not for oral, intravag, ophthal use

Sertraline (Zoloft)   WARNING: Closely monitor pts for worsening depression or emergence of suicidality, particularly in ped pts **Uses:** *Depression, panic disorders, OCD, posttraumatic stress disorder (PTSD),* social anxiety disorder, eating disorders, premenstrual disorders **Action:** ↓ Neuronal uptake of serotonin **Dose:** *Adults. Depression:* 50–200 mg/d PO. *PTSD:* 25 mg PO daily × 1 wk, then 50 mg PO daily, 200 mg/d max. *Peds 6–12 y:* 25 mg PO daily. *13–17 y:* 50 mg PO daily **Caution:** [C, ?/–] w/ Haloperidol (serotonin syndrome), sumatriptan, linezolid, hepatic impair **CI:** MAOI use w/in 14 d; concomitant pimozide **Disp:** Tabs 25, 50, 100, 150, 200 mg; 20 mg/mL oral **SE:** Activate manic/hypomanic state, ↓ wgt, insomnia, somnolence, fatigue, tremor, xerostomia, N/D, dyspepsia, ejaculatory dysfunction, ↓ libido, hepatotox

Sevelamer carbonate (Renvela)
Uses: *Control ↑ PO_4^{-3} in ESRD* **Action:** Phosphate binder **Dose:** *Initial:* PO_4^{-3} >5.5 and <7.5 mg/dL: 800 mg PO; ≥7.5 mg/dL: 1600 mg PO tid. *Switching from Sevelamer HCl:* g-per-g basis; titrate ↑/↓ 1 tab/meal 2-wk intervals PRN; take w/ food **Caution:** [C, ?] w/ Swallow disorders, bowel problems, may ↓ absorption of Vits D, E, K, ↓ ciprofloxacin & other medicine levels **CI:** ↓ PO_4, bowel obst **Disp:** Tab 800 mg **SE:** N/V/D, dyspepsia, Abd pain, flatulence, constipation **Notes:** Separate other meds 1 h before or 3 h after

Sevelamer HCl (Renagel)
Uses: *↓ PO_4^{-3} in ESRD* **Action:** Binds intestinal PO_4^{-3} **Dose:** 2–4 caps PO tid w/ meals; adjust based on PO_4^{-3}; max 4 g/dose **Caution:** [C, ?] May ↓ absorption of Vits D, E, K, ↓ ciprofloxacin & other medicine levels **CI:** ↓ PO_4^{-3}, bowel obst **Disp:** Tab 400, 800 mg **SE:** BP changes, N/V/D, dyspepsia, thrombosis **Notes:** Do not open/chew caps; separate other meds 1 h before or 3 h after; 800 mg sevelamer = 667 mg Ca acetate

Sibutramine (Meridia) [C-IV]
Uses: *Obesity* **Action:** Blocks uptake of norepinephrine, serotonin, dopamine **Dose:** 10 mg/d PO, may ↑ to 15 mg/d after 4 wk **Caution:** [C, –] w/ SSRIs, lithium, dextromethorphan, opioids **CI:** MAOI w/in 14 d, uncontrolled HTN, arrhythmias **Disp:** Caps 5, 10, 15 mg **SE:** HA, insomnia, xerostomia, constipation, rhinitis, tachycardia, HTN **Notes:** Use w/ low-calorie diet, monitor BP & HR; only for BMI >30 kg/m² or >27 kg/m² or CV risk factors

Sildenafil (Viagra, Revatio)
Uses: *Viagra:* *Erectile dysfunction*; *Revatio:* *Pulm artery HTN* **Action:** ↓ Phosphodiesterase type 5 (responsible for cyclic guanosine monophosphate [cGMP] breakdown); ↑ cGMP activity to relax smooth muscles & ↑ flow to corpus cavernosum and pulm vasculature; ? antiproliferative on pulm artery smooth muscle **Dose:** *ED:* 25–100 mg PO 1 h before sexual activity, max 1/d; ↓ if >65 y; avoid fatty foods w/ dose; *Revatio: Pulm HTN:* 20 mg PO tid **Caution:** [B, ?] w/ CYP3A4 inhibitors (Table 11), ↓ dose w/ ritonavir; retinitis pigmentosa; hepatic/severe renal impair; w/ sig hypo-/hypertension **CI:** w/ Nitrates or if sex not advised **Disp:** Tabs *Viagra* 25, 50, 100 mg, tabs *Revatio* 20 mg **SE:** HA; flushing; dizziness; blue haze visual change, hearing loss, priapism **Notes:** Cardiac events in absence of nitrates debatable; transient global amnesia reports

Silodosin (Rapaflo)
Uses: *BPH* **Action:** Antagonist of prostatic α_1 receptors (mostly α_{1A}) **Dose:** 8 mg/d; 4 mg/d w/ CrCl 30–50 mL/min; take w/ food

Caution: [B, ?], not for use in females; do not use w/other α-blockers or w/ cyclosporine; R/O PCa before use; IFIS possible w/ cataract surgery; avoid **CI:** Severe hepatic/renal impair (CrCl <30 mL/min), w/ CYP3A4 inhibitors (eg, ketoconazole, clarithromycin, itraconazole, ritonavir) **Disp:** Caps 4, 8 mg **SE:** Retrograde ejaculation, dizziness, D, syncope, somnolence, orthostatic ↓ BP, nasopharyngitis, nasal congestion **Notes:** Not for use as antihypertensive; no effect on QT interval

Silver Nitrate (Dey-Drop, others) **Uses:** *Removal of granulation tissue & warts; prophylaxis in burns* **Action:** Caustic antiseptic & astringent **Dose:** *Adults & Peds.* Apply to moist surface 2–3× wk for several wk or until effect **Caution:** [C, ?] **CI:** Do not use on broken skin **Disp:** Topical impregnated applicator sticks, soln 0.5, 10, 25, 50%; ophthal 1% amp; topical ointment 10% **SE:** May stain tissue black, usually resolves; local irritation, methemoglobinemia **Notes:** D/C if redness or irritation develop; no longer used in US for newborn prevention of gonococcus conjunctivitis

Silver Sulfadiazine (Silvadene, others) **Uses:** *Prevention & Rx of Infxn in 2nd- & 3rd-degree burns* **Action:** Bactericidal **Dose:** *Adults & Peds.* Aseptically cover the area w/ 1/16-inch coating bid **Caution:** [B unless near term, ?/–] **CI:** Infants <2 mo, PRG near term **Disp:** Cream 1% **SE:** Itching, rash, skin discoloration, blood dyscrasias, hep, allergy **Notes:** Systemic absorption w/ extensive application

Simethicone (Mylicon, others) [OTC] **Uses:** Flatulence **Action:** Defoaming, alters gas bubble surface tension action **Dose:** *Adult & Peds >12 y:* 40–125 mg PO pc & hs PRN; 500 mg/d max. *Peds <2 y:* 20 mg PO qid PRN. *2–12 y:* 40 mg PO qid PRN **Caution:** [C, ?] **CI:** GI Intestinal perforation or obst **Disp:** [OTC] Tabs 80, 125 mg; caps 125 mg; softgels 125, 166, 180 mg; susp 40 mg/0.6 mL; chew tabs 80, 125 mg **SE:** N/D **Notes:** Available in combo products OTC

Simvastatin (Zocor) **Uses:** ↓ Cholesterol **Action:** HMG-CoA reductase inhibitor **Dose:** *Adults.* 5–80 mg PO; w/ meals; ↓ in renal Insuff. *Peds 10–17 y:* 10 mg, 40 mg/d max **Caution:** [X, –] Avoid concurrent use of gemfibrozil **CI:** PRG, liver Dz **Disp:** Tabs 5, 10, 20, 40, 80 mg **SE:** HA, GI upset, myalgia, myopathy (muscle pain, tenderness or weakness with creatine kinase 10× ULN), hep **Notes:** Combo with ezetimibe/simvastatin; follow LFTs

Sirolimus [Rapamycin] (Rapamune) **WARNING:** Use only by physicians experienced in immunosuppression; immunosuppression associated w/ lymphoma, ↑ Infxn risk; do not use in lung transplant (fatal bronchial anastomotic dehiscence) **Uses:** *Prophylaxis of organ rejection in new Tx pts* **Action:** ↓ T-lymphocyte activation **Dose:** *Adults >40 kg:* 6 mg PO on day 1, then 2 mg/d PO. *Peds: <40 kg &≥13 y:* 3 mg/m² load, then 1 mg/m²/d (in H₂O/orange juice; no grapefruit juice w/ sirolimus); take 4 h after cyclosporine; ↓ in hepatic impair **Caution:** [C, ?/–] Grapefruit juice, ketoconazole **Disp:** Component allergy **Disp:** Soln 1 mg/mL, tab 1, 2 mg **SE:** HTN, edema, CP, fever, HA, insomnia, acne, rash, ↑ cholesterol, GI upset, ↑↓ K⁺, Infxns, blood dyscrasias, arthralgia, tachycardia, renal impair, hepatic artery thrombosis, graft loss & death in de novo liver transplant (↑ hepatic artery thrombosis), delayed wound healing *Notes:* Levels: *Trough:* 4–20 ng/mL; can vary based on assay and use of other immunosuppression agents

Sitagliptin (Januvia)   Uses: *Type 2 DM* Action: Dipeptidyl peptidase-4 (DDP-4) inhibitor, ↑ insulin synth/release Dose: 100 mg PO daily; ↓ w/ renal impair Caution: [B; ?] w/ Sulfonylurea may ↑ hypoglycemic risk CI: DKA, type 1 DM Disp: Tabs 25, 50, 100 SE: URI, HA, D, Abd pain, arthralgia

Sitagliptin/Metformin (Janumet)   WARNING: Associated w/ lactic acidosis Uses: *Adjunct to diet and exercise in type 2 DM* Action: See individual agents Dose: 1 tab PO bid, titrate; 100 mg sitagliptin & 2000 mg metformin/d max; take w/ meals Caution: [B, ?/–] CI: Type 1 DM, DKA, male Cr >15; female Cr >1.4 mg/dL Disp: Tabs 50/500, 50 mg/1000 mg SE: Nasopharyngitis, N/V/D, flatulence, Abd discomfort, dyspepsia, asthenia, HA Notes: Hold w/ contrast study; ✓ Cr, CBC

Smallpox Vaccine (Dryvax)   WARNING: Acute myocarditis and other infectious complications possible; CI in immunocompromised, eczema or exfoliative skin conditions, infants <1 y Uses: *Immunization against smallpox (variola virus)* Action: Active immunization (live attenuated cowpox virus) *Dose: Adults (routine nonemergency) or all ages (emergency):* 2–3 Punctures w/ bifurcated needle dipped in vaccine into deltoid, posterior triceps muscle; ✓ site for Rxn in 6–8 d; if major Rxn, site scabs, & heals, leaving scar; if mild/equivocal Rxn, repeat w/ 15 punctures Caution: [X, N/A] CI: *Nonemergency use,* febrile illness, immunosuppression, Hx eczema & their household contacts. *Emergency:* No absolute CI Disp: Vial for reconstitution: 100 million pock-forming units/mL SE: Malaise, fever, regional lymphadenopathy, encephalopathy, rashes, spread of inoculation to other sites administered; Stevens-Johnson syndrome, eczema vaccinatum w/ severe disability Notes: Avoid infant contact for 14 d; intradermal use only; restricted distribution

Sodium Bicarbonate [NaHCO₃]   Uses: *Alkalinization of urine,* RTA, *metabolic acidosis,* ↑ K⁺, TCA OD* Action: Alkalinizing agent Dose: *Adults.* *Cardiac arrest:* Initiate ventilation, 1 mEq/kg IV bolus; repeat 1/2 dose q10min PRN *(ECC 2005).* *Metabolic acidosis:* 2–5 mEq/kg IV over 8 h & PRN based on acid–base status. *Hyperkalemia:* 1 mg/kg IV over 5 min. *Alkalinize urine:* 4 g (48 mEq) PO, then 1–2 g q4h; adjust based on urine pH; 2 amp (100 mEq/1 L D₅W at 100–250 mL/h IV, monitor urine pH & serum bicarbonate. *Chronic renal failure:* 1–3 mEq/kg/d PO. *Distal RTA:* 1 mEq/kg/d PO. *Peds >1 y:* Cardiac arrest: See Adult dosage. *Peds <1 y:* *ECC 2005:* Initiate ventilation, 1:1 dilution 1 mEq/mL dosed 1 mEq/kg IV; can repeat w/ 0.5 mEq/kg in 10 min × 1 or based on acid–base status. *Chronic renal failure:* See Adult dosage. *Distal RTA:* 2–3 mEq/kg/d PO. *Proximal RTA:* 5–10 mEq/kg/d; titrate based on serum bicarbonate. *Urine alkalinization:* 84–840 mg/kg/d (1–10 mEq/kg/d) in ÷ doses; adjust based on urine pH

Caution: [C, ?] **CI:** Alkalosis, ↑ Na^+, severe pulm edema, ↓ Ca^{2+} **Disp:** Powder, tabs; 300 mg = 3.6 mEq; 325 mg = 3.8 mEq; 520 mg = 6.3 mEq; 600 mg = 7.3 mEq; 650 mg = 7.6 mEq; Inj 1 mEq/mL, 4.2% (5 mEq/10 mL), 7.5% (8.92 mEq/mL), 8.4% (10 mEq/10 mL) vial or amp **SE:** Belching, edema, flatulence, ↑ Na^+, metabolic alkalosis **Notes:** 1 g Neutralizes 12 mEq of acid; 50 mEq bicarb = 50 mEq Na; can make 3 amps in 1 L D_5W to = D5NS w/ 150 mEq bicarbonate

Sodium Citrate/Citric Acid (Bicitra, Oracit)   **Uses:** *Chronic metabolic acidosis, alkalinize urine; dissolve uric acid & cysteine stones* **Action:** Urinary alkalinizer **Peds:** 5–15 mL in 1–3 oz H_2O pc & hs. **Peds:** 5–15 mL in 1–3 oz H_2O pc & hs; best after meals **Caution:** [C, +] **CI:** Al-based antacids; severe renal impair or Na-restricted diets **Disp:** 15- or 30-mL unit dose: 16 (473 mL) or 4 (118 mL) fl oz **SE:** Tetany, metabolic alkalosis, ↑ K^+, GI upset; avoid use of multiple 50-mL amps; can cause ↑ Na^+/hyperosmolality **Notes:** 1 mL = 1 mEq Na & 1 mEq bicarbonate

Sodium Oxybate (Xyrem) [C-III]   **WARNING:** Known drug of abuse even at recommended doses; confusion, depression, resp depression may occur **Uses:** *Narcolepsy-associated cataplexy* **Action:** Inhibitory neurotransmitter **Dose:** *Adults & Peds >16 y:* 2.25 g PO qhs, 2nd dose 2.5–4 h later; may ↑ 9 g/d max **Caution:** [B, ?/–] EtOH **Disp:** 500 mg/mL (180-mL) PO soln **SE:** Confusion, depression, ↓ diminished level of consciousness, incontinence, sig V, resp depression, psychological Sxs **Notes:** May lead to dependence; synonym for γ-hydroxybutyrate (GHB), abused as a "date rape drug"; controlled distribution (prescriber & pt registration); must be administered when pt in bed

Sodium Phosphate (Visicol)   **Uses:** *Bowel preparation prior to colonoscopy,* short-term constipation **Action:** Hyperosmotic laxative **Dose:** 3 Tabs PO w/ at least 8 oz clear liq q15min (20 tabs total night before procedure); 3–5 h before colonoscopy, repeat) **Caution:** [C, ?] Renal impair, electrolyte disturbances **CI:** Megacolon, bowel obst, CHF, ascites, unstable angina, gastric retention, bowel perforation, colitis, hypomotility **Disp:** Tabs 0.398, 1.102 g **SE:** ↑ QT, ↑ PO^3, ↑ K^+, Na, D, flatulence, cramps, Abd bloating/pain

Sodium Polystyrene Sulfonate (Kayexalate)   **Uses:** *Rx of ↑ K^+* **Action:** Na^+/K^+ ion-exchange resin **Dose:** *Adults.* 15–60 g PO or 30–60 g PR q6h based on serum K^+. **Peds:** 1 g/kg/dose PO or PR q6h based on serum K^+ (given w/ agent, eg, sorbitol, to promote movement through the bowel) **Caution:** [C, M] **CI:** ↑ Na^+ **Disp:** Powder; susp 15 g/60 mL sorbitol **SE:** ↑ Na^+, ↓ K^+, Na retention, GI upset, fecal impaction **Notes:** Enema acts more quickly than PO; PO most effective, onset action >2 h

Solifenacin (Vesicare)   **Uses:** *OAB* **Action:** Antimuscarinic, ↓ detrusor contractions **Dose:** 5 mg PO daily, 10 mg/d max; ↓ w/ renal/hepatic impair **Caution:** [C, ?/–] BOO or GI obst, ulcerative colitis, MyG, renal/hepatic impair, QT prolongation risk **CI:** NAG, urinary/gastric retention **Disp:** Tabs 5, 10 mg

SE: Constipation, xerostomia, dyspepsia, blurred vision, drowsiness **Notes:** CYP3A4 substrate; azole antifungals ↑ levels; recent concern over cognitive effects

Sorafenib (Nexavar) **Uses:** *Advanced RCC* metastatic liver cancer **Action:** Kinase inhibitor **Dose:** *Adults.* 400 mg PO bid on empty stomach **Caution:** [D, –] w/ Irinotecan, doxorubicin, warfarin; avoid conception (male/female) **Disp:** Tabs 200 mg **SE:** Hand–foot syndrome; Tx-emergent hypertension; bleeding, ↑ INR, cardiac infarction/ischemia; ↑ pancreatic enzymes, hypophosphatemia, lymphopenia, anemia, fatigue, alopecia, pruritus, D, GI upset, HA, neuropathy **Notes:** Monitor BP 1st 6 wk; may require ↓ dose (daily or q other day); impaired metabolism in pt of Asian descent; minor effect on wound healing, D/C before major surgery

Sorbitol (generic) **Uses:** *Constipation* **Action:** Laxative **Dose:** 30–60 mL PO of a 20–70% soln PRN **Caution:** [B, +] **CI:** Anuria **Disp:** Liq 70% **SE:** Edema, electrolyte loss, lactic acidosis, GI upset, xerostomia **Notes:** May be vehicle for many liq formulations (eg, zinc, Kayexalate)

Sotalol (Betapace) **WARNING:** To minimize risk of induced arrhythmia, pts reinitiated/reinitiated on Betapace AF should be placed for a minimum of 3 d (on their maint) in a facility that can provide cardiac resuscitation, cont ECG monitoring, & calculations of CrCl. Betapace should not be substituted for Betapace AF because of labeling **Uses:** *Ventricular arrhythmias, AF* **Action:** β-Adrenergic-blocking agent **Dose:** *Adults. CrCl >60 mL/min:* 80 mg PO bid, may ↑ to 240–320 mg/d. *30–60 mL/min:* 80 mg q24h. *10–30 mL/min:* dose q36–48h 80 mg PO bid. *Peds Neonates:* 9 mg/m² tid. *1–19 mo:* 20.4 mg/m² tid. *20–23 mo:* 29.1 mg/m² tid. *≥2 y:* 30 mg/m² tid; to max dose of 90 mg/m² tid; ↓ w/ renal impair **Caution:** [B (1st tri) (D if 2nd or 3rd tri), +] **CI:** Asthma, COPD, bradycardia, ↑ prolonged QT interval, 2nd-/3rd-degree heart block w/o pacemaker, cardiogenic shock, uncontrolled CHF **Disp:** Tabs 80, 120, 160, 240 mg **SE:** Bradycardia, CP, palpitations, fatigue, dizziness, weakness, dyspnea **Notes:** Betapace should not be substituted for Betapace AF because of differences in labeling

Sotalol (Betapace AF) **WARNING:** See sotalol (Betapace) **Uses:** *Maintain sinus rhythm for symptomatic A fibrillation/flutter* **Action:** β-Adrenergic-blocking agent **Dose:** *Adults. CrCl >60 mL/min:* 80 mg PO q12h. *CrCl 40–60 mL/min:* 80 mg PO q24h; ↑ to 120 mg during hospitalization; monitor QT interval 2–4 h after each dose, dose reduction or D/C if QT interval ≥500 msec. *Peds Neonates:* 9 mg/m² tid. *1–19 mo:* 20 mg/m² tid. *20–23 mo:* 29.1 mg/m² tid. *≥2 y:* 30 mg/m² tid; can double all doses as max daily dose; allow ≈ 36 h between changes **Caution:** [B (1st tri; D if 2nd or 3rd tri), +] If converting from previous antiarrhythmic **CI:** Asthma, bradycardia, ↑ QT interval, 2nd- or 3rd-degree heart block w/o pacemaker, cardiogenic shock, uncontrolled CHF, CrCl <40 mL/min **Disp:** Tabs 80, 120, 160 mg **SE:** Bradycardia, CP, palpitations, fatigue, dizziness, weakness, dyspnea **Notes:** Follow renal Fxn & QT interval; Betapace should not be substituted for Betapace AF because of differences in labeling

Spironolactone (Aldactone)   Uses: *Hyperaldosteronism, HTN, ascites from cirrhosis* **Action:** Aldosterone antagonist; K+-sparing diuretic **Dose:** *Adults.* CHF (NYHA class III–IV) 12.5–25 mg/d (w/ ACE and loop diuretic) HTN 25–50 mg/d **Peds.** 1–3.3 mg/kg/24 h PO ÷ bid-qid. **Neonates:** 0.5–1 mg/kg/dose q8h; take w/ food **Disp:** [D, +] **CI:** ↑ K+, acute renal failure, anuria **Disp:** Tabs 25, 50, 100 mg **SE:** ↑ K+ & gynecomastia, arrhythmia, sexual dysfunction, confusion, dizziness, D/N/V, abnormal menstruation

Starch, topical, rectal (Tucks Suppositories [OTC])   Uses: *Temporary relief of anorectal disorders (itching, etc)* **Action:** Topical protectant **Dose:** *Adults & Peds ≥12 y:* Cleanse, rinse and dry, insert 1 sup rectally 6×/d × 7 d max. **Caution:** [?, ?] **CI:** None **Disp:** Supp **SE:** D/C w/ or if rectal bleeding occurs or if condition worsens or does not improve within 7 d

Stavudine (Zerit)   **WARNING:** Lactic acidosis & severe hepatomegaly w/ steatosis & pancreatitis reported **Uses:** *HIV in combo w/ other antiretrovirals* **Action:** Reverse transcriptase inhibitor **Dose:** *Adults >60 kg:* 40 mg bid. *<60 kg:* 30 mg bid. **Peds Birth–13 d:** 0.5 mg/kg q12h. *>14 d & <30 kg:* 1 mg/kg q12h. **≥30 kg:** Adult dose; ↓ w/ renal Insuff **Caution:** [C, +] **CI:** Allergy **Disp:** Caps 15, 20, 30, 40 mg; soln 1 mg/mL **SE:** Peripheral neuropathy, HA, chills, fever, malaise, rash, GI upset, anemias, lactic acidosis, ↑ LFTs, pancreatitis **Notes:** Take w/ plenty of H_2O

Steroids, Systemic (see also Table 3) The following relates only to the commonly used systemic glucocorticoids
Uses: *Endocrine disorders* (adrenal Insuff), *rheumatoid disorders, collagen–vascular Dzs, derm Dzs, allergic states, cerebral edema,* nephritis, nephrotic syndrome, immunosuppression for transplantation, ↑ Ca^{2+}, malignancies (breast, lymphomas), pre-op (in any pt who has been on steroids in the previous year, known hypoadrenalism, pre-op for adrenalectomy); Inj into joints/tissue **Action:** Glucocorticoid **Dose:** Varies w/ use & institutional protocols.

• *Adrenal Insuff, acute:* **Adults.** Hydrocortisone: 100 mg IV; then 300 mg/d ÷ q6h; convert to 50 mg PO q8h × 6 doses, taper to 30–50 mg/d ÷ bid. **Peds.** Hydrocortisone: 1–2 mg/kg IV, then 150–250 mg/d ÷ tid.
• *Adrenal Insuff, chronic (physiologic replacement):* May need mineralocorticoid supl such as Florinef. **Adults.** Hydrocortisone 20 mg PO q A.M., 10 mg PO q P.M.; cortisone 0.5–0.75 mg/kg/d ÷ bid; cortisone 0.25–0.35 mg/kg/d IM; dexamethasone 0.03–0.15 mg/kg/d or 0.6–0.75 mg/m²/d ÷ q6–12h PO, IM, IV. **Peds.** Hydrocortisone 0.5–0.75 mg/kg/d PO tid; hydrocortisone succinate 0.25–0.35 mg/kg/d IM.
• *Asthma, acute:* **Adults.** Methylprednisolone 60 mg PO/IV q6h or dexamethasone 12 mg IV q6h. **Peds.** Prednisolone 1–2 mg/kg/d or prednisone 1–2 mg/kg/d ÷ daily-bid for up to 5 d; methylprednisolone 2–4 mg/kg/d IV ÷ tid; dexamethasone 0.1–0.3 mg/kg/d divided q6h.

- *Congenital adrenal hyperplasia:* **Peds.** Initial *hydrocortisone* 30–36 mg/m²/d PO ÷ 1/3 dose q A.M., 2/3 dose q P.M.; maint 20–25 mg/m²/d ÷ bid.
- *Extubation/airway edema:* **Adults.** *Dexamethasone* 0.5–1 mg/kg/d IM/IV ÷ q6h (start 24 h prior to extubation; continue × 4 more doses). **Peds.** *Dexamethasone* 0.1–0.3 mg/kg/d ÷ q6h × 3–5 d (start 48–72 h before extubation)
- *Immunosuppressive/anti-inflammatory:* **Adults & Older Peds.** Hydrocortisone 15–240 mg PO, IM, IV q12h; *methylprednisolone* 4–48 mg/d PO, taper to lowest effective dose; *methylprednisolone Na succinate* 10–80 mg/d IM. **Adults.** *Prednisone* or *prednisolone* 5–60 mg/d PO ÷ daily-qid. **Infants & Younger Children.** *Hydrocortisone* 2.5–10 mg/kg/d PO ÷ q6–8h; 1–5 mg/kg/d IM/IV ÷ bid.
- *Nephrotic syndrome:* **Peds.** *Prednisolone* or *prednisone* 2 mg/kg/d PO tid-qid until urine is protein-free for 5 d, use up to 28 d; for persistent proteinuria, 4 mg/kg/dose PO q other day max 120 mg/d for an additional 28 d; maint 2 mg/kg/dose q other day for 28 d; taper over 4–6 wk (max 80 mg/d).
- *Septic shock (controversial):* **Adults.** *Hydrocortisone* 500 mg–1 g IM/IV q2–6h. **Peds.** *Hydrocortisone* 50 mg/kg IM/IV, repeat q4–24 h PRN.
- *Status asthmaticus:* **Adults & Peds.** *Hydrocortisone* 1–2 mg/kg/dose IV q6h; then ↓ by 0.5–1 mg/kg q6h.
- *Rheumatic Dz:* **Adults.** *Intraarticular:* Hydrocortisone acetate 25–37.5 mg large joint, 10–25 mg small joint; *methylprednisolone acetate* 20–80 mg large joint, 4–10 mg small joint. *Intrabursal:* Hydrocortisone acetate 25–37.5 mg. *Intraganglial:* Hydrocortisone acetate 25–37.5 mg. *Tendon sheath:* Hydrocortisone acetate 5–12.5 mg.
- *Perioperative steroid coverage:* Hydrocortisone 100 mg IV night before surgery, 1 h pre-op, intraoperative, & 4, 8, & 12 h post-op; post-op day No. 1 100 mg IV q6h; post-op day No. 2 100 mg IV q8h; post-op day No. 3 100 mg IV q12h; post-op day No. 4 50 mg IV q12h; post-op day No. 5 25 mg IV q12h; resume prior PO dosing if chronic use or D/C if only perioperative coverage required.
- *Cerebral edema:* Dexamethasone 10 mg IV; then 4 mg IV q4–6h **Caution:** [C, ?/–] **CI:** Active varicella Infxn, serious Infxn except TB, fungal Infxns **Disp:** Table 3 **SE:** ↑ Appetite, hyperglycemia, ↓ K⁺, osteoporosis, nervousness, insomnia, "steroid psychosis," adrenal suppression **Notes:** Hydrocortisone succinate for systemic, acetate for intraarticular; never abruptly D/C steroids, taper dose

Streptokinase (Streptase, Kabikinase)

Uses: *Coronary artery thrombosis, acute massive PE, DVT, & some occluded vascular grafts* **Action:** Activates plasminogen to plasmin that degrades fibrin **Dose:** *Adults.* **PE:** Load 250,000 units peripheral IV over 30 min, then 100,000 units/h IV for 24–72 h. *Coronary artery thrombosis:* 1.5 million units IV over 60 min. *DVT or arterial embolism:* Load as w/ PE, then 100,000 units/h for 72 h; 1.5 million Int Units in a 1-h Inf *(ECC 2005).* **Peds.** 3500–4000 units/kg over 30 min, then 1000–1500 units/kg/h.

Occluded catheter (controversial): 10,000–25,000 units in NS to final vol of catheter (leave in for 1 h, aspirate & flush w/ NS) **Caution:** [C, +] **CI:** Streptococcal Infxn or streptokinase in last 6 mo, active bleeding, CVA, TIA, spinal surgery/trauma in last month, vascular anomalies, severe hepatic/renal Dz, endocarditis, pericarditis, severe uncontrolled HTN **Disp:** Powder for Inj 250,000, 750,000, 1,500,000 units **SE:** Bleeding, ↓ BP, fever, bruising, rash, GI upset, hemorrhage, anaphylaxis **Notes:** If Inf inadequate to keep clotting time 2–5× control, see package for adjustments; antibodies remain 3–6 mo following dose

Streptomycin **WARNING:** Neuro-/oto-/renal tox possible; neuromuscular blockage w/ resp paralysis possible **Uses:** *TB combo therapy* streptococcal or enterococcal endocarditis **Action:** Aminoglycoside; ↓ protein synth **Dose:** *Adults.* *Endocarditis:* 1 g q12h 1–2 wk, then 500 mg q12h 1–4 wk; *TB:* 15 mg/kg/d (up to 1 g), directly observed therapy (DOT) 2× wk 20–30 mg/kg/dose (max 1.5 g), DOT 3× wk 25–30 mg/kg/dose (max 1 g). *Peds.* 15 mg/kg/d; DOT 2× wk 20–40 mg/kg/dose (max 1 g); DOT 3× wk 25–30 mg/kg/dose (max 1 g); ↓ w/ renal Insuff, either IM or IV over 30–60 min **Caution:** [D, +] **CI:** PRG **Disp:** Inj 400 mg/mL (1-g vial) **SE:** ↑ Incidence of vestibular & auditory tox, ↑ neurotx risk in pts w/ impaired renal fxn **Notes:** Monitor levels: *Peak:* 20–30 mcg/mL, *Trough:* <5 mcg/mL; *Toxic peak:* >50, *Trough:* >10; IV over 30–60 min

Streptozocin (Zanosar) **Uses:** *Pancreatic islet cell tumors* & carcinoid tumors **Action:** DNA–DNA (interstrand) cross-linking; DNA, RNA, & protein synth inhibitor **Dose:** Per protocol; ↓ in renal failure **Caution:** w/ Renal failure [D, ?/–] **CI:** w/ Rotavirus vaccine, PRG **Disp:** Inj 1 g **SE:** N/V/D, duodenal ulcers, depression, ↓ BM rare (20%) & mild; nephrotox (proteinuria & azotemia dose related), hypophosphatemia dose limiting; hypo-/hyperglycemia; Inj site Rxns **Notes:** Monitor Cr

Succimer (Chemet) **Uses:** *Lead poisoning (levels >45 mcg/mL)* **Action:** Heavy metal-chelating agent **Dose:** *Adults & Peds.* 10 mg/kg/dose q8h × 5 d, then 10 mg/kg/dose q12h for 14 d; ↓ in renal Insuff **Caution:** [C, ?] **CI:** Allergy **Disp:** Caps 100 mg **SE:** Rash, fever, GI upset, hemorrhoids, metallic taste, drowsiness, ↑ LFTs **Notes:** Monitor lead levels, maintain hydration, may open caps

Succinylcholine (Anectine, Quelicin, Sucostrin, others) **WARNING:** Risk of cardiac arrest from hyperkalemic rhabdomyolysis **Uses:** *Adjunct to general anesthesia, facilitates ET intubation; induce skeletal muscle relaxation during surgery or mechanical ventilation* **Action:** Depolarizing neuromuscular blocker; rapid onset, short duration (3–5 min) **Dose:** *Adults.* Rapid sequence intubation 1–2 mg/kg IV over 10–30 s or 2–4 mg/kg IM (*ECC 2005*). *Peds.* 1–2 mg/kg/dose IV, then by 0.3–0.6 mg/kg q5min; ↓ w/ severe renal/hepatic impair **Caution:** See warning [C, M] **CI:** w/ Malignant hyperthermia risk, myopathy, recent major burn, multiple trauma, extensive skeletal muscle denervation, NAG, pseudocholinesterase deficiency **Disp:** Inj 20, 50, 100 mg/mL

SE: Fasciculations, ↑ intraocular, intragastric, & intracranial pressure, salivation, myoglobinuria, malignant hyperthermia, resp depression, or prolonged apnea; multiple drugs potentiate; CV effects (arrhythmias, ↓ BP, brady/tachycardia) **Notes:** May be given IV push/Inf/IM deltoid; hyperkalemic rhabdomyolysis in children with undiagnosed myopathy such as Duchenne muscular dystrophy

Sucralfate (Carafate)
Uses: *Duodenal ulcers,* gastric ulcers, stomatitis, GERD, preventing stress ulcers, esophagitis **Action:** Forms ulcer-adherent complex that protects against acid, pepsin, & bile acid **Dose:** *Adults.* 1 g PO qid, 1 h prior to meals & hs. *Peds.* 40–80 mg/kg/d ÷ q6h; continue 4–8 wk unless healing demonstrated by x-ray or endoscopy; separate from other drugs by 2 h; take on empty stomach ac **Caution:** [B, +] **CI:** Component allergy **Disp:** Tabs 1 g; susp 1 g/10 mL **SE:** Constipation, D, dizziness, xerostomia **Notes:** Al may accumulate in renal failure

Sulfacetamide (Bleph-10, Cetamide, Sodium Sulamyd)
Uses: *Conjunctival Infxns* **Action:** Sulfonamide antibiotic **Dose:** 10% oint apply qid & hs; soln for keratitis apply q2–3h based on severity **Caution:** [C, M] **CI:** Sulfonamide sensitivity; age <2 mo **Disp:** Oint 10%; soln 10, 15, 30%; topical cream 10%; foam, gel, lotion, pad all 10% **SE:** Irritation, burning, blurred vision, brow ache, Stevens-Johnson syndrome, photosensitivity

Sulfacetamide & Prednisolone (Blephamide, others)
Uses: *Steroid-responsive inflammatory ocular conditions w/ Infxn or a risk of Infxn* **Action:** Antibiotic & anti-inflammatory **Dose:** *Adults & Peds >2 y:* Apply oint lower conjunctival sac daily-qid; soln 1–3 gtt 2–3 h while awake **Caution:** [C, ?/–] Sulfonamide sensitivity; age <2 mo **Disp:** *Oint:* sulfacetamide 10%/prednisolone 0.5%, sulfacetamide 10%/prednisolone 0.2%, sulfacetamide 10%/prednisolone 0.25%. *Susp:* sulfacetamide 10%/prednisolone 0.25%, sulfacetamide 10%/prednisolone 0.5%, sulfacetamide 10%/prednisolone 0.2% **SE:** Irritation, burning, blurred vision, brow ache, Stevens-Johnson syndrome, photosensitivity **Notes:** OK ophthal susp use as otic agent

Sulfasalazine (Azulfidine, Azulfidine EN)
Uses: *Ulcerative colitis, RA, juvenile RA,* active Crohn Dz, ankylosing spondylitis, psoriasis **Action:** Sulfonamide; actions unclear **Dose:** *Adults. Ulcerative colitis:* Initial, 1 g PO tid-qid; ↑ to a max of 8 g/d in 3–4 ÷ doses; maint 500 mg PO qid. *RA:* (EC tab) 0.5–1 g/d, ↑ weekly to maint 2 g/ ÷ bid. *Peds. Ulcerative colitis:* Initial: 40–60 mg/kg/24 h PO ÷ q4–6h; maint: 20–30 mg/kg/24 h PO ÷ q6h. *RA >6 y:* 30–50 mg/kg/d in 2 doses, start w/ 1/4–1/3 maint dose, ↑ weekly until dose reached at 1 mo, 2 g/d max; ↓ w/ renal Insuff **Caution:** [B (D if near term), M] **CI:** Sulfonamide or salicylate sensitivity, porphyria, GI or GU obst; avoid in hepatic impair **Disp:** Tabs 500 mg; EC DR tabs 500 mg **SE:** GI upset; discolors urine; dizziness, HA, photosensitivity, oligospermia, anemias, Stevens-Johnson syndrome **Notes:** May cause yellow-orange skin/contact lens discoloration; avoid sunlight exposure

Sulfinpyrazone   Uses: *Acute & chronic gout* Action: ↓ Renal tubular absorption of uric acid Dose: 100–200 mg PO bid for 1 wk, ↑ PRN to maint of 200–400 mg bid; max 800 mg/d; take w/ food or antacids, & plenty of fluids; avoid salicylates Caution: [C (D if near term), ?/–] CI: Renal impair, avoid salicylates; peptic ulcer; blood dyscrasias, near term PRG, allergy Disp: Tabs 100 mg; caps 200 mg SE: N/V, stomach pain, urolithiasis, leukopenia Notes: Take w/ plenty of H_2O

Sulindac (Clinoril)   WARNING: May ↑ risk of cardiovascular events & GI bleeding Uses: *Arthritis & pain* Action: NSAID; ↓ prostaglandins Dose: 150–200 mg bid, 400 mg max; w/ food Caution: [B (D if 3rd tri or near term), ?] CI: NSAID or ASA sensitivity, w/ ketorolac, ulcer, GI bleeding, post-op pain in coronary artery bypass graft Disp: Tabs 150, 200 mg SE: Dizziness, rash, GI upset, pruritus, edema, ↓ renal blood flow, renal failure (? fewer renal effects than other NSAIDs), peptic ulcer, GI bleeding

Sumatriptan (Imitrex)   Uses: *Rx acute migraine* Action: Vascular serotonin receptor agonist Dose: Adults. SQ: 6 mg SQ as a single-dose PRN; repeat PRN in 1 h to a max of 12 mg/24 h. PO: 25 mg, repeat in 2 h, PRN, 100 mg/d max PO dose; max 300 mg/d. Nasal spray: 1 spray into 1 nostril, repeat in 2 h to 40 mg/24 h max. Peds. Nasal spray: 6–9 y: 5–20 mg/d. 12–17 y: 5–20 mg, up to 40 mg/d Caution: [C, M] CI: Angina, ischemic heart Dz, uncontrolled HTN, severe hepatic impair, ergot use, MAOI use w/in 14 d Disp: OD tabs 25, 50, 100 mg; Inj 6, 8, 12 mg/mL; OD tabs 25, 50, 100 mg, orally disintegrating tabs 25, 50, 100 mg; nasal spray 5, 10, 20 mg/spray SE: Pain & bruising at site; dizziness, hot flashes, paresthesias, CP, weakness, numbness, coronary vasospasm, HTN

Sumatriptan & Naproxen Sodium (Treximet)   WARNING: ↑ Risk of serious CV (MI, stroke) serious GI events (bleeding, ulceration, perforation) of the stomach or intestines Uses: *Prevent migraines* Action: Anti-inflammatory NSAID w/ 5-HT₁ receptor agonist, constricts CNS vessels Dose: Adults. 1 tab PO; repeat PRN after 2 h; max 2 tabs/24 h, w/ or w/o food Caution: [C, –] CI: Significant CV Dz, severe hepatic impair, severe ↑ BP Disp: Tab naproxen/sumatriptan 500/85mg SE: Dizziness, somnolence, paresthesia, N, dyspepsia, dry mouth, chest/neck/throat/jaw pain, tightness, pressure Notes: Do not split/crush/chew

Sunitinib (Sutent)   Uses: *Advanced GI stromal tumor (GIST) refractory/intolerant of imatinib; advanced RCC* Action: Multi-TKI Dose: Adults. 50 mg PO daily × 4 wk, followed by 2 wk holiday = 1 cycle; ↓ to 37.5 mg w/ CYP3A4 inhibitors (Table 11), to ↑ 87.5 mg w/ CYP3A4 inducers CI: w/ Atazanavir Caution: [D, –] Multiple interactions require dose modification (eg, St. John's wort) Disp: Caps 12.5, 25, 50 mg SE: ↓ WBC & plt, bleeding, ↑ BP, ↓ ejection fraction, ↑ QT interval, pancreatitis, DVT, Szs, adrenal insufficiency, N/V/D, skin discoloration, oral ulcers, taste perversion, hypothyroidism Notes: Monitor left ventricular ejection fraction, ECG, CBC/plts, chemistries (K⁺/Mg²⁺/phosphate), TFT & LFTs periodically; ↓ dose in 12.5-mg increments if not tolerated

Tacrine (Cognex)   Uses: *Mild–mod Alzheimer dementia* Action: Cholinesterase inhibitor Dose: 10–40 mg PO qid to 160 mg/d; separate doses from food Caution: [C, ?] CI: Previous tacrine-induced jaundice Disp: Caps 10, 20, 30, 40 mg SE: ↑ LFTs, HA, dizziness, GI upset, flushing, confusion, ataxia, myalgia, bradycardia Notes: Serum conc >20 ng/mL have more SE; monitor LFTs

Tacrolimus [FK506] (Prograf, Protopic)   WARNING: ↑ Risk of Infxn and lymphoma Uses: *Prevent organ rejection,* eczema Action: Macrolide immunosuppressant Dose: *Adults. IV:* 0.05–0.1 mg/kg/d cont Inf. *PO:* 0.1–0.2 mg/kg/d ÷ 2 doses. *Peds. IV:* 0.03–0.05 mg/kg/d as cont Inf. *PO:* 0.15–0.2 mg/kg/d PO ÷ q 12 h. *Adults & Peds. Eczema:* Apply bid, continue 1 wk after clearing; take on empty stomach; ↓ w/ hepatic/renal impair Caution: [C, –] w/ Cyclosporine; avoid topical if <2 y of age CI: Component allergy, castor oil allergy w/ IV form Disp: Caps 0.5, 1, 5 mg; Inj 5 mg/mL; oint 0.03, 0.1% SE: Neuro- & nephrotox, HTN, edema, HA, insomnia, fever, pruritus, ↓/↑ K⁺, hyperglycemia, GI upset, anemia, leukocytosis, tremors, paresthesias, pleural effusion, Szs, lymphoma Notes: Monitor levels; *Trough* 5–20 ng/mL based on indication and time since transplant; reports of ↑ cancer risk; topical use for short-term/second-line

Tadalafil (Cialis)   Uses: *Erectile dysfunction* Action: PDE5 inhibitor, ↑ cyclic guanosine monophosphate & NO levels; relaxes smooth muscles, dilates cavernosal arteries Dose: *Adults. PRN:* 10 mg PO before sexual activity (5–20 mg max) 1 dose/72 h. *Daily dosing:* 2.5 mg q day w/o regard to timing of sex, may ↑ to 5 mg q day; w/o regard to meals; ↓ w/ renal/hepatic Insuff Caution: [B, –] w/ α-Blockers (except tamsulosin); use w/ CYP3A4 inhibitor (Table 11)(eg, ritonavir, ketoconazole, itraconazole) 2.5 mg/daily dose or 5 mg PRN dose; CrCl <30 mL/min/hemodialysis/severe hepatic impair do not use daily dosing CI: Nitrates, severe hepatic impair Disp: Tabs 5-, 10-, 20-mg SE: HA, flushing, dyspepsia, back/limb pain, myalgia, nasal congestion, urticaria, Stevens-Johnson syndrome, dermatitis, visual field defect, NIAON, sudden ↓/loss of hearing, tinnitus Notes: Longest acting of class (36 h); daily dosing may ↑ drug interactions; excessive EtOH may ↑ orthostasis; transient global amnesia reports

Talc (Sterile Talc Powder)   Uses: *↓ Recurrence of malignant pleural effusions (pleurodesis)* Action: Sclerosing agent Dose: Mix slurry: 50 mL NS w/ 5-g vial, mix, distribute 25 mL into two 60-mL syringes, vol to 50 mL/syringe w/ NS. Infuse each into chest tube, flush w/ 25 mL NS. Keep tube clamped; have pt change positions q15min for 2 h, unclamp tube Caution: [X, –] CI: Planned further surgery on site Disp: 5 g powder SE: Pain, Infxn Notes: May add 10–20 mL 1% lidocaine/syringe; must have chest tube placed, monitor closely while tube clamped (tension pneumothorax), not antineoplastic

Tamoxifen (generic)   WARNING: Cancer of the uterus, stroke, and blood clots can occur Uses: *Breast CA [postmenopausal, estrogen receptor(+)], ↓ risk of breast CA in high-risk, met male breast CA,* ductal carcinoma in situ, mastalgia, pancreatic CA, gynecomastia, ovulation induction Action: Nonsteroidal antiestrogen; mixed agonist–antagonist effect **Dose:** 20–40 mg/d; doses >20 mg ÷ bid. *Prevention:* 20 mg PO/d × 5 y **Caution:** [D, –] w/ ↓ WBC, ↓ plts, hyperlipidemia **CI:** PRG, undiagnosed Vag bleeding, Hx thromboembolism **Disp:** Tabs 10, 20 mg; oral soln 10 mg/5 mL **SE:** Uterine malignancy & thrombotic events noted in breast CA prevention trials; menopausal Sxs (hot flashes, N/V) in premenopausal pts; Vag bleeding & menstrual irregularities; skin rash, pruritus vulvae, dizziness, HA, peripheral edema; acute flare of bone metastasis pain & ↑ Ca²⁺; retinopathy reported (high dose) **Notes:** ↑ Risk of PRG in premenopausal women (induces ovulation); brand Nolvadex suspended in US

Tamsulosin (Flomax)
Uses: *BPH* **Action:** Antagonist of prostatic α-receptors **Dose:** 0.4 mg/d, may ↑ to 0.8 mg PO daily **Caution:** [B, ?] **CI:** Female gender **Disp:** Caps 0.4 mg **SE:** HA, dizziness, syncope, somnolence, ↓ libido, GI upset, retrograde ejaculation, rhinitis, rash, angioedema, IFIS **Notes:** Not for use as antihypertensive; do not open/crush/chew; approved for use w/ dutasteride for BPH

Tazarotene (Tazorac, Avage)
Uses: *Facial acne vulgaris; stable plaque psoriasis up to 20% BSA* **Action:** Keratolytic **Dose:** *Adults & Peds >12 y: Acne:* Cleanse face, dry, apply thin film qhs lesions. *Psoriasis:* Apply qhs **Caution:** [X, ?/–] **CI:** Retinoid sensitivity **Disp:** Gel 0.05, 0.1%; cream 0.05, 0.1% **SE:** Burning, erythema, irritation, rash, photosensitivity, desquamation, bleeding, skin discoloration **Notes:** D/C w/ excessive pruritus, burning, skin redness, or peeling until Sxs resolve

Telbivudine (Tyzeka)
WARNING: May cause lactic acidosis and severe hepatomegaly w/ steatosis when used alone or with antiretrovirals; D/C of the drug may lead to exacerbations of hep B; monitor LFTs **Uses:** *Rx chronic hep B* **Action:** Nucleoside RT inhibitor **Dose:** *CrCl >50 mL/min:* 600 mg PO daily; *CrCl 30–49 mL/min:* 600 mg q 48 h; *CrCl <30 mL/min:* 600 mg q 72 h; *ESRD:* 600 mg q96h; dose after hemodialysis **Caution:** [B; ?/–]; may cause myopathy; follow closely w/ other myopathy causing drugs **Disp:** Tabs 600 mg **SE:** Fatigue, Abd pain, N/V/D, HA, URI, nasopharyngitis, ↑ LFTs/creatine phosphokinase, myalgia/myopathy, flu-like Sxs, dizziness, insomnia, dyspepsia **Notes:** Use w/ PEG-interferon may ↑ peripheral neuropathy risk

Telithromycin (Ketek)
WARNING: CI in myasthenia gravis **Uses:** *Mild–mod CAP* **Action:** Unique macrolide, blocks ↓ protein synth; bactericidal. *Spectrum:* S. aureus, S. pneumoniae, H. influenzae, M. catarrhalis, C. pneumoniae, M. pneumoniae **Dose:** *CAP:* 800 mg (2 tabs) PO daily × 7–10 d **Caution:** [C, M] Pseudomembranous colitis, ↑ QTc interval, visual disturbances, hepatic dysfunction; dosing in renal impair unknown **CI:** Macrolide allergy, w/ pimozide; w/ MyG **Disp:** Tabs 300, 400 mg **SE:** N/V/D, dizziness, blurred vision **Notes:** A CYP450 inhibitor; multiple drug interactions; hold statins due to ↑ risk of myopathy

Telmisartan (Micardis)
Uses: *HTN, CHF* **Action:** Angiotensin II receptor antagonist **Dose:** 40–80 mg/d **Caution:** [C (1st tri; D 2nd & 3rd tri), ?/–]

CI: Angiotensin II receptor antagonist sensitivity **Disp:** Tabs 20, 40, 80 mg **SE:** Edema, GI upset, HA, angioedema, renal impair, orthostatic ↓ BP

Temazepam (Restoril) [C-IV] **Uses:** *Insomnia,* anxiety, depression, panic attacks **Action:** Benzodiazepine **Dose:** 15–30 mg PO hs PRN; ↓ in elderly **Caution:** [X, ?/–] Potentiates CNS depressive effects of opioids, barbs, EtOH, antihistamines, MAOIs, TCAs **CI:** NAG **Disp:** Caps 7.5, 15, 22.5, 30 mg **SE:** Confusion, dizziness, drowsiness, hangover **Notes:** Abrupt D/C after >10 d use may cause withdrawal

Temsirolimus (Torisel) **Uses:** *Advanced RCC* **Action:** Multikinase inhibitor, ↓ mTOR (mammalian target of rapamycin), ↓ hypoxic-induced factors, ↓ VEGF **Dose:** 25 mg IV 30–60 min 1×/wk. Hold w/ ANC <1000/mm³, plt <75,000/mm³, or National Cancer Institute (NCI) grade 3 tox. Resume when tox grade 2 or less, restart w/ dose ↓ 5 mg/wk not <15 mg/wk. w/ CYP3A4 Inhibitors: ↓ 12.5 mg/wk. w/ CYP3A4 Inducers ↑ 50 mg/wk **Caution:** [D, –] Avoid live vaccines, ↓ wound healing, avoid perioperatively **CI:** None **Disp:** Inj 25 mg/mL w/ 250 mL diluent **SE:** Rash, asthenia, mucositis, N, bowel perforation, anorexia, edema, ↑ lipids, ↑ glucose, ↑ triglycerides, ↑ LFTs, ↑ Cr, ↓ WBC, ↓ HCT, ↓ plt, ↓ PO₄ **Notes:** Premedicate w/ antihistamine; ✓ lipids, CBC, plt, Cr, glucose; w/ sunitinib dose-limiting tox likely; females use w/ contraception

Tenecteplase (TNKase) **Uses:** *Restore perfusion & ↓ mortality w/ AMI* **Action:** Thrombolytic; TPA **Dose:** 30–50 mg; see table below **Caution:** [C, ?], ↑ Bleeding w/ NSAIDs, ticlopidine, clopidogrel, GPIIb/IIIa antagonists **CI:** Bleeding, CVA, CNS neoplasm, uncontrolled ↑ BP, major surgery (intracranial, intraspinal) or trauma w/in 2 mo **Disp:** Inj 50 mg, reconstitute w/ 10 mL sterile H₂O only **SE:** Bleeding, allergy **Notes:** Do not shake w/ reconstitution; start ASA ASAP, IV heparin ASAP w/ aPTT 50–70 s

Tenecteplase Dosing

Weight (kg)	TNKase (mg)	TNKaseᵃ Volume (mL)
<60	30	6
60–69	35	7
70–79	40	8
80–89	45	9
≥90	50	10

ᵃFrom one vial of reconstituted TNKase.
Based on data in Haist SA and Robbins JB: *Internal Medicine on Call*, 4th ed, 2005 McGraw-Hill). See also www.fda.gov.

Tenofovir (Viread) WARNING: Lactic acidosis & severe hepatomegaly with steatosis, including fatal cases, have been reported with the use of nucleoside analogs alone or in combo w/ other antiretrovirals. Not OK w/ chronic hep; effects in pts coinfected with hep B & HIV unknown Uses: *HIV Infxn* Action: Nucleotide RT inhibitor Dose: 300 mg PO daily Δ to w/ or w/o meal; CrCl Δ ≥50 mL/min Δ q24h, CrCl 30–49 mL/min q48H, CrCl 10–29 mL/min 2×/wk Caution: [B, ?/–] Didanosine (separate administration times), lopinavir, ritonavir w/ known risk factors for liver Dz CI: Hypersensitivity Disp: Tabs 300 mg SE: GI upset, metabolic syndrome, hepatotox; separate didanosine doses by 2 h Notes: Combo product w/ emtricitabine is Truvada

Tenofovir/Emtricitabine (Truvada) WARNING: Lactic acidosis & severe hepatomegaly with steatosis, including fatal cases, have been reported with the use of nucleoside analogs alone or in combo w/ other antiretrovirals. Not OK w/ chronic hep; effects in pts coinfected with hep B & HIV unknown Uses: *HIV Infxn* Action: Dual nucleotide RT inhibitor Dose: 300 mg PO daily w/ or w/o a meal; adjust w/ renal impair Caution: [B, ?/–] w/ Known risk factors for liver Dz CI: CrCl <30 mL/min; Disp: Tabs 200 mg emtricitabine/300 mg tenofovir SE: GI upset, rash, metabolic syndrome, hepatotox

Terazosin (Hytrin) Uses: *BPH & HTN* Action: α₁-Blocker (blood vessel & bladder neck/prostate) Dose: Initial, 1 mg PO hs; ↑ 20 mg/d max; may ↓ w/ diuretic or other BP medicine Caution: [C, ?] w/ β Blocker, CCB, ACE inhibitor CI: α-Antagonist sensitivity Disp: Tabs 1, 2, 5, 10 mg; caps 1, 2, 5, 10 mg SE: ↓ BP, & syncope following 1st dose; dizziness, weakness, nasal congestion, peripheral edema, palpitations, GI upset Notes: Caution w/ 1st dose syncope; if for HTN, combine w/ thiazide diuretic

Terbinafine (Lamisil, Lamisil AT) Uses: *Onychomycosis, athlete's foot, jock itch, ringworm,* cutaneous candidiasis, pityriasis versicolor Action: ↓ Squalene epoxidase resulting in fungal death Dose: *PO:* 250 mg/d PO for 6–12 wk. *Topical:* Apply to area *tinea pedis* bid, *tinea cruris & corporus* q day-bid, *tinea versicolor* soln bid; ↓ PO in renal/hepatic impair Caution: [B, –] PO ↑ effects of drug metabolism by CYP2D6, w/ liver/renal impair CI: CrCl <50 mL/min, WBC <1000, severe liver Dz Disp: Tabs 250 mg; *Lamisil AT* [OTC] cream, gel, soln 1% SE: HA, dizziness, rash, pruritus, alopecia, GI upset, taste perversion, neutropenia, retinal damage, Stevens–Johnson syndrome, ↑ LFTs Notes: Effect may take months due to needed for new nail growth; topical not for nails; do not use occlusive dressings; PO follow CBC/LFTs

Terbutaline (Brethine) Uses: *Reversible bronchospasm (asthma, COPD); inhibit labor* Action: Sympathomimetic; tocolytic Dose: *Adults. Bronchodilator:* 2.5–5 mg PO qid or 0.25 mg SQ; repeat in 15 min PRN; max 0.5 mg in 4 h. *Metered-dose inhaler:* 2 Inh q4–6h. *Premature labor:* Acutely 2.5–10 mg/min/IV, gradually ↑ as tolerated q10–20min; maint 2.5–5 mg PO q4–6h until term. *Peds. PO:* 0.05–0.15 mg/kg/dose PO tid; max 5 mg/24h; ↓ in renal failure Caution:

[B, +] ↑ Tox w/ MAOIs, TCAs; DM, HTN, hyperthyroidism, CV Dz, DM, convulsive disorders, ↓ K⁺ **CI:** Component allergy **Disp:** Tabs 2.5, 5 mg; Inj 1 mg/mL; metered-dose inhaler **SE:** HTN, hyperthyroidism, β₁-adrenergic effects w/ high dose, nervousness, trembling, tachycardia, HTN, dizziness

Terconazole (Terazol 7)
Uses: *Vag fungal Infxns* **Action:** Topical triazole antifungal **Dose:** 1 applicator-full or 1 supp intravag hs × 3–7 d **Caution:** [C, ?] **CI:** Component allergy **Disp:** Vag cream 0.4, 0.8%, Vag supp 80 mg **SE:** Vulvar/Vag burning **Notes:** Insert high into vagina

Teriparatide (Forteo)
WARNING: ↑ Osteosarcoma risk in animals, therefore only use in pts for whom the potential benefits outweigh risks **Uses:** *Severe/refractory osteoporosis* **Action:** PTH (recombinant) **Dose:** 20 mcg SQ daily in thigh or abdomen **Caution:** [C, ?/–] **CI:** w/ Paget Dz, prior radiation, bone metastases, ↑ Ca²⁺; caution in urolithiasis **Disp:** 3-mL Prefilled device (discard after 28 d) **SE:** Orthostatic ↓ BP on administration, N/D, ↑ Ca²⁺; leg cramps **Notes:** 2 y Max use; osteosarcoma in animals

Testosterone (AndroGel, Androderm, Striant, Testim) [CIII]
Uses: *Male hypogonadism* **Action:** Testosterone replacement; ↑ lean body mass, libido **Dose:** All daily AndroGel: 5-g gel. Androderm: Two 2.5-mg or one 5-mg patch daily. Striant: 30-mg Buccal tabs bid. Testim: One 5-g gel tube. **Caution:** [N/A, N/A] **CI:** PCa, male breast CA **Disp:** AndroGel, Testim: 5-g gel (50-mg test); Androderm: 2.5-, 5-mg patches; Striant: 30-mg Buccal tabs **SE:** Site Rxns, acne, edema, wgt gain, gynecomastia, HTN, ↑ sleep apnea, prostate enlargement **Notes:** IM testosterone enanthate (Delatestryl; Testro-L.A.) & cypionate (Depo-Testosterone) dose q14–28d with highly variable serum levels; PO agents (methyl-testosterone & oxandrolone) associated w/ hep/hepatic tumors; transdermal/mucosal forms preferred

Tetanus Immune Globulin
Uses: *Passive tetanus immunization* (suspected contaminated wound w/ unknown immunization status, see also Table 8) **Action:** Passive immunization **Dose:** Adults & Peds. 250–500 units IM (higher dose w/ delayed Rx) **Caution:** [C, ?] **CI:** Thimerosal sensitivity **Disp:** Inj 250-unit vial/syringe **SE:** Pain, tenderness, erythema at site; fever, angioedema, muscle stiffness, anaphylaxis **Notes:** May begin active immunization series at different Inj site if required

Tetanus Toxoid
Uses: *Tetanus prophylaxis* **Action:** Active immunization **Dose:** Based on previous immunization, Table 8 **Caution:** [C, ?] **CI:** Chloramphenicol use, neurologic Sxs w/ previous use, active Infxn w/ routine primary immunization **Disp:** Inj tetanus toxoid, fluid, 4–5 Lf units/0.5 mL; tetanus toxoid, adsorbed, 5, 10 Lf units/0.5 mL **SE:** Local erythema, induration, sterile abscess, chills, fever, neurologic disturbances

Tetracycline (Achromycin V, Sumycin)
Uses: *Broad-spectrum antibiotic* **Action:** Bacteriostatic; ↓ protein synth. Spectrum: Gram(+): Staphylococcus, Streptococcus. Gram(–): H. pylori. Atypicals: Chlamydia, Rickettsia, &

Mycoplasma **Dose:** *Adults.* 250–500 mg PO bid-qid. *Peds >8 y:* 25–50 mg/kg/24 h
PO q6–12h; ↓ w/ renal/hepatic impair, w/o food preferred **Caution:** [D, +] **CI:**
PRG, antacids, w/ dairy products, children <8 y **Disp:** Caps 100, 250, 500 mg; tabs
250, 500 mg; PO susp 250 mg/5 mL **SE:** Photosensitivity, GI upset, renal failure,
pseudotumor cerebri, hepatic impair **Notes:** Can stain tooth enamel & depress
bone formation in children

Thalidomide (Thalomid)   WARNING: Restricted use; use associated w/
severe birth defects and ↑ risk of venous thromboembolism **Uses:** *Erythema
nodosum leprosum (ENL),* *GVHD;* aphthous ulceration in HIV(+) **Action:** ↓ Neutrophil chemotaxis, ↓ monocyte phagocytosis **Dose:** *GVHD:* 100–1600 mg PO
daily. *Stomatitis:* 200 mg bid for 5 d, then 200 mg daily up to 8 wk. *Erythema
nodosum leprosum:* 100–300 mg PO qhs **Cautions:** [X, –] May ↑ HIV viral load;
Hx Szs **CI:** PRG; sexually active males not using latex condoms, or females not
using 2 forms of contraception **Disp:** 50, 100, 200 mg caps **SE:** Dizziness, drowsiness, rash, fever, orthostasis, Stevens-Johnson syndrome, peripheral neuropathy,
Szs **Notes:** MD must register per STEPS risk-management program; informed consent necessary; immediately D/C if rash develops

Theophylline (Theo24, Theochron)   **Uses:** *Asthma, bronchospasm*
Action: Relaxes smooth muscle of the bronchi & pulm blood vessels **Dose:** *Adults.*
900 mg PO ÷ q6h; SR products may be ÷ q8–12h (maint). *Peds.* 16–22 mg/kg/24 h
PO ÷ q6h; SR products may be ÷ q8–12h (maint); ↓ in hepatic failure **Caution:**
[C, +] Multiple interactions (eg, caffeine, smoking, carbamazepine, barbiturates,
β-blockers, ciprofloxacin, E-mycin, INH, loop diuretics) **CI:** Arrhythmia, hyperthyroidism, uncontrolled Szs **Disp:** Elixir 80, 15 mL; soln 80 mg/15 mL; syrup 80,
150 mg/15 mL; caps 100, 200, 250 mg; tabs 100, 125, 200, 250, 300 mg; SR caps
100, 125, 200, 250, 260, 300 mg; SR tabs 100, 200, 300, 400, 450, 600 mg **SE:**
N/V, tachycardia, Szs, nervousness, arrhythmias **Notes:** Levels IV: Sample 12–24 h
after Inf started; *Therapeutic:* 5–15 mcg/mL; *Toxic:* >20 mcg/mL. Levels PO:
Trough; just before next dose; *Therapeutic:* 5–15 mcg/mL

Thiamine [Vitamin B1]   **Uses:** *Thiamine deficiency (beriberi),* alcoholic neuritis, Wernicke encephalopathy* **Action:** Dietary suppl **Dose:** *Adults.*
Deficiency: 100 mg/d IM for 2 wk, then 5–10 mg/d PO for 1 mo. *Wernicke
encephalopathy:* 100 mg IV single dose, then 100 mg/d IM for 2 wk. *Peds.* 10–25
mg/d IM for 2 wk, then 5–10 mg/d/24 h PO for 1 mo **Caution:** [A (C if doses exceed
RDA), +] **CI:** Component allergy **Disp:** Tabs 5, 10, 25, 50, 100, 250, 500 mg; Inj
100, 200 mg/mL **SE:** Angioedema, paresthesias, rash, anaphylaxis w/ rapid IV
Notes: IV use associated w/ anaphylactic Rxn; give IV slowly

Thiethylperazine (Torecan)   **Uses:** *N/V* **Action:** Antidopaminergic
antiemetic **Dose:** 10 mg PO, PR, or IM daily-tid; ↓ in hepatic failure **Caution:** [X,
?] **CI:** Phenothiazine & sulfite sensitivity, PRG **Disp:** Tabs 10 mg; supp 10 mg; Inj
5 mg/mL **SE:** EPS, xerostomia, drowsiness, orthostatic ↓ BP, tachycardia,
confusion

6-Thioguanine [6-TG] (Tabloid) Uses: *AML, ALL, CML* Action: Purine-based antimetabolite (substitutes for natural purines interfering w/ nucleotide synth) Dose: 2–3 mg/kg/d; ↓ in severe renal/hepatic impair Caution: [D, –] CI: Resistance to mercaptopurine Disp: Tabs 40 mg SE: ↓ BM (leucopenia/ thrombocytopenia), N/V/D, anorexia, stomatitis, rash, hyperuricemia, rare hepatotox

Thioridazine (Mellaril) WARNING: Dose-related QT prolongation Uses: *Schizophrenia,* psychosis Action: Phenothiazine antipsychotic Dose: Adults. Initial, 50–100 mg PO tid; maint 200–800 mg/24 h PO in 2–4 ÷ doses. Peds >2 y: 0.5–3 mg/kg/24 h PO in 2–3 ÷ doses Caution: [C, ?] Phenothiazines, QTc-prolonging agents, AI CI: Phenothiazine sensitivity Disp: Tabs 10, 15, 25, 50, 100, 150, 200 mg; PO conc 30, 100 mg/mL SE: Low incidence of EPS; ventricular arrhythmias; ↓ BP, dizziness, drowsiness, neuroleptic malignant syndrome, Szs, skin discoloration, photosensitivity, constipation, sexual dysfunction, blood dyscrasias, pigmentary retinopathy, hepatic impair Notes: Avoid EtOH, dilute PO conc in 2–4 oz liq

Thiothixene (Navane) WARNING: Not for dementia-related psychosis; increased mortality risk in elderly on antipsychotics Uses: *Psychosis* Action: ?; antagonizes dopamine receptors Dose: Adults & Peds >12 y: Mild–mod psychosis: 2 mg PO tid, up to 20–30 mg/d. Severe psychosis: 5 mg PO bid; ↑ to max of 60 mg/24 h PRN. IM use: 16–20 mg/24 h ÷ bid-qid; max 30 mg/d. Peds <12 y: 0.25 mg/kg/24 h PO ÷ q6–12h Caution: [C, ?] Avoid w/ ↑ QT interval or meds that can ↑ QT CI: Phenothiazine sensitivity Disp: Caps 1, 2, 5, 10, 20 mg; PO conc 5 mg/mL; Inj 10 mg/mL SE: Drowsiness, EPS most common; ↓ BP, dizziness, drowsiness, neuroleptic malignant syndrome, Szs, skin discoloration, photosensitivity, constipation, sexual dysfunction, blood dyscrasias, pigmentary retinopathy, hepatic impair Notes: Dilute PO conc immediately before use

Tiagabine (Gabitril) Uses: *Adjunct in partial Szs,* bipolar disorder Action: Antiepileptic, enhances activity of GABA Dose: Adults & Peds ≥12 y: Initial 4 mg/d PO, ↑ by 4 mg during 2nd wk; ↑ PRN by 4–8 mg/d based on response, 56 mg/d max; take w/ food Caution: [C, M] May ↑ suicidal risk CI: Component allergy Disp: Tabs 2, 4, 12, 16, 20 mg SE: Dizziness, HA, somnolence, memory impair, tremors Notes: Use gradual withdrawal; used in combo w/ other anticonvulsants

Ticarcillin/Potassium Clavulanate (Timentin) Uses: *Infxns of the skin, bone, resp & urinary tract, abdomen, sepsis* Action: Carboxy-PCN; bactericidal; ↓ cell wall synth; clavulanic acid blocks β-lactamase. Spectrum: Good gram(+), not MRSA; good gram(–) & anaerobes Dose: Adults. 3.1 g IV q4–6h max 24 g ticarcillin component/d. Peds. 200–300 mg/kg/d IV ÷ q4–6h; ↓ in renal failure Caution: [B, +/–] PCN sensitivity Disp: Inj ticarcillin/clavulanate acid 3.1 g/0.1 g vial SE: Hemolytic anemia, false + proteinuria Notes: Often used in combo w/ aminoglycosides; penetrates CNS with meningeal irritation

Ticlopidine (Ticlid) **WARNING:** Neutropenia/agranulocytosis, TTP, aplastic anemia reported **Uses:** *↓ Risk of thrombotic stroke,* protect grafts status post-coronary artery bypass graft, diabetic microangiopathy, ischemic heart Dz, DVT prophylaxis, graft prophylaxis after renal transplant **Action:** Plt aggregation inhibitor **Dose:** 250 mg PO bid w/ food **Caution:** [B, ?/–], ↑ tox of ASA, anticoagulation, NSAIDs, theophylline **CI:** Bleeding, hepatic impair, neutropenia, thrombocytopenia **Disp:** Tabs 250 mg **SE:** Bleeding, GI upset, rash, ↑ on LFTs **Notes:** Follow CBC 1st 3 mo

Tigecycline (Tygacil) **Uses:** *Rx complicated skin & soft-tissue Infxns & complicated intra-Abd Infxns* **Action:** New class: related to tetracycline; *Spectrum:* Broad gram(+), gram(–), anaerobic, some mycobacterial; *E. coli, E. faecalis* (vancomycin-susceptible isolates), *S. aureus* (methicillin-susceptible/resistant), *Streptococcus* (*agalactiae, anginosus* grp, *pyogenes*), *Citrobacter freundii, Enterobacter cloacae, B. fragilis* group, *C. perfringens, Peptostreptococcus* **Dose:** *Adults.* 100 mg, then 50 mg q12h IV over 30–60 min q12h **Caution:** [D, ?] Hepatic impair, monotherapy w/ intestinal perforation, not OK in peds; w/ tetracycline allergy **CI:** Component sensitivity **Disp:** Inj 50 mg vial **SE:** N/V, Inj site Rxn

Timolol (Blocadren) **WARNING:** Exacerbation of ischemic heart Dz w/ abrupt D/C **Uses:** *HTN & MI* **Action:** β-Adrenergic receptor blocker, β₁, β₂ **Dose:** *HTN:* 10–20 mg bid, up to 60 mg/d. *MI:* 10 mg bid **Caution:** [C (1st tri; D 2nd or 3rd tri), +] **CI:** CHF, cardiogenic shock, bradycardia, heart block, COPD, asthma **Disp:** Tabs 5, 10, 20 mg **SE:** Sexual dysfunction, arrhythmia, dizziness, fatigue, CHF

Timolol, ophthalmic (Timoptic) **Uses:** *Glaucoma* **Action:** β-Blocker **Dose:** 0.25% 1 gt bid; ↓ to daily when controlled; use 0.5% if needed; 1-gtt/d gel **Caution:** [C (1st tri; D 2nd or 3rd), ?/+] **Disp:** Soln 0.25/0.5%; Timoptic XE (0.25, 0.5%) gel-forming soln **SE:** Local irritation

Tinidazole (Tindamax) **WARNING:** Off-label use discouraged (animal carcinogenicity w/ other drugs in class) **Uses:** *Adults/children >3 y:* *Trichomoniasis & giardiasis; intestinal amebiasis or amebic liver abscess* **Action:** Antiprotozoal nitroimidazole; *Spectrum:* *Trichomonas vaginalis, Giardia duodenalis, Entamoeba histolytica* **Dose:** *Adults.* Trichomoniasis: 2 g PO; Rx partner. Giardiasis: 2 g PO. Amebiasis: 2 g PO daily × 3 d. Amebic liver abscess: 2 g PO daily × 3–5 d. *Peds.* Trichomoniasis: 50 mg/kg PO, 2 g/d max. Giardiasis: 50 mg/kg PO, 2 g max. Amebiasis: 50 mg/kg PO daily × 3 d, 2 g/d max. Amebic liver abscess: 50 mg/kg PO daily × 3–5 d, 2 g/d max; take w/ food **Caution:** [C, D in 1st tri; –] May be cross-resistant with metronidazole; Sz/peripheral neuropathy may require D/C; w/ CNS/hepatic impair **CI:** Metronidazole allergy, 1st tri PRG, w/ EtOH use **Disp:** Tabs 250, 500 **SE:** CNS disturbances; blood dyscrasias, taste disturbances, N/V, darkens urine **Notes:** D/C EtOH during & 3 d after Rx; potentiates warfarin & lithium; clearance ↓ w/ other drugs; crush & disperse in cherry syrup for peds; removed by HD

Tinzaparin (Innohep)   **WARNING:** Risk of spinal/epidural hematomas development w/ spinal anesthesia or lumbar puncture **Uses:** *Rx of DVT w/ or w/o PE* **Action:** LMW heparin **Dose:** 175 units/kg SQ daily at least 6 d until warfarin dose stabilized **Caution:** [B, ?] Pork allergy, active bleeding, mild–mod renal impair, morbid obesity **CI:** Allergy to sulfites, heparin, benzyl alcohol; HIT **Disp:** Inj 20,000 units/mL **SE:** Bleeding, bruising, ↓ plts, Inj site pain, ↑ LFTs **Notes:** Monitor via anti-Xa levels; no effect on bleeding time, plt Fxn, PT, aPTT

Tioconazole (Vagistat)   **Uses:** *Vag fungal Infxns* **Action:** Topical antifungal **Dose:** 1 Applicator-full Intravag hs (single dose) **Caution:** [C, ?] **CI:** Component allergy **Disp:** Vag oint 6.5% **SE:** Local burning, itching, soreness, polyuria **Notes:** Insert high into vagina

Tiotropium (Spiriva)   **Uses:** *Bronchospasm w/ COPD, bronchitis, emphysema* **Action:** Synthetic anticholinergic like atropine **Dose:** 1 Caps/d inhaled using HandiHaler, *do not* use w/ spacer **Caution:** [C, ?/–] BPH, NAG, MyG, renal impair **CI:** Acute bronchospasm **Disp:** Inh caps 18 mcg **SE:** URI, xerostomia **Notes:** Monitor FEV1 or peak flow

Tirofiban (Aggrastat)   **Uses:** *Acute coronary syndrome* **Action:** Glycoprotein IIB/IIIa inhibitor **Dose:** Initial 0.4 mcg/kg/min for 30 min, followed by 0.1 mcg/kg/min 12–24h; use in combo w/ heparin; *ACS or PCI:* 0.4 mcg/kg/min IV for 30 min, then 0.1 mcg/kg/min *(ECC 2005);* ↓ in renal Insuff **Caution:** [B, ?/–] **CI:** Bleeding, intracranial neoplasm, vascular malformation, stroke/surgery/trauma w/in last 30 d, severe HTN **Disp:** Inj 50, 250 mcg/mL **SE:** Bleeding, bradycardia, coronary dissection, pelvic pain, rash

Tobramycin (Nebcin)   **Uses:** *Serious gram(−) Infxns* **Action:** Aminoglycoside; ↓ protein synth. **Spectrum:** Gram(−) bacteria (including *Pseudomonas*) **Dose:** *Adults.* Conventional dosing: 1–2.5 mg/kg/dose IV q8–12h. *Once-daily dosing:* 5–7 mg/kg/dose q24h. *Peds.* 2.5 mg/kg/dose IV q8h; ↓ w/ renal Insuff **Caution:** [C, M] **CI:** Aminoglycoside sensitivity **Disp:** Inj 10, 40 mg/mL **SE:** Nephro- & ototox **Notes:** Follow CrCl & levels. Levels: *Peak:* 30 min after Inf; *Trough* <0.5 h before next dose; *Therapeutic Conventional: Peak* 5-10 mcg/mL, *Trough* <2 mcg/mL

Tobramycin Ophthalmic (AKTob, Tobrex)   **Uses:** *Ocular bacterial Infxns* **Action:** Aminoglycoside **Dose:** 1–2 gtt q4h; oint bid–tid; if severe, use oint q3–4h, or 2 gtt q30–60 min, then less frequently **Caution:** [C, M] **CI:** Aminoglycoside sensitivity **Disp:** Oint & soln tobramycin 0.3% **SE:** Ocular irritation

Tobramycin & Dexamethasone Ophthalmic (TobraDex) **Uses:** *Ocular bacterial Infxns associated w/ sig inflammation* **Action:** Antibiotic w/ anti-inflammatory **Dose:** 0.3% Oint apply q3–8h or soln 0.3% apply 1–2 gtt q1–4h **Caution:** [C, M] **CI:** Aminoglycoside sensitivity **Disp:** Oint & susp 0.3%, 5 & 10 mL tobramycin 0.3% & dexamethasone 0.1% **SE:** Local irritation/edema **Notes:** Use under ophthalmologist's direction

Tolazamide (Tolinase)   **Uses:** *Type 2 DM* **Action:** Sulfonylurea; ↑ pancreatic insulin release; ↑ peripheral insulin sensitivity; ↓ hepatic glucose output **Dose:** 100–500 mg/d (no benefit >1 g/d) **Caution:** [C, +/–] Elderly, hepatic or renal impair **Disp:** Tabs 100, 250, 500 mg **SE:** HA, dizziness, GI upset, rash, hyperglycemia, photosensitivity, blood dyscrasias

Tolazoline (Priscoline) Uses: *Peripheral vasospastic disorders, persistent pulm hypertension of newborn* **Action:** Competitively blocks α-adrenergic receptors **Dose:** *Adults.* 10–50 mg IM/IV/SQ qid. *Neonates.* 1–2 mg/kg IV over 10–15 min, then 1–2 mg/kg/h (adjust w/ ↓ renal Fxn) **Caution:** [C, ?] Avoid alcohol, w/ CAD, renal impair, CVA, PUD, ↓ BP **CI:** CAD **Disp:** Inj 25 mg/mL **SE:** ↓ BP, peripheral vasodilation, tachycardia, arrhythmias, GI upset & bleeding, blood dyscrasias, renal failure

Tolbutamide (Orinase) Uses: *Type 2 DM* **Action:** Sulfonylurea; ↑ pancreatic insulin release; ↑ peripheral insulin sensitivity; ↓ hepatic glucose output **Dose:** 500–1000 mg bid; 3 g/d max; ↓ in hepatic failure **Caution:** [C, +] **CI:** Sulfonylurea sensitivity **Disp:** Tabs 250, 500 mg **SE:** HA, dizziness, GI upset, rash, photosensitivity, blood dyscrasias, hypoglycemia, heartburn

Tolcapone (Tasmar) WARNING: Cases of fulminant liver failure resulting in death have occurred Uses: *Adjunct to carbidopa/levodopa in Parkinson Dz* **Action:** Catechol-*O*-methyltransferase inhibitor slows levodopa metabolism **Dose:** 100 mg PO tid w/ first daily levodopa/carbidopa dose, then dose 6 & 12 h later; ↓ /w renal Insuff **Caution:** [C, ?] **CI:** Hepatic impair; w/ nonselective MAOI **Disp:** Tabs 100 mg, 200 mg **SE:** Constipation, xerostomia, vivid dreams, hallucinations, anorexia, N/D, orthostasis, liver failure, Rhabdomyolysis **Notes:** Do not abruptly D/C or ↓ dose; monitor LFTs

Tolmetin (Tolectin) WARNING: May ↑ risk of cardiovascular events & GI bleeding Uses: *Arthritis & pain* **Action:** NSAID; ↓ prostaglandins **Dose:** 200–600 mg PO tid; 2000 mg/d max **Caution:** [C (D in 3rd tri or near term), +] **CI:** NSAID or ASA sensitivity; use for pain post-coronary artery bypass graft **Disp:** Tabs 200, 600 mg; caps 400 mg **SE:** Dizziness, rash, GI upset, edema, GI bleeding, renal failure

Tolnaftate (Tinactin) [OTC] Uses: *Tinea pedis, cruris, corporis, manus, versicolor* **Action:** Topical antifungal **Dose:** Apply to area bid for 2–4 wk **Caution:** [C, ?] **CI:** Nail & scalp Infxns **Disp:** OTC 1% liq; gel; powder; topical cream; ointment, powder, and spray soln **SE:** Local irritation **Notes:** Avoid ocular contact, Infxn should improve in 7–10 d

Tolterodine (Detrol, Detrol LA) Uses: *OAB (frequency, urgency, incontinence)* **Action:** Anticholinergic **Dose:** *Detrol* 1–2 mg PO bid; *Detrol LA* 2–4 mg/d **Caution:** [C, ?/–] w/ CYP2D6 & 3A3/4 inhibitor (Table 11) **CI:** Urinary retention, gastric retention, or uncontrolled NAG **Disp:** Tabs 1, 2 mg; *Detrol LA* tabs 2, 4 mg **SE:** Xerostomia, blurred vision, headache, constipation **Notes:** LA form may see "intact" pill in stool

Topiramate (Topamax) Uses: *Adjunctive Rx for complex partial Szs & tonic–clonic Szs,* bipolar disorder, neuropathic pain, migraine prophylaxis

Action: Anticonvulsant **Dose:** **Adults.** *Seizures:* Total dose 400 mg/d; see insert for 8-wk titration schedule. *Migraine prophylaxis:* titrate 100 m/d total. *Peds 2–16 y:* **Initial:** 1–3 mg/kg/d PO qhs; titrate per insert to 5–9 mg/kg/d; ↓ w/ renal impair **Caution:** [C, ?/–] **CI:** Component allergy **Disp:** Tabs 25, 50, 100, 200 mg; caps sprinkles 15, 25, 50 mg **SE:** Wgt loss, memory impair, metabolic acidosis, kidney stones, fatigue, dizziness, psychomotor slowing, paresthesias, GI upset, tremor, nystagmus, acute glaucoma requiring D/C **Notes:** Metabolic acidosis responsive to ↓ dose or D/C; D/C w/ taper

Topotecan (Hycamtin) **WARNING:** Chemotherapy precautions, for use by physicians familiar with chemotherapeutic agents, BM suppression possible **Uses:** *Ovarian CA (cisplatin-refractory), cervical CA, NSCLC,* sarcoma, ped NSCLC **Action:** Topoisomerase I inhibitor; ↓ DNA synth **Dose:** 1.5 mg/m²/d as a 1-h IV Inf × 5 d, repeat q3wk; ↓ w/ renal impair **Caution:** [D, –] **CI:** PRG, breast-feeding **Disp:** Inj 4-mg vials **SE:** ↓ BM, N/V/D, drug fever, skin rash

Torsemide (Demadex) **Uses:** *Edema, HTN, CHF, & hepatic cirrhosis* **Action:** Loop diuretic; ↓ reabsorption of Na⁺ & Cl⁻ in ascending loop of Henle & distal tubule **Dose:** 5–20 mg/d PO or IV; 200 mg/d max **Caution:** [B, ?] **CI:** Sulfonylurea sensitivity **Disp:** Tabs 5, 10, 20, 100 mg; Inj 10 mg/mL **SE:** Orthostatic ↓ BP, HA, dizziness, photosensitivity, electrolyte imbalance, blurred vision, renal impair **Notes:** 10–20 mg torsemide = 40 mg furosemide = 1 mg bumetanide

Tramadol (Ultram, Ultram ER) **Uses:** *Mod–severe pain* **Action:** Centrally acting analgesic **Dose:** **Adults.** 50–100 mg PO q4–6h PRN, start 25 mg PO q A.M., ↑ q3d to 25 mg PO qid; ↑ 50 mg/d max, 400 mg/d max (300 mg if >75 y); ER 100–300 mg PO daily. **Peds.** 0.5–1 mg/kg PO q4–6h PRN; ↓ w/ renal Insuff **Caution:** [C, ?/–] **CI:** Opioid dependency; w/ MAOIs; sensitivity to codeine **Disp:** Tabs 50 mg; ER 10, 20, 30 mg **SE:** Dizziness, HA, somnolence, GI upset, resp depression, anaphylaxis **Notes:** ↓ Sz threshold; tolerance/dependence may develop

Tramadol/Acetaminophen (Ultracet) **Uses:** *Short-term Rx acute pain (<5 d)* **Action:** Centrally acting analgesic; nonnarcotic analgesic **Dose:** 2 tabs PO q4–6h PRN; 8 tabs/d max. *Elderly/renal impair:* Lowest possible dose; 2 tabs q12h max if CrCl <30 **Caution:** [C, –] Szs, hepatic/renal impair, or Hx addictive tendencies **CI:** Acute intoxication **Disp:** Tab 37.5 mg tramadol/325 mg APAP **SE:** SSRIs, TCAs, opioids, MAOIs ↑ risk of Szs; dizziness, somnolence, tremor, HA, N/V/D, constipation, xerostomia, liver tox, rash, pruritus, ↑ sweating, physical dependence **Notes:** Avoid EtOH

Trandolapril (Mavik) **WARNING:** Use in PRG in 2nd/3rd tri can result in fetal death **Uses:** *HTN,* heart failure, LVD, post-AMI **Action:** ACE inhibitor **Dose:** *HTN:* 1–4 mg/d. *Heart failure/LVD:* Start 1 mg/d, titrate to 4 mg/d; ↓ w/ severe renal/hepatic impair **Caution:** [D, +] ACE inhibitor sensitivity, angioedema w/ ACE inhibitors **Disp:** Tabs 1, 2, 4 mg **SE:** ↓ BP, bradycardia, dizziness, ↑ K⁺, GI upset, renal impair, cough, angioedema **Notes:** African Americans minimum dose is 2 mg vs 1 mg in whites

Trastuzumab (Herceptin)   WARNING: Can cause cardiomyopathy and ventricular dysfunction; Inf Rxns and pulm tox reported **Uses:** *Metastases breast CA that overexpress the HER2/neu protein,* breast CA adjuvant, w/ doxorubicin, cyclophosphamide, and paclitaxel if pt HER2/neu(+) **Action:** MoAb; binds human epidermal growth factor receptor 2 protein (HER2); mediates cellular cytotoxicity **Dose:** Per protocol, typical 2 mg/kg/IV/wk **Caution:** [B, ?] CV dysfunction, allergy/Inf Rxns **CI:** Live vaccines **Disp:** Inj form 21 mg/mL **SE:** Anemia, cardiomyopathy, nephrotic syndrome, pneumonitis **Notes:** Inf-related Rxns minimized w/ acetaminophen, diphenhydramine, & meperidine

Trazodone (Desyrel)   WARNING: Closely monitor for worsening depression or emergence of suicidality, particularly in pts <24 y **Uses:** *Depression,* hypnotic, augment other antidepressants **Action:** Antidepressant; ↓ reuptake of serotonin & norepinephrine **Dose:** *Adults & Adolescents.* 50–150 mg PO daily–qid; max 600 mg/d. *Sleep:* 50 mg PO, qhs, PRN **Caution:** [C, ?/–] **CI:** Component allergy **Disp:** Tabs 50, 100, 150, 300 mg **SE:** Dizziness, HA, sedation, N, xerostomia, syncope, confusion, tremor, hep, EPS **Notes:** Takes 1–2 wk for Sx improvement; may interact with CYP3A4 inhibitors to ↑ trazodone concentrations, carbamazepine to ↓ trazodone concentrations

Treprostinil Sodium (Remodulin)   Uses: *NYHA class II–IV pulm arterial HTN* **Action:** Vasodilation, inhibits plt aggregation **Dose:** 0.625–1.25 ng/kg/min cont Inf, titrate to effect, limited experience w/ dose >40 mg/min **Caution:** [B, ?/–] **CI:** Component allergy **Disp:** 1, 2.5, 5, 10 mg/mL Inj **SE:** Additive effects w/ anticoagulants, antihypertensives; Inf site Rxns; D (25%), N (22%), HA (27%), ↓ BP **Notes:** Initiate in monitored setting; do not D/C or ↓ dose abruptly

Tretinoin, Topical [Retinoic Acid] (Retin-A, Avita, Renova, Retin-A Micro)   Uses: *Acne vulgaris, sun-damaged skin, wrinkles* (photo aging), some skin CAs **Action:** Exfoliant retinoic acid derivative **Dose:** *Adults & Peds >12 y:* Apply daily hs (w/ irritation, ↓ frequency). *Photoaging:* Start w/ 0.025%, ↑ to 0.1% over several mo (apply only q3d if on neck area; dark skin may require bid use) **Caution:** [C, ?] **CI:** Retinoid sensitivity **Disp:** Cream 0.02, 0.025, 0.05, 0.1%; gel 0.01, 0.025, microformulation gel 0.1, 0.04%; liq 0.05% **SE:** Avoid sunlight; edema; skin dryness, erythema, scaling, changes in pigmentation, stinging, photosensitivity

Triamcinolone (Azmacort)   Uses: *Chronic asthma* **Actions:** Topical steroid **Dose:** 2-Inhs tid-qid or 4 Inh bid **Caution:** [C, ?] **CI:** Component allergy **Disp:** Aerosol, metered inhaler 100-mcg spray **SE:** Cough, oral candidiasis **Notes:** Instruct pts to rinse mouth after use; not for acute asthma

Triamcinolone & Nystatin (Mycolog-II)   Uses: *Cutaneous candidiasis* **Action:** Antifungal & anti-inflammatory **Dose:** Apply lightly to area bid; max 25 mg/d **Caution:** [C, ?] **CI:** Varicella; systemic fungal Infxns **Disp:** Cream & oint 15, 30, 60, 120 mg **SE:** Local irritation, hypertrichosis, pigmentation changes **Notes:** For short-term use (<7 d)

Triamterene (Dyrenium)   Uses: *Edema associated w/ CHF, cirrhosis* **Action:** K+-sparing diuretic **Dose:** *Adults.* 100–300 mg/24 h PO ÷ daily-bid. *Peds. HTN:* 2–4 mg/kg/d in 1–2 ÷ doses; ↓ w/ renal/hepatic impair **Caution:** [B (manufacturer; D end. opinion), ?/–] **CI:** ↑ K+, renal impair; caution w/ other K+-sparing diuretics **Disp:** Caps 50, 100 mg **SE:** ↓ K+, blood dyscrasias, liver damage, other Rxns

Triazolam (Halcion) [C-IV]   Uses: *Short-term management of insomnia* **Action:** Benzodiazepine **Dose:** 0.125–0.25 mg/d PO hs PRN; ↓ in elderly **Caution:** [X, ?/–] **CI:** NAG; cirrhosis; concurrent amprenavir, ritonavir, nelfinavir, itraconazole, ketoconazole, nefazodone **Disp:** Tabs 0.125, 0.25 mg **SE:** Tachycardia, CP, drowsiness, fatigue, memory impair, GI upset **Notes:** Additive CNS depression w/ EtOH & other CNS depressants, avoid abrupt D/C, do not prescribe >1 mo supply

Triethanolamine (Cerumenex) [OTC]   Uses: *Cerumen (ear wax) removal* **Action:** Ceruminolytic agent **Dose:** Fill ear canal & insert cotton plug; irrigate w/ H2O after 15 min; repeat PRN **Caution:** [C, ?] **CI:** Perforated tympanic membrane, otitis media **Disp:** Soln 10, 16, 12 mL **SE:** Local dermatitis, pain, erythema, pruritus

Triethylenethiophosphoramide (Thio-Tepa, Tespa, TSPA)   Uses: *Hodgkin Dz & NHLs; leukemia; breast, ovarian CAs, preparative regimens for allogeneic & ABMT w/ high doses, intravesical for bladder CA* **Action:** Polyfunctional alkylating agent **Dose:** 0.5 mg/kg q1–4wk, 6 mg/m² IM or IV × 4 d q2–4wk, 15–35 mg/m² by cont IV Inf over 48 h; 60 mg into the bladder & retained 2 h q1–4wk; 900–125 mg/m² in ABMT regimens (highest dose w/o ABMT is 180 mg/m²); 1–10 mg/m² (typically 15 mg) IT 1 or 2×/wk; 0.8 mg/kg in 1–2 L of soln may be instilled intraperitoneally; ↓ in renal failure **Caution:** [D, –] **CI:** Component allergy **Disp:** Inj 15, 30 mg **SE:** ↓ BM, N/V, dizziness, HA, allergy, paresthesias, alopecia **Notes:** Intravesical use in bladder CA infrequent today

Trifluoperazine (Stelazine)   Uses: *Psychotic disorders* **Action:** Phenothiazine; blocks postsynaptic CNS dopaminergic receptors **Dose:** *Adults.* 2–10 mg PO bid. *Peds 6–12 y:* 1 mg PO daily-bid initial, gradually ↑ to 15 mg/d; ↓ in elderly/debilitated pts **Caution:** [C, ?/–] **CI:** Hx blood dyscrasias; phenothiazine sensitivity **Disp:** Tabs 1, 2, 5, 10 mg; PO conc 10 mg/mL; Inj 2 mg/mL **SE:** Orthostatic ↓ BP, EPS, dizziness, neuroleptic malignant syndrome, skin discoloration, lowered Sz threshold, photosensitivity, blood dyscrasias **Notes:** PO conc must be diluted to 60 mL or more prior to administration; requires several wk for onset of effects

Trifluridine Ophthalmic (Viroptic)   Uses: *Herpes simplex keratitis & conjunctivitis* **Action:** Antiviral **Dose:** 1 gtt q2h, max 9 gtt/d; ↓ to 1 gtt q4h after healing begins; Rx up to 21 d **Caution:** [C, M] **CI:** Component allergy **Disp:** Soln 1% **SE:** Local burning, stinging

Trihexyphenidyl (Artane) Uses: *Parkinson Dz* Action: Blocks excess acetylcholine at cerebral synapses Dose: 2–5 mg PO daily-qid Caution: [C, +] CI: NAG, GI obst, MyG, bladder obsts Disp: Tabs 2, 5 mg; elixir 2 mg/5 mL SE: Dry skin, constipation, xerostomia, photosensitivity, tachycardia, arrhythmias

Trimethobenzamide (Tigan) Uses: *N/V* Action: ↓ Medullary chemoreceptor trigger zone Dose: Adults. 300 mg PO or 200 mg IM tid-qid PRN. Peds. 20 mg/kg/24 h PO in 3–4 ÷ doses Caution: [C, ?] CI: Benzocaine sensitivity Disp: Caps 300 mg; Inj 100 mg/mL SE: Drowsiness, ↓ BP, dizziness; hepatic impair, blood dyscrasias, Szs, parkinsonian-like syndrome Notes: In the presence of viral Infxns, may mask emesis or mimic CNS effects of Reye syndrome

Trimethoprim (Primsol, Proloprim) Uses: *UTI due to susceptible gram(+) & gram(−) organisms; Rx PCP w/ dapsone* suppression of UTI Action: ↓ Dihydrofolate reductase. Spectrum: Many gram(+) & (−) except Bacteroides, Branhamella, Brucella, Chlamydia, Clostridium, Mycobacterium, Mycoplasma, Nocardia, Neisseria, Pseudomonas, & Treponema Dose: Adults. 100 mg PO bid or 200 mg PO q day; PCP 5 mg/kg tid × 21 d w/ dapsone. Peds. Mg/kg/d in 2 ÷ doses; ↓ w/ renal failure Caution: [C, +] CI: Megaloblastic anemia due to folate deficiency Disp: Tabs 100 mg; PO soln 50 mg/5 mL SE: Rash, pruritus, megaloblastic anemia, hepatic impair Notes: Take w/ plenty of H₂O

Trimethoprim (TMP)–Sulfamethoxazole (SMX) [Co-Trimoxazole] (Bactrim, Septra) Uses: *UTI Rx & prophylaxis, otitis media, sinusitis, bronchitis* Action: SMX ↓ synth of dihydrofolic acid, TMP ↓ dihydrofolate reductase to impair protein synth. Spectrum: Includes Shigella, PCP, & Nocardia Infxns, Mycoplasma, Enterobacter sp, Staphylococcus, Streptococcus, & more Dose: Adults. 1 DS tab PO bid or 5–20 mg/kg/24 h (based on TMP) IV in 3–4 ÷ doses. Nocardia: 10–15 mg/kg/d IV or PO (TMP) in 4 ÷ doses. UTI prophylaxis: 1 PO daily. Peds. 8–10 mg/kg/24 h (TMP) PO ÷ into 2 doses or 3–4 doses IV; do not use in newborns; ↓ in renal failure; maintain hydration Caution: [B (D if near term), +] CI: Sulfonamide sensitivity, porphyria, megaloblastic anemia w/ folate deficiency, sig hepatic impair Disp: Regular tabs 80 mg TMP/400 mg SMX; DS tabs 160 mg TMP/800 mg SMX; PO susp 40 mg TMP/200 mg SMX/5 mL; Inj 80 mg TMP/400 mg SMX/5 mL SE: Allergic skin Rxns, photosensitivity, GI upset, Stevens-Johnson syndrome, blood dyscrasias, hep Notes: Synergistic combo, interacts w/ warfarin

Trimetrexate (NeuTrexin) WARNING: Must be used w/ leucovorin to avoid tox Uses: *Mod–severe PCP* Action: ↓ Dihydrofolate reductase Dose: 45 mg/m² IV q24h for 21 d; administer w/ leucovorin 20 mg/m² IV q6h for 24 d; ↓ in hepatic impair Caution: [D, ?/−] CI: MTX sensitivity Disp: Inj 25, 200 mg/vial SE: Sz, fever, rash, GI upset, anemias, ↑ LFTs, peripheral neuropathy, renal impair Notes: Use cytotoxic cautions; Inf over 60 min

Triptorelin (Trelstar Depot, Trelstar LA) Uses: *Palliation of advanced PCa* **Action:** LHRH analog; ↓ GNRH w/ cont dosing; transient ↑ in LH, FSH, testosterone, & estradiol 7–10 d after first dose; w/ chronic/cont use (usually 2–4 wk), sustained ↓ LH & FSH w/ ↓ testicular & ovarian steroidogenesis similar to surgical castration **Dose:** 3.75 mg IM monthly or 11.25 mg IM q3mo **Caution:** [X, N/A] **CI:** Not indicated in females **Disp:** Inj Depot 3.75 mg; LA 11.25 mg **SE:** Dizziness, emotional lability, fatigue, HA, insomnia, HTN, D, V, ED, retention, UTI, pruritus, anemia, Inj site pain, musculoskeletal pain, osteoporosis, allergic Rxns

Trospium (Sanctura, Sanctura XR) Uses: *OAB w/ Sx of urge incontinence, urgency, frequency* **Action:** Muscarinic antagonist, ↓ bladder smooth muscle tone **Dose:** 20 mg tab PO bid; 60 mg ER caps PO q day A.M., 1 h ac or on empty stomach. ↓ w/ CrCl <30 mL/min and elderly **Caution:** [C, +/–] w/ EtOH use, in hot environments, ulcerative colitis, MyG, renal/hepatic impair **CI:** Urinary/gastric retention, NAG **Disp:** Tab 20 mg; caps ER 60 mg **SE:** Dry mouth, constipation, HA, rash

Urokinase (Abbokinase) Uses: *PE, DVT, restore patency to IV catheters* **Action:** Converts plasminogen to plasmin; causes clot lysis **Dose:** *Adults & Peds. Systemic effect:* 4400 units/kg IV over 10 min, then 4400–6000 units/kg/h for 12 h. *Restore catheter patency:* Inject 5000 units into catheter & aspirate up to 2 doses **Caution:** [B, +] **CI:** Do not use w/in 10 d of surgery, delivery, or organ biopsy; bleeding, CVA, vascular malformation **Disp:** Powder for Inj, 250,000-unit vial **SE:** Bleeding, ↓ BP, dyspnea, bronchospasm, anaphylaxis, cholesterol embolism **NOTES:** aPTT should be <2× nl before use and before starting anticoagulants after

Valacyclovir (Valtrex) Uses: *Herpes zoster; genital herpes; herpes labialis* **Action:** Prodrug of acyclovir; ↓ viral DNA replication. *Spectrum:* Herpes simplex I & II **Dose:** *Zoster:* 1 g PO tid × 7 d. *Genital herpes(initial episode):* 1 g bid × 7–10 d, *(recurrent)* 500 mg PO bid × 3 d or 1 g PO q day × 5 d. *Herpes prophylaxis:* 500–1000 mg/d. *Herpes labialis:* 2 g PO q12h × 1 d ↓ w/ renal failure **Caution:** [B, +] **Disp:** Caplets 500, 1000 mg **SE:** HA, GI upset, dizziness, pruritus, photophobia

Valganciclovir (Valcyte) **WARNING:** Granulocytopenia, anemia, and thrombocytopenia reported. Carcinogenic, teratogenic, and may cause aspermatogenesis Uses: *CMV retinitis and CMV prophylaxis in solid-organ transplantation* **Action:** Ganciclovir prodrug; ↓ viral DNA synth **Dose:** *CMV Retinitis induction:* 900 mg PO bid w/ food × 21 d, then 900 mg PO daily; *CMV prevention:* 900 mg PO q day × 100 d posttransplant, ↓ w/ renal dysfunction **Caution:** [C, ?/–] Use w/ imipenem/cilastatin, nephrotoxic drugs **CI:** Allergy to acyclovir, ganciclovir, valganciclovir; ANC <500; plt <25 K; Hgb <8 g/dL **Disp:** Tabs 450 mg **SE:** BM suppression, headache, GI upset **Notes:** Monitor CBC & Cr

Valproic Acid (Depakene, Depakote)   WARNING: Fatal hepatic failure, teratogenic effects, and life-threatening pancreatitis reported **Uses:** *Rx epilepsy, mania; prophylaxis of migraines,* Alzheimer behavior disorder **Action:** Anticonvulsant; ↑ availability of GABA **Dose:** *Adults & Peds. Szs:* 30–60 mg/kg/24 h PO ÷ tid (after initiation of 10–15 mg/kg/24 h). *Mania:* 750 mg in 3 ÷ doses, ↑ 60 mg/kg/d max. *Migraines:* 250 mg bid, ↑ 1000 mg/d max; ↓ w/ hepatic impair **Caution:** [D, +] **CI:** Severe hepatic impair **Disp:** Caps 250 mg; caps w/ coated particles 125 mg; tabs DR 125, 250, 500 mg; tabs ER 250, 500 mg; syrup 250 mg/5 mL; Inj 100 mg/mL **SE:** Somnolence, dizziness, GI upset, diplopia, ataxia, rash, thrombocytopenia, hep, pancreatitis, ↑ bleeding times, alopecia, wgt ↑, hyperammonemic encephalopathy in pts w/ urea cycle disorders **Notes:** Monitor LFTs & levels: *Trough:* Just before next dose; *Therapeutic: Peak:* 50–100 mcg/mL; *Toxic Trough:* >100 mcg/mL. *Half-life:* 5–20 h; phenobarbital & phenytoin may alter levels

Valsartan (Diovan)   WARNING: Use during 2nd/3rd tri of PRG can cause fetal harm **Uses:** HTN, CHF, DN **Action:** Angiotensin II receptor antagonist **Dose:** 80–160 mg/d, max 320 mg/d **Caution:** [D, ?/–] w/ K⁺-sparing diuretics or K⁺ supls **CI:** Severe hepatic impair, biliary cirrhosis/obst, primary hyperaldosteronism, bilateral RAS **Disp:** Tabs 40, 80, 160, 320 mg **SE:** ↓ BP, dizziness, HA, viral Infxn, fatigue, Abd pain, D, arthralgia, fatigue, back pain, hyperkalemia, cough, ↑ Cr

Vancomycin (Vancocin, Vancoled)   **Uses:** *Serious MRSA Infxns;* enterococcal Infxns; PO Rx of *S. aureus* and *C. difficile* pseudomembranous colitis* **Action:** ↓ Cell wall synth. *Spectrum:* Gram(+) bacteria & some anaerobes (includes MRSA, *Staphylococcus, Enterococcus, Streptococcus* sp, *C. difficile*) **Dose:** *Adults.* 1 g IV q12h or 15–20 mg/kg/dose; *C. difficile:* 125–500 mg PO q6h × 7–10 d. *Peds.* 40–60 mg/kg/d IV in ÷ doses q6–12 h; *C. difficile:* 40–60 mg/kg/d PO × 7–10 d. *Neonates.* 10–15 mg/kg/dose q12h; ↓ w/ renal Insuff **Caution:** [C, M] **CI:** Component allergy; avoid in Hx hearing loss **Disp:** Caps 125, 250 mg; powder 250 mg/5 mL, 500 mg/6 mL for PO soln; powder for Inj 500 mg, 1000 mg, 10 g/vial **SE:** Oto-/nephrotoxic, GI upset (PO), ↓ WBC **Notes:** Not absorbed PO, effect in gut only; give IV slowly (over 1–3 h) to prevent "red-man syndrome" (flushing of head/neck/upper torso); IV product PO for colitis. Levels: *Peak:* 1 h after Inf; *Trough:* <0.5 h before next dose; *Therapeutic: Peak:* 20–40 mcg/mL; *Trough:* 10–20 mcg/mL; *Toxic Peak:* >50 mcg/mL; *Trough:* >20 mcg/mL. *Half-life:* 6–8 h

Vardenafil (Levitra)   **Uses:** *ED* **Action:** PDE5 inhibitor, increases cyclic guanosine monophosphate (cGMP) NO levels; relaxes smooth muscles; dilates cavernosal arteries **Dose:** 10 mg PO 60 min before sexual activity; titrate; max × 1 = 20 mg; 2.5 mg w/ CYP3A4 inhibitors (Table 11); **Caution:** [B, –] w/ CV, hepatic, or renal Dz or if sex activity not advisable **CI:** w/ nitrates **Disp:** Tabs 2.5, 5, 10, 20 mg tabs **SE:** ↑ QT interval ↓ BP, HA, dyspepsia, priapism, flushing, rhinitis, sinusitis, flu syndrome, sudden ↓/loss of hearing, tinnitus, NIAON. **Notes:** Concomitant α-blockers may cause ↓ BP; transient global amnesia reports

Varenicline (Chantix) **Uses:** *Smoking cessation* **Action:** Nicotine receptor partial agonist **Dose:** *Adults.* 0.5 mg PO daily × 3 d, 0.5 mg bid × 4 d, then 1 mg PO bid for 12 wk total; after meal w/ glass of water **Caution:** [C, ?/–] ↓ Dose w/ renal impair **Disp:** Tabs 0.5, 1 mg **SE:** Serious psychological disturbances, N, V, insomnia, flatulence, unusual dreams **Notes:** Slowly ↑ dose to ↓ N; initiate 1 wk before desired smoking cessation date; monitor for changes in behavior

Varicella Virus Vaccine (Varivax) **Uses:** *Prevent varicella (chickenpox)* **Action:** Active immunization; live attenuated virus **Dose:** *Adults & Peds.* 0.5 mL SQ, repeat 4–8 wk **Caution:** [C, M] **CI:** Immunocompromise; neomycinanaphylactoid Rxn, blood dyscrasias; immunosuppressive drugs; avoid PRG for 3 mo after **Disp:** Powder for Inj **SE:** Mild varicella Infxn; fever, local Rxns, irritability, GI upset **Notes:** OK for all children & adults who have not had chickenpox

Vasopressin [Antidiuretic Hormone, ADH] (Pitressin) **Uses:** *DI; Rx post-op Abd distention*; adjunct Rx of GI bleeding & esophageal varices; asystole and pulseless electrical activity, pulseless VT & VF, adjunct systemic vasopressor (IV drip) **Action:** Posterior pituitary hormone, potent GI, and peripheral vasoconstrictor **Dose:** *Adults & Peds. DI:* 2.5–10 units SQ or IM tid-qid. *GI hemorrhage:* 0.2–0.4 units/min; ↓ in cirrhosis; caution in vascular Dz. *VT/VF:* 40 units IV push × 1. *Vasopressor:* 0.01–0.04 units/min **Caution:** [B, +] **CI:** Allergy **Disp:** Inj 20 units/mL **SE:** HTN, arrhythmias, fever, vertigo, GI upset, tremor **Notes:** Addition of vasopressor to concurrent norepinephrine or epi Infs

Vecuronium (Norcuron) **WARNING:** To be administered only by appropriately trained individuals **Uses:** *Skeletal muscle relaxation* **Action:** Nondepolarizing neuromuscular blocker; onset 2–3 min **Dose:** *Adults & Peds.* 0.1–0.2 mg/kg IV bolus (also rapid intubation (*ECC 2005*); maint 0.010–0.015 mg/kg after 25–40 min; additional doses q12–15min PRN; ↓ in severe renal/hepatic impair **Caution:** [C, ?] Drug interactions cause ↑ effect (eg, aminoglycosides, tetracycline, succinylcholine) **Disp:** Powder for Inj 10, 20 mg **SE:** Bradycardia, ↓ BP, itching, rash, tachycardia, CV collapse **Notes:** Fewer cardiac effects than succinylcholine

Venlafaxine (Effexor, Effexor XR) **WARNING:** Monitor for worsening depression or emergence of suicidality, particularly in ped pts **Uses:** *Depression, generalized anxiety,* social anxiety disorder; panic disorder,* OCD, chronic fatigue syndrome, ADHD, autism **Action:** Potentiation of CNS neurotransmitter activity **Dose:** 75–225 mg/d ÷ into 2–3 equal doses (IR) or q day (ER); 375 mg IR or 225 mg ER max/d ↓ w/ renal/hepatic impair **Caution:** [C, ?/–] **CI:** MAOIs **Disp:** Tabs IR 25, 37.5, 50, 75, 100 mg; ER caps 37.5, 75, 150 mg **SE:** HTN, ↑ HR, HA, somnolence, GI upset, sexual dysfunction; actuates mania or Szs **Notes:** Avoid EtOH

Verapamil (Calan, Isoptin, Verelan) Uses: *Angina, HTN, PSVT, AF, atrial flutter,* migraine prophylaxis, hypertrophic cardiomyopathy, bipolar Dz **Action:** CCB **Dose:** *Adults. Arrhythmias:* 2nd line for PSVT w/ narrow QRS complex & adequate BP 2.5–5 mg IV over 1–2 min; repeat 5–10 mg in 15–30 min PRN (30 mg max). *Angina:* 80–120 mg PO tid, ↑ 480 mg/24 h max. *HTN:* 80–180 mg PO tid or SR tabs 120–240 mg PO daily to 240 mg bid; 2.5–5.0 mg IV over 1–2 min; repeat 5–10 mg, in 5–30 min PRN; or 5-mg bolus q15min (max 30 mg) *(ECC 2005).* *Peds <1 y:* 0.1–0.2 mg/kg IV over 2 min (may repeat in 30 min). *1–16 y:* 0.1–0.3 mg/kg IV over 2 min (may repeat in 30 min); 5 mg max. *PO: 1–5 y:* 4–8 mg/kg/d in 3 ÷ doses. *>5 y:* 80 mg q6–8h; ↓ in renal/hepatic impair **Caution:** [C, +] Amiodarone/β-blockers/flecainide can cause bradycardia; statins, midazolam, tacrolimus, theophylline levels may be ↑; w/ elderly pts **CI:** Conduction disorders, cardiogenic shock; β-blocker/thiazide combo, dofetilide, pimozide, ranolazine **Disp:** Tabs 40, 80, 120 mg; tabs ER 120, 180, 240 mg; tabs ER 24-h 180, 240, mg; caps SR 120, 180, 240, 360 mg; caps ER 100, 200, 300 mg; Inj 5 mg/2 mL **SE:** Gingival hyperplasia, constipation, ↓ BP, bronchospasm, HR or conduction disturbances

Vinblastine (Velban, Velbe) WARNING: Chemotherapeutic agent; handle w/ caution Uses: *Hodgkin Dz & NHLs, mycosis fungoides, CAs (testis, renal cell, breast, NSCLC), AIDS-related Kaposi sarcoma,* choriocarcinoma, histiocytosis **Action:** ↓ Microtubule assembly **Dose:** 0.1–0.5 mg/kg/wk (4–20 mg/m²); ↓ in hepatic failure **Caution:** [D, ?] **CI:** Intrathecal use **Disp:** Inj 1 mg/mL in 10 mg vial **SE:** ↓ BM (especially leukopenia), N/V, constipation, neurotox, alopecia, rash, myalgia, tumor pain

Vincristine (Oncovin, Vincasar PFS) WARNING: Chemotherapeutic agent; handle w/ caution; fatal if administered intrathecally Uses: *ALL, breast & small-cell lung CA, sarcoma (eg, Ewing tumor, rhabdomyosarcoma), Wilms tumor, Hodgkin Dz & NHLs, neuroblastoma, multiple myeloma* **Action:** Promotes disassembly of mitotic spindle, causing metaphase arrest **Dose:** 0.4–1.4 mg/m² (single doses 2 mg/max); ↓ in hepatic failure **Caution:** [D, ?] **CI:** Intrathecal use **Disp:** Inj 1 mg/mL, 5 mg vial **SE:** Neurotox commonly dose limiting, jaw pain (trigeminal neuralgia), fever, fatigue, anorexia, constipation & paralytic ileus, bladder atony; no sig ↓ BM w/ standard doses; tissue necrosis w/ extrav

Vinorelbine (Navelbine) WARNING: Chemotherapeutic agent; handle w/ caution Uses: *Breast CA & NSCLC* (alone or w/ cisplatin) **Action:** ↓ Polymerization of microtubules, impairing mitotic spindle formation; semisynthetic vinca alkaloid **Dose:** 30 mg/m²/wk; ↓ in hepatic failure **Caution:** [D, ?] **CI:** Intrathecal use, granulocytopenia (<1000/mm³) **Disp:** Inj 10 mg **SE:** ↓ BM (leukopenia), mild GI, neurotox (6–29%); constipation/paresthesias (rare); tissue damage from extrav

Vitamin B₁ See Thiamine (page 224)
Vitamin B₆ See Pyridoxine (page 200)

Vitamin B$_{12}$ See Cyanocobalamin (page 77)
Vitamin K See Phytonadione (page 192)
Vitamin, multi See Multivitamins (Table 13)
Voriconazole (VFEND) Uses: *Invasive aspergillosis, candidemia, serious fungal Infxns* Action: ↓ Ergosterol synth. Spectrum: Candida, Aspergillus, Scedosporium, Fusarium sp Dose: **Adults & Peds >12 y:** IV: 6 mg/kg q12h × 2, then 4 mg/kg bid; may ↓ to 3 mg/kg/dose. PO: <40 kg: 100 mg q12h, up to 150 mg; >40 kg: 200 mg q12h, up to 300 mg; ↓ w/ mild–mod hepatic impair; IV w/ renal impair × 1 dose; PO w/o food Caution: [D, ?/–] CI: Severe hepatic impair, w/ CYP3A4 substrates (see Table 11) Disp: Tabs 50, 200 mg; susp 200 mg/5 mL; 200 mg Inj SE: Visual changes, fever, rash, GI upset, ↑ LFTs Notes: √ for multiple drug interactions (eg, ↑ dose w/ phenytoin)

Vorinostat (Zolinza) Uses: *Rx cutaneous manifestations in cutaneous T-cell lymphoma* Action: Histone deacetylase inhibitor Dose: 400 mg PO daily w/ food; if intolerant ↓ 300 mg PO d × 5 consecutive days each wk Caution: [D; ?/–] w/ Warfarin(↑ INR) Disp: Caps 100 mg SE: N/V/D, dehydration, fatigue, anorexia, dysgeusia, DVT, PE, ↓ plt, anemia, hyperglycemia, QTc prolongation, Notes: Monitor CBC, lytes (K, Mg, CA), glucose, & SCr q2wk × 2 mo then monthly; baseline, periodic ECGs; drink 2 L fluid/d

Warfarin (Coumadin) WARNING: Caw cause major or fatal bleeding Uses: *Prophylaxis & Rx of PE & DVT, AF w/ embolization,* other post-op indications Action: ↓ Vit K-dependent clotting factors in order: VII-IX-X-II Dose: **Adults.** Titrate, INR 2.0–3.0 for most; mechanical valves INR is 2.5–3.5. American College of Chest Physicians guidelines: 5 mg initial, may use 7.5–10 mg; ↓ if pt elderly or w/has other bleeding risk factors; maint 2–10 mg/d PO, follow daily INR initial to adjust dosage (Table 9). **Peds.** 0.05–0.34 mg/kg/24 h PO or IV; follow PT/INR to adjust dosage; monitor vit K intake; ↓ w/ hepatic impair/elderly Caution: [X, +] CI: Severe hepatic/renal Dz, bleeding, peptic ulcer, PRG Disp: Tabs 1, 2, 2.5, 3, 4, 5, 6, 7.5, 10 mg; Inj SE: Bleeding due to over-anticoagulation or injury & therapeutic INR; bleeding, alopecia, skin necrosis, purple toe syndrome Notes: Monitor vit K intake (↓ effect); INR preferred test; to rapidly correct overanticoagulation: vit K, fresh-frozen plasma, or both; highly teratogenic. Caution pt on taking w/ other meds, especially ASA. Common warfarin interactions: Potentiated by: APAP, EtOH (w/ liver Dz), amiodarone, cimetidine, ciprofloxacin, cotrimoxazole, erythromycin, fluconazole, flu vaccine, isoniazid, itraconazole, metronidazole, omeprazole, phenytoin, propranolol, quinidine, tetracycline. Inhibited by: barbiturates, carbamazepine, chlordiazepoxide, cholestyramine, dicloxacillin, nafcillin, rifampin, sucralfate, high–vit K foods. Consider genotyping for VKORC1 & CYP2C9

Witch Hazel (Tucks Pads, others [OTC]) Uses: After bowel movement cleansing to decrease local irritation or relieve hemorrhoids; after anorectal surgery, episiotomy, Vag hygiene Dose: Apply PRN Caution: [?, ?] External use only CI: None Supplied: Presoaked pads SE: Mild itching or burning

Zafirlukast (Accolate)   Uses: *Adjunctive Rx of asthma* Action: Selective & competitive inhibitor of leukotrienes Dose: Adults & Peds >12 y: 20 mg bid. Peds 5–11 y: 10 mg PO bid (empty stomach) Caution: [B, –] Interacts w/ warfarin, ↑ INR CI: Component allergy SE: Tabs 10, 20 mg SE: Hepatic dysfunction, usually reversible on D/C; HA, dizziness, GI upset; Churg-Strauss syndrome Notes: Not for acute asthma

Zaleplon (Sonata) [C-IV]   Uses: *Insomnia* Action: A nonbenzodiazepine sedative/hypnotic, a pyrazolopyrimidine Dose: 5–20 mg hs PRN; not w/ high-fat meal; ↓ w/ renal/hepatic Insuff, elderly Caution: [C, ?/–] w/ Mental/psychological conditions CI: Component allergy Disp: Caps 5, 10 mg SE: HA, edema, amnesia, somnolence, photosensitivity Notes: Take immediately before desired onset

Zanamivir (Relenza)   Uses: *Influenza A & B w/ Sxs <2 d; prophylaxis for influenza* Action: ↓ Viral neuraminidase Dose: Adults & Peds >7 y: 2 Inh (10 mg) bid × 10 d, initiate w/in 48 h of Sxs. Prophylaxis Household: 10 mg q day × 10 d. Adults & Peds >12 y: Prophylaxis Community: 10 mg q day × 28 d Caution: [C, M] Not ok for pt w/ airway Dz CI: Pulm Dz Disp: Powder for Inh 5 mg SE: Bronchospasm, HA, GI upset, allergic Rxn, abnormal behavior, ear, nose, throat Sx Notes: Uses a Diskhaler for administration; dose same time each day

Ziconotide (Prialt)   WARNING: Psychological, cognitive, neurologic impair may develop over several wk; monitor frequently; may necessitate D/C Uses: *IT Rx of severe, refractory, chronic pain* Action: N-type CCB in spinal cord Dose: 2.4 mcg/d IT at 0.1 mcg/h; may ↑ 2.4 mcg/d 2–3×/wk to max 19.2 mcg/d (0.8 mcg/h) by day 21 Caution: [C, ?/–] w/ Neuro-/psychological impair CI: Psychosis Disp: Inj 25, 100 mcg/mL SE: Dizziness, N/V, confusion, psych disturbances, abnormal vision, meningitis; may require dosage adjustment Notes: May D/C abruptly; uses specific pumps; do not ↑ more frequently than 2–3×/wk

Zidovudine (Retrovir)   WARNING: Neutropenia, anemia, lactic acidosis, myopathy & hepatomegaly w/ steatosis Uses: *HIV Infxn, prevent maternal HIV transmission* Action: ↓ RT Dose: Adults. 200 mg PO tid or 300 mg PO bid or 1 mg/kg/dose IV q4h. PRG: 100 mg PO 5×/d until labor; during labor 2 mg/kg IV over 1 h then 1 mg/kg/h until cord clamped. Peds. 160 mg/m²/dose q8h; ↓ in renal failure Caution: [C, ?/–] CI: Allergy Disp: Caps 100 mg; tabs 300 mg; syrup 50 mg/5 mL; Inj 10 mg/mL SE: Hematologic tox, HA, fever, rash, GI upset, malaise, myopathy, fat redistribution

Zidovudine & Lamivudine (Combivir)   WARNING: Neutropenia, anemia, lactic acidosis, myopathy & hepatomegaly w/ steatosis Uses: *HIV Infxn* Action: Combo of RT inhibitors Dose: Adults & Peds >12 y: 1 tab PO bid; ↓ in renal failure Caution: [C, ?/–] CI: Component allergy Disp: Tab zidovudine 300 mg/ lamivudine 150 mg SE: Hematologic tox, HA, fever, rash, GI upset, malaise, pancreatitis Notes: Combo product ↓ daily pill burden

Zileuton (Zyflo, Zyflo CR) Uses: *Chronic Rx asthma* Action: Leukotriene inhibitor (↓ 5-lipoxygenase) Dose: *Adults & Peds >12 y:* 600 mg PO qid; CR 1200 mg bid w/in 1 h of A.M./P.M. meal Caution: [C, ?/–] CI: Hepatic impair Disp: Tabs 600 mg; CR tabs 600 mg SE: Hepatic damage, HA, GI upset, leukopenia Notes: Monitor LFTs q mo × 3, then q2–3mo; take regularly; not for acute asthma; do not chew/crush CR

Ziprasidone (Geodon) WARNING: ↑ Mortality in elderly with dementia-related psychosis Uses: *Schizophrenia, acute agitation* Action: Atypical antipsychotic Dose: 20 mg PO bid, may ↑ in 2-d intervals up to 80 mg bid; agitation 10–20 mg IM PRN up to 40 mg/d; separate 10 mg doses by 2 h & 20 mg doses by 4 h (w/ food) Caution: [C, –] w/ ↓ Mg²⁺, ↓ K⁺ CI: QT prolongation, recent MI, uncompensated HF, ↑ QT interval Disp: Caps 20, 40, 60, 80 mg; susp 10 mg/mL; Inj 20 mg/mL SE: Bradycardia; rash, somnolence, resp disorder, EPS, wgt gain, orthostatic ↓ BP Notes: ✓ Lytes

Zoledronic Acid (Zometa, Reclast) Uses: *↑ Ca²⁺ of malignancy (HCM), skeletal-related events in CAP, multiple myeloma, & metastatic bone lesions (Zometa)*; *postmenopausal osteoporosis, Paget Dz (Reclast)* Action: Bisphosphonate; ↓ osteoclastic bone resorption Dose: *Zometa HCM:* 4 mg IV over ≥15 min; may retreat in 7 d w/ adequate renal Fxn. *Zometa Bone lesions/myeloma:* 4 mg IV over >15 min, repeat q3–4wk PRN; extend w/ ↑ Cr. *Reclast:* 5 mg IV annually Caution: [C, ?/–] Diuretics, aminoglycosides; ASA-sensitive asthmatics; avoid invasive dental procedures CI: Bisphosphonate allergy; urticaria, angioedema, w/ dental procedures Disp: Vial 4 mg, 5 mg SE: All ↑ w/ renal dysfunction; fever, flu-like syndrome, GI upset, insomnia, anemia; electrolyte imbalance, bone, joint, muscle pain, a-fib, osteonecrosis of jaw Notes: Requires vigorous prehydration; do not exceed recommended doses/Inf duration to ↓ renal dysfunction; follow Cr; effect prolonged w/ Cr ↑; avoid oral surgery; dental exam recommended prior to therapy; give Ca²⁺ and vit D supls

Zolmitriptan (Zomig, Zomig XMT, Zomig Nasal) Uses: *Acute Rx migraine* Action: Selective serotonin agonist; causes vasoconstriction Dose: Initial 2.5 mg PO, may repeat after 2 h, 10 mg max in 24 h; nasal 5 mg; if HA returns, repeat after 2 h, 10 mg max 24 h Caution: [C, ?/–] CI: Ischemic heart Dz, Prinzmetal angina, uncontrolled HTN, accessory conduction pathway disorders, ergots, MAOIs Disp: Tabs 2.5, 5 mg; rapid tabs (XMT) 2.5, 5 mg; nasal 5 mg, SE: Dizziness, hot flashes, paresthesias, chest tightness, myalgia, diaphoresis

Zolpidem (Ambien, Ambien CR) [C-IV] Uses: *Short-term Rx of insomnia* Action: Hypnotic agent Dose: 5–10 mg or 12.5 mg CR PO hs PRN; ↓ in elderly (use 6.25 mg) Caution: [B, –/–] CI: Breast-feeding Disp: Tabs 5, 10 mg; CR 6.25, 12.5 mg SE: HA, dizziness, drowsiness, N, myalgia Notes: May be habit forming; CR only if able to get 7–8 h sleep

Zonisamide (Zonegran) WARNING: ↑ Risk of suicidal thoughts or behavior Uses: *Adjunct Rx complex partial Szs* Action: Anticonvulsant

Dose: Initial 100 mg/d PO; may ↑ to 400 mg/d **Caution:** [C, –] ↑ tox w/ CYP3A4 inhibitor; ↓ levels w/ carbamazepine, phenytoin, phenobarbital, valproic acid **CI:** Allergy to sulfonamides; oligohydrosis & hypothermia in peds **Disp:** Caps 25, 50, 100 mg **SE:** Dizziness, drowsiness, confusion, ataxia, memory impair, paresthesias, psychosis, nystagmus, diplopia, tremor, anemia, leukopenia; GI upset, nephrolithiasis, Stevens-Johnson syndrome; monitor for ↓ sweating & ↑ body temperature **Notes:** Swallow caps whole

Zoster vaccine, live (Zostavax)   Uses: *Prevent varicella zoster in adults >60 y* **Action:** Active immunization (live vaccine) to herpes zoster **Dose:** *Adults.* 0.65 mL SQ × 1 **CI:** Gelatin, neomycin anaphylaxis; untreated TB, immunocompromise **Caution:** [C, ?/–] Not for peds **Disp:** SD Vial **SE:** Inj site Rxn, HA

NATURAL AND HERBAL AGENTS

The following is a guide to some common herbal products. These may be sold separately or in combo with other products. According to the FDA, "Manufacturers of dietary supplements can make claims about how their products affect the structure or function of the body, but they may not claim to prevent, treat, cure, mitigate, or diagnose a disease without prior FDA approval."

Black Cohosh Uses: Sx of menopause (eg, hot flashes), PMS, hypercholesterolemia, peripheral arterial Dz; has anti-inflammatory & sedative effects **Efficacy:** May have short-term benefit on menopausal Sx **Dose:** 20–40 mg bid **Caution:** May further ↓ lipids &/or BP w/ prescription meds **CI:** PRG (miscarriage, prematurity reports); lactation **SE:** w/ OD, N/V, dizziness, nervous system & visual changes, bradycardia, & (possibly) Szs, liver damage/failure

Chamomile Uses: Antispasmodic, sedative, anti-inflammatory, astringent, antibacterial. **Dose:** 10–15 g PO daily (3 g dried flower heads tid-qid between meals; can steep in 250 mL hot H$_2$O) **Caution:** w/ Allergy to chrysanthemums, ragweed, asters (family *Compositae*) **SE:** Contact dermatitis; allergy, anaphylaxis **Interactions:** w/ Anticoagulants, additive w/ sedatives (benzodiazepines); delayed ↓ gastric absorption of meds if taken together (↓ GI motility)

Cranberry (*Vaccinium macrocarpon*) Uses: Prevention & Rx UTI. **Efficacy:** Possibly effective **Dose:** 300–400 mg bid in 6 oz. juice qid; *tincture* 1/2–1 tsp up to 3×/d, *tea* 2–3 tsps of dried flowers/cup; *creams* apply topically 2–3×/d PO **Caution:** May ↑ kidney stones in some susceptible individuals, V **SE:** None known **Interactions:** May potentiate warfarin

Dong Quai (*Angelica polymorpha, sinensis*) Uses: Uterine stimulant; anemia, menstrual cramps, irregular menses, & menopausal Sx; anti-inflammatory, vasodilator, CNS stimulant, immunosuppressant, analgesic, antipyretic, antiasthmatic **Efficacy:** Possibly effective for menopausal Sx **Dose:** 3–15 g daily, 9–12 g PO tab bid. **Caution:** Avoid in PRG & lactation **SE:** D, photosensitivity, skin cancer **Interactions:** Anticoagulants (↑ INR w/ warfarin)

Echinacea (*Echinacea purpurea*) Uses: Immune system stimulant; prevention/Rx URI of colds, flu; supportive care in chronic Infxns of the resp/lower urinary tract **Efficacy:** Not established; may ↓ severity & duration of URI

(Adapted from Haist SA and Robbins JB: *Internal Medicine on Call*, 4th ed., 2005 McGraw-Hill).

Dose: Caps 500 mg, 6–9 mL expressed juice or 2–5 g dried root PO **Caution:** Do not use w/ progressive systemic or immune Dzs (eg, TB, collagen–vascular disorders, MS); may interfere w/ immunosuppressive therapy, not OK w/ PRG; do not use >8 consecutive wk; possible immunosuppression; 3 different commercial forms **SE:** N; rash **Interactions:** Anabolic steroids, amiodarone, MTX, corticosteroids, cyclosporine

Ephedra/Ma Huang
Uses: Stimulant, aid in wgt loss, bronchial dilation. **Dose:** Not OK due to reported deaths (>100 mg/d can be life-threatening); US sales banned by FDA in 2004; bitter orange w/ similar properties has replaced this compound in most wgt-loss supls **Caution:** Adverse cardiac events, strokes, death **SE:** Nervousness, HA, insomnia, palpitations, V, hyperglycemia **Interactions:** Digoxin, antihypertensives, antidepressants, diabetic meds

Fish Oil Supplements (omega-3 polyunsaturated fatty acid)
Uses: CAD, hypercholesterolemia, hypertriglyceridemia, type 2 DM, arthritis **Efficacy:** No definitive data on ↓ cardiac risk in general population; may ↓ lipids and help w/ secondary MI prevention **Dose:** One FDA approved (see Lovaza, page 179); OTC 1500–3000 mg/d; American Heart Association recommends 1 g/d **Caution:** Mercury contamination possible, some studies suggest ↑ cardiac events **SE:** ↑ Bleeding risk, dyspepsia, belching, aftertaste **Interactions:** Anticoagulants

Evening Primrose Oil
Uses: PMS, diabetic neuropathy, ADHD **Efficacy:** Possibly for PMS, not for menopausal Sx **Dose:** 2–4 g/d PO **SE:** Indigestion, N, soft stools, HA **Interactions:** ↑ Phenobarbital metabolism, ↓ Sz threshold

Feverfew (Tanacetum parthenium)
Uses: Prevent/Rx migraine; fever; menstrual disorders; arthritis; toothache; insect bites **Efficacy:** Weak for migraine prevention **Dose:** 125 mg PO of dried leaf (standardized to 0.2% of parthenolide) PO **Caution:** Do not use in PRG **SE:** Oral ulcers, gastric disturbance, swollen lips, Abd pain; long-term SE unknown **Interactions:** ASA, warfarin

Garlic (Allium sativum)
Uses: Antioxidant; hyperlipidemia, HTN; anti-infective (antibacterial, antifungal); tick repellant (oral) **Efficacy:** ↓ Cholesterol by 4–6%; soln ↓ BP; possible ↓ GI/CAP risk **Dose:** 2–5 g, fresh garlic; 0.4–1.2 g of dried powder; 2–5 mg oil; 300–1000 mg extract or other formulations = to 2–5 mg of allicin daily, 400–1200 mg powder (2–5 mg allicin) PO **Caution:** Do not use in PRG (abortifacient); D/C 7 d pre-op (bleeding risk) **SE:** ↑ Insulin levels, ↑ insulin/lipid/cholesterol levels, anemia, oral burning sensation, N/V/D **Interactions:** Warfarin & ASA (↓ plt aggregation), additive w/ DM agents (↑ hypoglycemia). CYP450 3A4 inducer (may ↑ cyclosporine, HIV antivirals, oral contraceptives)

Ginger (Zingiber officinale)
Uses: Prevent motion sickness; N/V due to anesthesia **Efficacy:** Benefit in ↓ N/V w/motion or PRG; weak for post-op or chemotherapy **Dose:** 1–4 g rhizome or 0.5–2 g powder PO daily **Caution:** Pt w/ gallstones; excessive dose (↑ depression, & may interfere w/ cardiac Fxn or anticoagulants) **SE:** Heartburn **Interactions:** Excessive consumption may interfere with cardiac, DM, or anticoagulant meds **Dose:** Ginger

powder tabs or caps or fresh-cut ginger in doses of 1–4 g daily PO, divided into smaller doses

Ginkgo Biloba
Uses: Memory deficits, dementia, anxiety, improvement Sx peripheral vascular Dz, vertigo, tinnitus, asthma/bronchospasm, antioxidant, premenstrual Sx (especially breast tenderness), impotence, SSRI-induced sexual dysfunction **Dose:** 60–80 mg standardized dry extract PO bid-tid **Efficacy:** Small cognition benefit w/ dementia; no other demonstrated benefit in healthy adults **Caution:** ↑ Bleeding risk (antagonism of plt-activating factor), concerning w/ antiplatelet agents (D/C 3 d pre-op); reports of ↑ Sz risk **SE:** GI upset, HA, dizziness, heart palpitations, rash **Interactions:** ASA, salicylates, warfarin

Ginseng
Uses: "Energy booster" general; also for pt undergoing chemotherapy, stress reduction, improve brain activity & physical endurance (adaptogenic), antioxidant, aid to control type 2 DM; Panax ginseng being studied for ED **Efficacy:** Not established **Dose:** 1–2 g of root or 100–300 mg of extract (7% ginsenosides) PO tid **Caution:** w/ Cardiac Dz, DM, ↑ BP, HTN, mania, schizophrenia, w/ corticosteroids; avoid in PRG; D/C 7 d pre-op (bleeding risk) **SE:** Controversial "ginseng abuse syndrome" w/ high dose (nervousness, excitation, HA, insomnia); palpitations, Vag bleeding, breast nodules, hypoglycemia **Interactions:** Warfarin, antidepressants & caffeine (↑ stimulant effect), DM meds (↑ hypoglycemia)

Glucosamine Sulfate (Chitosamine) and Chondroitin Sulfate
Uses: Osteoarthritis (glucosamine: rate-limiting step in glycosaminoglycan synth), ↑ cartilage rebuilding; *Chondroitin:* biological polymer, flexible matrix between protein filaments in cartilage; draws fluids/nutrients into joint, "shock absorption") **Efficacy:** Controversial **Dose:** Glucosamine 500 PO tid, chondroitin 400 mg PO tid **Caution:** Many forms come from shellfish, so avoid if have shellfish allergy **SE:** ↑ Insulin resistance in DM; concentrated in cartilage, theoretically unlikely to cause toxic/teratogenic effects **Interactions:** *Glucosamine:* None. *Chondroitin:* Monitor anticoagulant therapy

Kava Kava (Kava Kava Root Extract, *Piper methysticum*)
Uses: Anxiety, stress, restlessness, insomnia **Efficacy:** Possible mild anxiolytic **Dose:** Standardized extract (70% kavalactones) 100 mg PO bid-tid **Caution:** Hepatotox risk, banned in Europe/Canada. Not OK in PRG, lactation. D/C 24 h pre-op (may ↑ sedative effect of anesthetics) **SE:** Mild GI disturbances; rare allergic skin/rash Rxns, may ↑ cholesterol; ↑ LFTs/jaundice; vision changes, red eyes, puffy face, muscle weakness **Interactions:** Avoid w/ sedatives, alcohol, stimulants, barbiturates (may potentiate CNS effect)

Melatonin
Uses: Insomnia, jet lag, antioxidant, immunostimulant **Efficacy:** Sedation most pronounced w/ elderly pts with ↑ endogenous melatonin levels; some evidence for jet lag **Dose:** 1–3 mg 20 min before HS (w/ CR 2 h before hs) **Caution:** Use synthetic rather than animal pineal gland, "heavy head," HA, depression, daytime sedation, dizziness **Interactions:** β-Blockers, steroids, NSAIDs, benzodiazepines

Milk Thistle (*Silybum marianum*)   Uses: Prevent/Rx liver damage (eg, from alcohol, toxins, cirrhosis, chronic hep); preventive w/ chronic toxin exposure (painters, chemical workers, etc) **Efficacy:** Use before exposure more effective than use after damage has occurred **Dose:** 80–200 mg PO tid **SE:** GI intolerance **Interactions:** None

Saw Palmetto (*Serenoa repens*)   Uses: Rx BPH, hair tonic, PCa prevention (weak 5α-reductase inhibitor like finasteride, dutasteride) **Efficacy:** Small, no significant benefit for prostatic Sx **Dose:** 320 mg daily **Caution:** Possible hormonal effects, avoid in PRG, w/ women of childbearing years **SE:** Mild GI upset, mild HA, D w/ large amounts **Interactions:** ↑ Iron absorption; ↑ estrogen replacement effects

St. John's wort (*Hypericum perforatum*)   Uses: Mild–mod depression, anxiety, gastritis, insomnia, vitiligo; anti-inflammatory; immune stimulant/anti-HIV/antiviral **Efficacy:** Variable; benefit w/ mild–mod depression in several trials, but not always seen in clinical practice *Dose:* 2–4 g of herb or 0.2–1 mg of total hypericin (standardized extract) daily. *Common preparations:* 300 mg PO tid (0.3% hypericin) **Caution:** Excess doses may potentiate MAOI, cause allergic Rxn, not OK in PRG **SE:** Photosensitivity, xerostomia, dizziness, constipation, confusion, fluctuating mood w/ chronic use **Interactions:** CYP 3A enzyme inducer; do not use w/ Rx antidepressants(especially MAOI); ↓ cyclosporine efficacy (may cause rejection), digoxin (may ↑ CHF), protease inhibitors, theophylline, OCP; potency varies between products/batches

Valerian (*Valeriana officinalis*)   Uses: Anxiolytic, sedative, restlessness, dysmenorrhea **Efficacy:** Probably effective sedative (reduces sleep latency) **Dose:** 2–3 g in extract PO daily-bid added to 2/3 cup boiling H_2O, tincture 15–20 drops in H_2O, oral 400–900 mg hs (combined w/ OTC sleep product Alluna) **Caution:** None known **SE:** Sedation, hangover effect, HA, cardiac disturbances, GI upset **Interactions:** Caution w/ other sedating agents (eg, alcohol, or prescription sedatives): may cause drowsiness w/ impaired Fxn

Yohimbine (*Pausinystalia yohimbe*) Yocon, Yohimex   Uses: Improve sexual vigor, Rx ED **Efficacy:** Variable **Dose:** 1 tab = 5.4 mg PO tid (use w/ physician supervision) **Caution:** Do not use w/ renal/hepatic Dz; may exacerbate schizophrenia/mania (if pt predisposed). α₂-Adrenergic antagonist (↓ BP, Abd distress, weakness w/ high doses), OD can be fatal; salivation, dilated pupils, arrhythmias **SE:** Anxiety, tremors, dizziness, high BP, ↑ HR **Interactions:** Do not use w/ antidepressants (eg, MAOIs or similar agents)

Unsafe Herbs with Known Toxicity

Agent	Toxicities
Aconite	Salivation, N/V, blurred vision, cardiac arrhythmias
Aristolochic acid	Nephrotox
Calamus	Possible carcinogenicity
Chaparral	Hepatotox, possible carcinogenicity, nephrotox
"Chinese herbal mixtures"	May contain Ma Huang or other dangerous herbs
Coltsfoot	Hepatotox, possibly carcinogenic
Comfrey	Hepatotox, carcinogenic
Ephedra/Ma Huang	Adverse cardiac events, stroke, Sz
Juniper	High allergy potential, D, Sz, nephrotox
Kava kava	Hepatotox
Licorice	Chronic daily amounts (>30 g/mo) can result in ↓ K+, Na/fluid retention w/ HTN, myoglobinuria, hyporeflexia
Life root	Hepatotox, liver cancer
Ma Huang/Ephedra	Adverse cardiac events, stroke, Sz
Pokeweed	GI cramping, N/D/V, labored breathing, ↓ BP, Sz
Sassafras	V, stupor, hallucinations, dermatitis, abortion, hypothermia, liver cancer
Usnic acid	Hepatotox
Yohimbine	Hypotension, Abd distress, CNS stimulation (mania/& psychosis in predisposed individuals)

Tables

TABLE 1
Quick Guide to Dosing of Acetaminophen Based on the Tylenol Product Line

	Suspension[a] Drops and Original Drops 80 mg/0.8 mL Dropperful	Chewable[a] Tablets 80-mg tablets	Suspension[a] Liquid and Original Elixir 160 mg/5 mL	Junior[a] Strength 160-mg Caplets/ Chewables	Regular[b] Strength 325-mg Caplets/ Tablets	Extra Strength[b] 500-mg Caplets/ Gelcaps
Birth–3 mo/ 6–11 lb/ 2.5–5.4 kg	$\frac{1}{2}$ dppr[c] (0.4 mL)					
4–11 mo/ 12–17 lb/ 5.5–7.9 kg	1 dppr[c] (0.8 mL)		$\frac{1}{2}$ tsp			
12–23 mo/ 18–23 lb/ 8.0–10.9 kg	1$\frac{1}{2}$ dppr[c] (1.2 mL)		$\frac{3}{4}$ tsp			
2–3 y/24–35 lb/ 11.0–15.9 kg	2 dppr[c] (1.6 mL)	2 tab	1 tsp			
4–5 y/36–47 lb/ 16.0–21.9 kg		3 tab	1$\frac{1}{2}$ tsp			

6–8 y/48–59 lb/ 22.0–26.9 kg	4 tab	2 tsp		2 cap/tab
9–10 y/60–71 lb/ 27.0–31.9 kg	5 tab	2½ tsp		2½ cap/ tab
11 y/72–95 lb/ 32.0–43.9 kg	6 tab	4 tsp		3 cap/tab
Adults & children ≥ 12 y ≥ 96 lb ≥ 44.0 kg	4 cap/tab		1 or 2 cap/ tab	2 cap/ gel

[a]Doses should be administered 4 or 5 times daily. Do not exceed 5 doses in 24 h.

[b]No more than 8 dosage units in any 24-h period. Not to be taken for pain for more than 10 days or for fewer for more than 3 days unless directed by a physician.

[c]Dropperful.

TABLE 2
Local Anesthetic Comparison Chart for Commonly Used Injectable Agents

Agent	Proprietary Names	Onset	Duration	Maximum Dose mg/kg	Maximum Dose Volume in 70-kg Adult[a]
Bupivacaine	Marcaine	7–30 min	5–7 h	3	70 mL of 0.25% solution
Lidocaine	Xylocaine, Anestacon	5–30 min	2 h	4	28 mL of 1% solution
Lidocaine with epinephrine (1:200,000)		5–30 min	2–3 h	7	50 mL of 1% solution
Mepivacaine	Carbocaine	5–30 min	2–3 h	7	50 mL of 1% solution
Procaine	Novocaine	Rapid	30 min–1 h	10–15	70–105 mL of 1% solution

[a]To calculate the maximum dose if not a 70-kg adult, use the fact that a 1% solution has 10 mg/ml drug.

TABLE 3
Comparison of Systemic Steroids (See also page 214)

Drug	Relative Equivalent Dose (mg)	Relative Mineralo-corticoid Activity	Duration (h)	Route
Betamethasone	0.75	0	36–72	PO, IM
Cortisone (Cortone)	25	2	8–12	PO, IM
Dexamethasone (Decadron)	0.75	0	36–72	PO, IV
Hydrocortisone (Solu-Cortef, Hydrocortone)	20	2	8–12	PO, IM, IV
Methylprednisolone acetate (Depo-Medrol)	4	0	36–72	PO, IM, IV
Methylprednisolone succinate (Solu-Medrol)	4	0	8–12	PO, IM, IV
Prednisone (Deltasone)	5	1	12–36	PO
Prednisolone (Delta-Cortef)	5	1	12–36	PO, IM, IV

TABLE 4
Topical Steroid Preparations

Agent	Common Trade Names	Potency	Apply
Alclometasone dipropionate	Aclovate cream, oint 0.05%	Low	bid/tid
Amcinonide	Cyclocort cream, lotion, oint 0.1%	High	bid/tid
Betamethasone			
Betamethasone valerate	Valisone cream, lotion 0.01%	Low	qd/bid
Betamethasone valerate	Valisone cream 0.01, 0.1%, oint, lotion 0.1%	Intermediate	qd/bid
Betamethasone dipropionate	Diprosone cream 0.05% Diprosone aerosol 0.1%	High	qd/bid
Betamethasone dipropionate, augmented	Diprolene oint, gel 0.05%	Ultrahigh	qd/bid
Clobetasol propionate	Temovate cream, gel, oint, scalp, soln 0.05%	Ultrahigh	bid (2 wk max)
Clocortolone pivalate	Cloderm cream 0.1%	Intermediate	qd–qid
Desonide	DesOwen cream, oint, lotion 0.05%	Low	bid–qid
Desoximetasone			
Desoximetasone 0.05%	Topicort LP cream, gel 0.05%	Intermediate	
Desoximetasone 0.25%	Topicort cream, oint	High	bid–qid
Dexamethasone base	Aeroseb-Dex aerosol 0.01% Decadron cream 0.1%	Low	bid–qid
Diflorasone diacetate	Psorcon cream, oint 0.05%	Ultrahigh	bid/qid
Fluocinolone			
Fluocinolone acetonide 0.01%	Synalar cream, soln 0.01%	Low	bid/tid
Fluocinolone acetonide 0.025%	Synalar oint, cream 0.025%	Intermediate	bid/tid

252

Drug	Formulation	Potency	Frequency
Fluocinolone acetonide 0.2%	Synalar-HP cream 0.2%	High	bid/tid
Fluocinonide 0.05%	Lidex anhydrous cream, gel, soln 0.05%	High	bid/tid oint
	Lidex-E aqueous cream 0.05%		
Flurandrenolide	Cordran cream, oint 0.025% cream, lotion, oint 0.05% tape, 4 mcg/cm²	Intermediate Intermediate Intermediate	bid/tid bid/tid qd
Fluticasone propionate	Cutivate cream 0.05%, oint 0.005%	Intermediate	bid
Halobetasol	Ultravate cream, oint 0.05%	Very high	bid
Halcinonide	Halog cream 0.025%, emollient base 0.1%, cream, oint, sol 0.1%	High	qd/tid
Hydrocortisone	Cortizone, Caldecort, Hycort, Hytone, etc. aerosol 1%; cream 0.5, 1, 2.5%; gel 0.5%; oint 0.5, 1, 2.5%; lotion 0.5, 1, 2.5%; paste 0.5%; soln 1%	Low	tid/qid
Hydrocortisone acetate	Corticaine cream, oint 0.5, 1%	Low	tid/qid
Hydrocortisone butyrate	Locoid oint, soln 0.1%	Intermediate	bid/tid
Hydrocortisone valerate	Westcort cream, oint 0.2%	Intermediate	bid/tid

TABLE 4 (continued)
Topical Steroid Preparations

Agent	Common Trade Names	Potency	Apply
Mometasone furoate	Elocon cream, oint, lotion 0.1%	Intermediate	qd
Prednicarbate	Dermatop cream 0.1%	Intermediate	bid
Triamcinolone			
Triamcinolone acetonide 0.025%	Aristocort, Kenalog cream, oint, lotion 0.025%	Low	tid/qid
Triamcinolone acetonide 0.1%	Aristocort, Kenalog cream, oint, lotion 0.1%	Intermediate	tid/qid
	Aerosol 0.2-mg/2-sec spray		
Triamcinolone acetonide 0.5%	Aristocort, Kenalog cream, oint 0.5%	High	tid/qid

TABLE 5
Comparison of Insulins (See also page 134)

Type of Insulin	Onset (h)	Peak (h)	Duration (h)
Ultra Rapid			
Apidra (glulisine)	Immediate	0.5–1.5	3–5
Humalog (lispro)	Immediate	0.5–1.5	3–5
NovoLog (insulin aspart)	Immediate	0.5–1.5	3–5
Rapid			
Regular Iletin II	0.25–0.5	2–4	5–7
Humulin R	0.5	2–4	6–8
Novolin R	0.5	2.5–5	5–8
Velosulin	0.5	2–5	6–8
Intermediate			
NPH Iletin II	1–2	6–12	18–24
Lente Iletin II	1–2	6–12	18–24
Humulin N	1–2	6–12	14–24
Novulin L	2.5–5	7–15	18–24
Novulin 70/30	0.5	7–12	24
Prolonged			
Ultralente	4–6	14–24	28–36
Humulin U	4–6	8–20	24–28
Lantus (insulin glargine)	4–6	No peak	24
Combination Insulins			
Humalog Mix (lispro protamine/ lispro)	0.25–0.5	1–4	24

TABLE 6
Commonly Used Oral Contraceptives (See also page 180 for a discussion of specific oral contraceptive dosing) (Note: 21 = 21 Active Pills; 28 = 21 Active Pills + 7 Placebo[9])

Drug (Manufacturer)	Estrogen (mcg)	Progestin (mg)	Iron/Other
Monophasics			
Alesse 21, 28 (Wyeth)	Ethinyl estradiol (20)	Levonorgestrel (0.1)	
Apri 28 (Barr)	Ethinyl estradiol (30)	Desogestrel (0.15)	
Aviane 28 (Barr)	Ethinyl estradiol (20)	Levonorgestrel (0.1)	
Brevicon 28 (Watson)	Ethinyl estradiol (35)	Norethindrone (0.5)	
Cryselle 28 (Barr)	Ethinyl estradiol (30)	Norgestrel (0.3)	
Demulen 1/35 21, 28 (Pfizer)	Ethinyl estradiol (35)	Ethynodiol diacetate (1)	
Demulen 1/50 21, 28 (Pfizer)	Ethinyl estradiol (50)	Ethynodiol diacetate (1)	
Desogen 28 (Organon)	Ethinyl estradiol (30)	Desogestrel (0.15)	
Femcon Fe (Warner-Chilcott)	Ethinyl estradiol (35)	Norethindrone (0.4)	75 mg Fe × 7 d
Junel Fe 1/20 28 (Barr)	Ethinyl estradiol (20)	Norethindrone acetate (1)	75 mg × 7 d in 28 d
Junel Fe 1.5/30 28 (Barr)	Ethinyl estradiol (30)	Norethindrone acetate (1.5)	75 mg × 7 d in 28 d
Kariva 28 (Barr)	Ethinyl estradiol (20, 0, 10)	Desogestrel (0.15)	+2 inert +2 ethinyl estradiol (10)
Kelnor 1/35 28 (Barr)	Ethinyl estradiol (35)	Ethynodiol diacetate (1)	
Lessina 28 (Barr)	Ethinyl estradiol (20)	Levonorgestrel (0.1)	
Levlen 21, 28 (Bayer)	Ethinyl estradiol (30)	Levonorgestrel (0.15)	
Levlite 28 (Bayer)	Ethinyl estradiol (20)	Levonorgestrel (0.1)	
Levora 28 (Watson)	Ethinyl estradiol (30)	Levonorgestrel (0.15)	
Loestrin Fe 24 (Warner-Chilcott)	ethinyl estradiol (20)	Norethindrone (1)	4 inert 28-d pack
Loestrin Fe 1.5/30 21, 28 (Warner-Chilcott)	Ethinyl estradiol (30)	Norethindrone acetate (1.5)	75 mg × 7 d in 28 d

256

Product	Estrogen	Progestin	Iron
Loestrin Fe 1/20 21, 28 (Warner-Chilcott)	Ethinyl estradiol (20)	Norethindrone acetate (1)	75 mg × 7 d in 28 d
Lo/Ovral 21, 28 (Wyeth)	Ethinyl estradiol (30)	Norgestrel (0.3)	
Low-Ogestrel 28 (Watson)	Ethinyl estradiol (30)	Norgestrel (0.3)	
Microgestin Fe 1/20 21, 28 (Watson)	Ethinyl estradiol (20)	Norethindrone acetate (1)	75 mg × 7 d in 28 d
Microgestin Fe 1.5/30 21, 28 (Watson)	Ethinyl estradiol (30)	Norethindrone acetate (1.5)	75 mg × 7 d in 28 d
Mircette 28 (Organon)	Ethinyl estradiol (20, 0, 10)	Desogestrel (0.15)	
Modicon 28 (Ortho-McNeil)	Ethinyl estradiol (35)	Norethindrone (0.5)	
MonoNessa 28 (Watson)	Ethinyl estradiol (35)	Norgestimate (0.25)	
Necon 1/50 28 (Watson)	Mestranol (50)	Norethindrone (1)	
Necon 1/35 28 (Watson)	Ethinyl estradiol (35)	Norethindrone (0.5)	
Necon 1/35 28 (Watson)	Ethinyl estradiol (35)	Norethindrone (1)	
Nordette 21, 28 (King)	Ethinyl estradiol (30)	Levonorgestrel (0.15)	
Nortrel 0.5/35 28 (Barr)	Ethinyl estradiol (35)	Norethindrone (0.5)	
Nortrel 1/35 21, 28 (Barr)	Ethinyl estradiol (35)	Norethindrone (1)	
Norinyl 1/35 28 (Watson)	Ethinyl estradiol (35)	Norethindrone (1)	
Norinyl 1/50 28 (Watson)	Mestranol (50)	Norethindrone (1)	
Ogestrel 0.05/50 28 (Watson)	Ethinyl estradiol (50)	Norgestrel (0.5)	
Ortho-Cept 28 (Ortho-McNeil)	Ethinyl estradiol (30)	Desogestrel (0.15)	
Ortho-Cyclen 28 (Ortho-McNeil)	Ethinyl estradiol (35)	Norgestimate (0.25)	
Ortho-Novum 1/35 28 (Ortho-McNeil)	Ethinyl estradiol (35)	Norethindrone (1)	
Ortho-Novum 1/50 28 (Ortho-McNeil)	Mestranol (50)	Norethindrone (1)	
Ovcon 35 21, 28 (Warner-Chilcott)	Ethinyl estradiol (35)	Norethindrone (0.4)	
Ovcon 35 Fe (Warner-Chilcott)	Ethinyl estradiol (35)	Norethindrone (0.4)	75 mg × 7 d in 28 d

TABLE 6 (continued)
Commonly Used Oral Contraceptives (See also page 180 for a discussion of specific oral contraceptive dosing) (Note: 21 = 21 Active Pills; 28 = 21 Active Pills + 7 Placebo[a])

Drug (Manufacturer)	Estrogen (mcg)	Progestin (mg)	Iron/Other
Ovcon 50 28 (Warner-Chilcott)	Ethinyl estradiol (50)	Norethindrone (1)	
Ovral 21, 28 (Wyeth-Ayerst)	Ethinyl estradiol (50)	Norgestrel (0.5)	
Portia 28 (Barr)	Ethinyl estradiol (30)	Levonorgestrel (0.15)	
Sprintec 28 (Barr)	Ethinyl estradiol (35)	Norgestimate (0.25)	
Yasmin 28 (Bayer)	Ethinyl estradiol (30)	Drospirenone (3.0)	
Yaz (Bayer) 28 day [b,d]	Ethinyl estradiol (20)	Drospirenone (3.0)	4 inert
Zovia 1/50E 28 (Watson)	Ethinyl estradiol (50)	Ethynodiol diacetate (1.0)	
Zovia 1/35E 28 (Watson)	Ethinyl estradiol (35)	Ethynodiol diacetate (1.0)	
Multiphasics			
Aranelle 28 (Barr)	Ethinyl estradiol (35)	Norethindrone (0.5, 1, 0.5)	
Cyclessa 28 (Organon)	Ethinyl estradiol (25)	Desogestrel (0.1, 0.125, 0.15)	
Enpresse 28 (Barr)	Ethinyl estradiol (30, 40, 30)	Levonorgestrel (0.05, 0.075, 0.125)	
Estrostep Fe 28 (Warner-Chilcott)b	Ethinyl estradiol (20, 30, 35)	Norethindrone acetate (1)	75 mg Fe × 7 d
Leena 28 (Watson)	Ethinyl estradiol (35)	Norethindrone (0.5, 1, 0.5)	
Necon 10/11 21, 28 (Watson)	Ethinyl estradiol (35)	Norethindrone (0.5, 1.0)	
Necon 7/7/7 (Watson)	Ethinyl estradiol (35)	Norethindrone (0.5, 0.75, 1.0)	
Nortrel 7/7/7 28 (Barr)	Ethinyl estradiol (35)	Norethindrone (0.5, 0.75, 1.0)	
Ortho-Novum 10/11 21 (Ortho-McNeil)	Ethinyl estradiol (35, 35)	Norethindrone (0.5, 1.0)	
Ortho-Novum 7/7/7 21 (Ortho-McNeil)	Ethinyl estradiol (35, 35, 35)	Norethindrone (0.5, 0.75, 1.0)	

258

Ortho Tri-Cyclen 21, 28 (Ortho-McNeil)[b]	Ethinyl estradiol (25)	Norgestimate (0.18, 0.215, 0.25)	
Ortho Tri-Cyclen Lo 21, 28 (Ortho-McNeil)	Ethinyl estradiol (35, 35, 35)	Norgestimate (0.18, 0.215, 0.25)	
Tilia Fe 28 (Watson)	Ethinyl estradiol (20, 30, 35)	Norethindrone (1)	75 mg Fe × 7 d
Tri-Legest 21 (Barr)	Ethinyl estradiol (20, 30, 35)	Norethindrone (1)	
Tri-Legest Fe 28 (Barr)	Ethinyl estradiol (20, 30, 35)	Norethindrone (1)	75 mg Fe × 7 d
Tri-Levlen 28 (Bayer)	Ethinyl estradiol (30, 40, 30)	Levonorgestrel (0.05, 0.075, 0.125)	
TriNessa 28 (Watson)	Ethinyl estradiol (35)	Norgestimate (0.18, 0.215, 0.25)	
Tri-Norinyl 21, 28 (Watson)	Ethinyl estradiol (35, 35, 35)	Norethindrone (0.5, 1.0, 0.5)	
Tri-Previfem 28 (Teva)	Ethinyl estradiol (35)	Norgestimate (0.18, 0.215, 0.25)	
Tri-Sprintec (Barr)	Ethinyl estradiol (35)	Norgestimate (0.18, 0.215, 0.25)	
Triphasil 21, 28 (Wyeth)	Ethinyl estradiol (30, 40, 30)	Levonorgestrel (0.05, 0.075, 0.125)	
Trivora-28 (Watson)	Ethinyl estradiol (30, 40, 30)	Levonorgestrel (0.05, 0.075, 0.125)	
Velivet (Barr)	Ethinyl estradiol (25)	Desogestrel (0.1, 0.125, 0.15)	

Progestin Only (AKA "mini-pills")

Camila (Barr)	None	Norethindrone (0.35)	
Errin (Barr)	None	Norethindrone (0.35)	
Jolivette 28 (Watson)	None	Norethindrone (0.35)	
Micronor 28 (Ortho-McNeil)	None	Norethindrone (0.35)	
Nor-QD (Watson)	None	Norethindrone (0.35)	
Nora-BE 28 (Ortho-McNeil)	None	Norethindrone (0.35)	

259

TABLE 6 (continued)

Commonly Used Oral Contraceptives (See also page 180 for a discussion of specific oral contraceptive dosing)

[Note: 21 = 21 Active Pills; 28 = 21 Active Pills + 7 Placebo[a]]

Drug	Estrogen (mg)	Progestin (mcg)	additional pills
Extended-Cycle Combination (aka COCP [combined oral contraceptive pills])			
Jolessa (Barr) 91-day pack	Levonorgestrel (0.15)	Ethinyl estradiol (30)	7 inert
Lybrel (Wyeth) 28-day pack[c]	Ethinyl estradiol (20)	Levonorgestrel (0.9)	None
Seasonique (Duramed) 91-day pack	Ethinyl estradiol (30)	Levonorgestrel (0.15)	7 (10 mcg ethinyl estradiol)
Seasonale (Duramed) 91 day	Ethinyl estradiol (30)	Levonorgestrel (0.15)	7 inert
Quasense (Watson)	Ethinyl estradiol (30)	Levonorgestrel (0.15)	7 inert

[a] The designations 21 and 28 refer to number of days in regimen available.

[b] Also approved for acne.

[c] First FDA approved pill for 365-d dosing.

[d] Approved for premenstrual dysphoric disorder (PMDD) in women who use contraception for birth control.

[e] Avoid in patients with hyperkalemia risk.

Based in part on data published in the Medical Letter, Volume 49 (Issue 1266) 2007. manufacturers insert and websites as of September 29, 2008

TABLE 7
Some Common Oral Potassium Supplements (See also page 196)

Brand Name	Salt	Form	mEq Potassium/ Dosing Unit
Glu-K	Gluconate	Tablet	2 mEq/tablet
Kaochlor 10%	KCl	Liquid	20 mEq/15 mL
Kaochlor S-F 10% (sugar-free)	KCl	Liquid	20 mEq/15 mL
Kaochlor Eff	Bicarbonate/ KCl/citrate	Effervescent tablet	20 mEq/tablet
Kaon elixir	Gluconate	Liquid	20 mEq/15 mL
Kaon	Gluconate	Tablet	5 mEq/tablet
Kaon-Cl	KCl	Tablet, SR	6.67 mEq/tablet
Kaon-Cl 20%	KCl	Liquid	40 mEq/15 mL
KayCiel	KCl	Liquid	20 mEq/15 mL
K-Lor	KCl	Powder	15 or 20 mEq/packet
Klorvess	Bicarbonate/ KCl	Liquid	20 mEq/15 mL
Klotrix	KCl	Tablet, SR	10 mEq/tablet
K-Lyte	Bicarbonate/ citrate	Effervescent tablet	25 mEq/tablet
K-Tab	KCl	Tablet, SR	10 mEq/tablet
Micro-K	KCl	Capsule, SR	8 mEq/capsule
Slow-K	KCl	Tablet, SR	8 mEq/tablet
Tri-K	Acetate/bicarbonate and citrate	Liquid	45 mEq/15 mL
Twin-K	Citrate/gluconate	Liquid	20 mEq/5 mL

SR = sustained release.

TABLE 8
Tetanus Prophylaxis (See also page 223)

History of Absorbed Tetanus Toxoid Immunization	Clean, Minor Wounds		All Other Wounds[a]	
	Td[b]	TIG[c]	Td[d]	TIG[c]
Unknown or <3 doses	Yes	No	Yes	Yes
=3 doses	No[e]	No	No[f]	No

[a]Such as, but not limited to, wounds contaminated with dirt, feces, soil, saliva, etc; puncture wounds; avulsions; and wounds resulting from missiles, crushing, burns, and frostbite.

[b]Td = tetanus-diphtheria toxoid (adult type), 0.5 mL IM.
  • For children <7 y, DPT (DT, if pertussis vaccine is contraindicated) is preferred to tetanus toxoid alone.
  • For persons >7 y, Td is preferred to tetanus toxoid alone.
  • DT = diphtheria-tetanus toxoid (pediatric), used for those who cannot receive pertussis.

[c]TIG = tetanus immune globulin, 250 units IM.

[d]If only 3 doses of fluid toxoid have been received, then a fourth dose of toxoid, preferably an adsorbed toxoid, should be given.

[e]Yes, if >10 y since last dose.

[f]Yes, if >5 y since last dose.

Based on guidelines from the Centers for Disease Control and Prevention and reported in *MMWR*.

TABLE 9
Oral Anticoagulant Standards of Practice (See also warfarin page 237)

Thromboembolic Disorder	INR	Duration
Deep Venous Thrombosis & Pulmonary Embolism		
Treatment single episode		
Transient risk factor	2–3	3 mo
Idiopathic	2–3	6–12 mo
Recurrent systemic embolism	2–3	Indefinite
Prevention of Systemic Embolism		
Atrial fibrillation (AF)[a]	2–3	Indefinite
AF: cardioversion	2–3	3 wk prior; 4 wk post sinus rhythm
Valvular heart disease	2–3	Indefinite
Cardiomyopathy	2–3	Indefinite
Acute Myocardial Infarction		
High-risk patients[c]	2–3 + lowdose aspirin	3 mo
Prosthetic Valves		
Tissue heart valves	2–3	3 mo
Bileaflet mechanical valves in aortic position	2–3	Indefinite
Other mechanical prosthetic valves[b]	2.5–3.5	Indefinite

[a]With high-risk factors or multiple moderate risk factors.

[b]May add aspirin 81 mg to warfarin in patients with caged ball or caged disk valves or with additional risk factors.

[c]Large anterior MI, significant heart failure, intracardiac thrombus, and/or history of thromboembolic event.

INR = international normalized ratio.

Based on data published in *Chest* 2004 Sep; 126 (Suppl): 163S–696S.

TABLE 10
Antiarrhythmics: Vaughn Williams Classification

Class I: Sodium Channel Blockade

A. **Class Ia:** Lengthens duration of action potential (↑ the refractory period in atrial and ventricular muscle, in SA and AV conduction systems, and Purkinje fibers)
   1. Amiodarone (also class II, III, IV)
   2. Disopyramide (Norpace)
   3. Imipramine (MAO inhibitor)
   4. Procainamide (Pronestyl)
   5. Quinidine
B. **Class Ib:** No effect on action potential
   1. Lidocaine (Xylocaine)
   2. Mexiletine (Mexitil)
   3. Phenytoin (Dilantin)
   4. Tocainide (Tonocard)
C. **Class Ic:** Greater sodium current depression (blocks the fast inward Na⁺ current in heart muscle and Purkinje fibers, and slows the rate of ↑ of phase 0 of the action potential)
   1. Flecainide (Tambocor)
   2. Propafenone

Class II: β Blocker

D. Amiodarone (also class Ia, III, IV)
E. Esmolol (Brevibloc)
F. Sotalol (also class III)

Class III: Prolong Refractory Period via Action Potential

G. Amiodarone (also class Ia, II, IV)
H. Sotalol

Class IV: Calcium Channel Blocker

I. Amiodarone (also class Ia, II, III)
J. Diltiazem (Cardizem)
K. Verapamil (Calan)

TABLE 11
Cytochrome P-450 Isoenzymes and Common Drugs
They Metabolize, Inhibit, and Induce[a]

CYP1A2

Substrates:	Acetaminophen, caffeine, clozapine, imipramine, theophylline, propranolol
Inhibitors:	Most fluoroquinolone antibiotics, fluvoxamine, cimetidine
Inducers:	Tobacco smoking, charcoal-broiled foods, cruciferous vegetables, omeprazole

CYP2C9

Substrates:	Most NSAIDs (including COX-2), warfarin, phenytoin
Inhibitors:	Fluconazole
Inducers:	Barbiturates, rifampin

CYP2C19

Substrates:	Diazepam, lansoprazole, omeprazole, phenytoin, pantoprazole
Inhibitors:	Omeprazole, isoniazid, ketoconazole
Inducers:	Barbiturates, rifampin

CYP2D6

Substrates:	Most β-blockers, codeine, clomipramine, clozapine, codeine, encainide, flecainide, fluoxetine, haloperidol, hydrocodone, 4-methoxy-amphetamine, metoprolol, mexiletine, oxycodone, paroxetine, propafenone, propoxyphene, risperidone, selegiline (deprenyl), thioridazine, most tricyclic antidepressants, timolol
Inhibitors:	Fluoxetine, haloperidol, paroxetine, quinidine
Inducers:	Unknown

CYP3A

Substrates:	**Anticholinergics:** Darifenacin, oxybutynin, solifenacin, tolterodine
	Benzodiazepines: Alprazolam, midazolam, triazolam
	Ca channel blockers: Diltiazem, felodipine, nimodipine, nifedipine, nisoldipine, verapamil

(continued)

**TABLE 11 (continued)
Cytochrome P-450 Isoenzymes and Common Drugs
They Metabolize, Inhibit, and Induce[a]**

	Chemotherapy: Cyclophosphamide, erlotinib, ifosfamide, paclitaxel, tamoxifen, vinblastine, vincristine
	HIV protease inhibitors: Amprenavir, atazanavir, indinavir, nelfinavir, ritonavir, saquinavir
	HMG-CoA reductase inhibitors: Atorvastatin, lovastatin, simvastatin
	Immunosuppressive agents: Cyclosporine, tacrolimus
	Macrolide-type antibiotics: Clarithromycin, erythromycin, telithromycin, troleandomycin
	Opioids: Alfentanyl, cocaine, fentanyl, sufentanil
	Steroids: Budesonide, cortisol, 17-β-estradiol, progesterone
	Others: Acetaminophen, amiodarone, carbamazepine, delavirdine, efavirenz, nevirapine, quinidine, repaglinide, sildenafil, tadalafil, trazodone, vardenafil
Inhibitors:	Amiodarone, amprenavir, atazanavir, ciprofloxacin, cisapride, clarithromycin, diltiazem, erythromycin, fluconazole, fluvoxamine, grapefruit juice (in high ingestion), indinavir, itraconazole, ketoconazole, nefazodone, nelfinavir, norfloxacin, ritonavir, telithromycin, troleandomycin, verapamil, voriconazole
Inducers:	Carbamazepine, efavirenz, glucocorticoids, macrolide antibiotics, nevirapine, phenytoin, phenobarbital, rifabutin, rifapentine, rifampin, St. John's wort

[a]Increased or decreased (primarily hepatic cytochrome P-450) metabolism of medications may influence the effectiveness of drugs or result in significant drug-drug interactions. Understanding the common cytochrome P-450 isoforms (eg, CYP2C9, CYP2D9, CYP2C19, CYP3A4) and common drugs that are metabolized by (aka "substrates"), inhibit, or induce activity of the isoform helps minimize significant drug interactions. CYP3A is involved in the metabolism of >50% of drugs metabolized by the liver.

Based on data from Katzung B (ed): *Basic and Clinical Pharmacology*, 9th ed. McGraw-Hill, New York, 2004; *The Medical Letter*, Volume 47, July 4, 2004; http://www.fda.gov/cder/drug/drugreactions (accessed September 16, 2006).

TABLE 12
SSRIs/SNRI/Triptan and Serotonin Syndrome

A life-threatening condition, when selective serotonin reuptake inhibitors (SSRIs) and 5-hydroxytryptamine receptor agonists (triptans) are used together. However, many other drugs have been implicated (see below). Signs and symptoms of serotonin syndrome include the following:

Restlessness, coma, N/V/D, hallucinations, loss of coordination, overactive reflexes, ↑ HR/temperature, rapid changes in BP, increased body temperature

Class	Drugs
Antidepressants	MAOIs, TCAs, SSRIs, SNRIs, mirtazapine, venlafaxine
CNS stimulants	Amphetamines, phentermine, methylphenidate, sibutramine
5-HT$_1$ agonists	Triptans
Illicit drugs	Cocaine, methylenedioxymethamphetamine (ecstasy), lysergic acid diethylamide (LSD)
Opioids	Tramadol, pethidine, oxycodone, morphine, meperidine
Others	Buspirone, chlorpheniramine, dextromethorphan, linezolid, lithium, selegiline, tryptophan, St John's Wort

Management includes removal of the precipitating drugs and supportive care. To control agitation serotonin antagonists (cyproheptadine or methysergide) can be used. When symptoms are mild, discontinuation of the medication or medications, and the control of agitation with benzodiazepines may be needed. Critically ill patients may require sedation and mechanical ventilation as well as control of hyperthermia. (Boyer EW, Shannon M: "The Serotonin Syndrome". *N Engl J Med.* 2005; 352 (11): 1112–20)
MOAI = monoamine oxidase inhibitor
TCA = tricyclic antidepressant
SNRI = serotonin-norepinephrine reuptake inhibitors

TABLE 13

Composition of Selected Multivitamins and Multivitamins with Mineral and Trace Element Supplements. Listings show vitamin content (Part 1) and then mineral trace element and other components (Part 2) of popular US brands. Values listed are a percentage of Daily Value. (See also page 168)

Part 1. Vitamins

	Fat Soluble				Water Soluble								
	A	D	E	K	C	B₁	B₂	B₃	B₆	Folate	B₁₂	Biotin	B₅
Centrum[a]	70	100	100	31	150	100	100	100	100	125	100	10	100
Centrum Performance[a]	70	200	200	31	200	300	300	200	300	100	300	17	100
Centrum Silver[a]	50	125	167	38	150	100	100	100	150	125	417	10	100
Nature Made Multi Complete	50	250	167	100	300	100	100	100	100	100	100	10	100
Nature Made Multi Daily	60	100	100	0	100	100	100	100	100	100	100	0	100
Nature Made Multi Max	60	100	500	50	500	3333	2941	250	2500	100	833	17	500
Nature Made Multi 50+	60	100	200	13	200	200	200	100	200	100	417	10	100

One-A-Day 50 Plus	50	100	110	25	200	300	200	100	300	100	417	10	150
One-A-Day Essential	60	100	100	0	100	100	100	100	100	100	100	0	100
One-A-Day Maximum[b]	50	100	100	31	100	100	100	100	100	100	100	10	100
Therapeutic Vitamin	100	100	100	0	150	200	200	100	100	100	150	10	100
Theragran-M Advanced High Protein	100	100	200	35	150	200	200	100	300	100	200	10	100
Theragran-M Premier High Potency	70	100	200	31	200	267	235	125	200	100	150	10	100
Theragran-M Premier 50 Plus High Potency	70	100	200	13	125	200	176	125	300	100	500	12	150
Therapeutic Vitamin + Minerals[b]	100	100	200	0	200	100	100	100	100	100	100	10	100
Unicap M	100	100	100	0	100	100	100	100	100	100	100	0	100
Unicap Sr.	100	50	50	NA	100	80	82	80	110	50	50	0	100
Unicap T	100	100	100	0	833	667	588	500	300	100	300	0	250

TABLE 13 (continued)

Composition of Selected Multivitamins and Multivitamins with Mineral and Trace Element Supplements. Listings show vitamin content (Part 1) and then mineral trace element and other components (Part 2) of popular US brands. Values listed are a percentage of Daily Value. (See also page 168)

Part 2. Minerals, trace elements, and other components

	Minerals							Trace Elements					Other
	Ca	P	Mg	Fe	Zn	I	Se	K	Mn	Cu	Cr	Mo	
Centrum[a]	20	11	25	100	73	100	79	2	115	45	29	60	Lutein, lycopene
Centrum Performance[a]	10	5	10	100	73	100	100	2	200	45	100	100	Gingko, ginseng
Centrum Silver[a]	22	11	13	0	73	100	79	2	115	45	38	60	Lutein, lycopene
Nature Made Multi Complete[a]	16	NA	25	100	100	100	35	NA	200	100	100	100	
Nature Made Multi Daily	45	0	0	100	100	0	0	0	0	0	0	0	
Nature Made Multi Max	10	4	6	50	100	100	100	1	100	100	100	0	Lutein
Nature Made Multi 50+	20	5	25	0	100	100	71	2	100	100	100	33	Lutein
One-A-Day 50 Plus	12	0	25	0	150	100	150	1	200	100	150	120	Lutein
One-A-Day Essential	5	0	0	100	100	100	0	0	0	0	0	0	
One-A-Day Maximum	16	11	25	100	100	100	29	2	175	100	54	213	

270

Therapeutic Vitamin[b]	0	0	0	0	0	0	0	0	0	0	0	0
Theragran-M Advanced High Potency	4	3	25	50	100	100	100	1	100	100	42	100
Theragran-M Premier High Potency	17	11	25	100	100	100	286	2	175	100	107	Lutein, lycopene, coenzyme Q10
Theragran-M Premier 50 Plus High Potency	20	5	25	0	113	100	286	2	100	21	100	Lutein, coenzyme Q10
Therapeutic Vitamin + Minerals[b]	4	3	10	50	100	50	36	<1	100	100	42	100
Unicap M	6	5	0	100	100	0	<1	50	0	0	0	
Unicap Sr.	10	8	8	56	100	0	<1	50	0	0	0	
Unicap T	0	0	0	100	100	14	<1	50	0	0	0	

Common multivitamins available without a prescription are listed. Most chain drug stores have generic versions of many of the multivitamin supplements listed above; thus, specific generic brands are not listed. Many specialty vitamin combinations are available, but not included in this list (examples are B vitamins plus C, supplements for a specific condition or organ, pediatric and infant formulations, and prenatal vitamins). Values are listed as percentages of the Daily Value (also known as %DV) based on Recommended Dietary Allowances of vitamins and minerals based on Dietary Reference Intakes (Food and Nutrition Board, Institute of Medicine, National Academy of Science). Additional information may be available for many other supplements from the NIH Dietary Supplements Labels Database http://dietarysupplements.nlm.nih.gov/dietary

[a]New formulation October 2007.

[b]Formulations may vary. Consult with pharmacy for current product.

[c]Common generic brands (when other than the store name itself) are: Osco Drug Central-Vite (Albertson's); Spectravite (CVS); Kirkland Signature Daily Multivitamin (Costco); Whole Source, PharmAssure (Rite Aid); Central-Vite (Safeway); Member's Mark (Sam's Club); Vitasmart (Kmart); Century (Target); A thru Z Select, Super Aytinal, Ultra Choice (Walgreens); Equate Complete or Spring Valley Sentury-Vite (Wal-Mart).

Vitamins: B₁ = Thiamine; B₂ = Riboflavin; B₃ = Niacin; B₅ = Pantothenic Acid; B₆ = Pyridoxine; B₁₂ = Cyanocobalamin. Elements: Ca = calcium; Cr = chromium; Cu = copper; Fe = iron; I = iodine; K = potassium; Mg = magnesium; Mn = manganese; Mo = molybdenum; P = phosphorus; Se = selenium; Zn = zinc; 0 = not applicable or not available.

Index

Page numbers followed by *t* indicate tables.

Generic (Trade) — Adult Dose (Continued)

Generic (Trade)	Adult Dose (Continued)
Magnesium Sulfate	VF/pulseless VT arrest with torsade de pointes: 1–2 g IV push (2–4 mL 5% solution) in 10 mL D₅W. If pulse present then 1–2 g in 50–100 mL D₅W over 5–60 min.
Metoprolol	5 mg slow IV q5min, total 15 mg.
Morphine	2–4 mg IV (over 1–5 min) then give 2–8 mg IV q5–15min as needed.
Nitroglycerin	IV bolus: infuse at 10–20 mcg/min every 3–5 min PRN. SL: 0.3–0.4 mg, repeat q5min. Aerosol spray: Spray 0.5–1 s at 5-min intervals.
Nitroprusside	0.1–0.3 mcg/kg/min start, titrate max dose 10 mcg/kg/min).
Procainamide	Stable monomorphic VT, HR control in a fib, AV reentrant narrow complex tachycardia: 20 mg/min IV until one of these: arrhythmia stopped, hypotension, QRS widens >50%, total 17 mg/kg; then maintenance infusion of 1–4 mg/min.
Propranolol (Inderal)	0.1 mg/kg slow IV push, ÷ 3 equal doses q2–3min, max 1 mg/min; repeat in 2 min PRN.
Reteplase recombinant (Retavase)	10 Units IV bolus over 2 min; 30 min later, 10 units IV bolus over 2 min NS flush before and after each dose.
Sodium Bicarbonate	1 mEq/kg IV bolus; repeat ½ dose q10min PRN.
Sotalol (Betapace)	1–1.5 mg/kg IV over 5 min then 10 mg/min.
Streptokinase	AMI: 1.5 million Int Units over 1 h.
Tirofiban (Aggrastat)	ACS or PCI: 0.4 mcg/kg/min IV for 30 min, then 0.1 mcg/kg/min.
Verapamil	2.5–5 mg IV over 1–2 min; repeat 5–10 mg, in 15–30 min PRN max of 20 mg; or 5 mg bolus q15min (max 30 mg).

Based on 2005 American Heart Association Guidelines for Cardiopulmonary Resuscitation and Emergency Cardiovascular Care. *Circulation* 2005;112(24 Suppl). Available online at: http://circ.ahajournals.org/content/vol112/24_suppl (accessed September 28, 2008)

Generic (Trade)	Adult Dose
Calcium Chloride	**Hyperkalemia/hypermagnesemia/CCB overdose:** 8–16 mg/kg; 10% solution, 5–10 mL over 2–5 min.
Clopidogrel	**ACS:** 300-mg loading dose then 75 g/d.
Diltiazem (Cardizem)	**Acute Rate Control:** 0.25 mg/kg (15–20 mg) over 2 min followed in 15 min by 0.35 mg/kg (20–25 mg) over 2 min mainf int 5–15 mg/h.
Dobutamine (Dobutrex)	0.5–1.0 mcg/kg/min; titrate to HR not >10% of baseline.
Dopamine	2–20 mcg/kg/min; **Bradycardia:** 2–10 mcg/kg/min.
Epinephrine	1-mg IV push, repeat q3–5min (0.2 mg/kg max) if 1 mg dose fails. Inf. 30 mg (30 mL of 1:1000 solution) in 250 mL NS or D5W, at 100 mL/h, titrate. ET 2–2.5 mg in 20 mL NS. **Profound bradycardia/hypotension:** 2–10 mg/min (1 mg of 1:1000; in 500 mL NS, infuse 1–5 mL/min).
Eptifibatide (Integrilin)	**ACS:** 180 mcg/kg/min IV bolus over 1–2 min then 2 mcg/kg/min.
Esmolol (Brevibloc)	0.5 mg/kg over 1 min, then 0.05 mg/kg/min for 4 min; if no response 2nd bolus of 0.5 mg/kg with maintenance of 0.1 mg/kg/min with maximum of 0.3 mg/kg/min.
Glucagon	**β-Blocker or CCB overdose:** 3 mg initially followed by 3 mg/h: **Hypoglycemia:** 1 mg IM, or sub Q
Heparin (Unfractionated)	Bolus 80 Int Units/kg (max 4000 Int Units); then 18 Int Units/kg/h (max 1000 Int Units/h for patients >70 kg) round to nearest 50 U; keep PTT 1.5–2× control 48 h or until angiography. If adjunct with fibrin specific lytics then 60 IU/kg bolus then 12 Int Units/kg/h.
Ibutilide	Adults ≥60 kg, 1 mg (10 mL) over 10 min; a second dose may be used; <60 kg 0.01 mg/kg.
Labetalol (Tandate)	10 mg IV over 1–2 min; repeat or double dose q10min (150 mg max); or initial bolus, then 2–8 mg/min.
Lidocaine	**Cardiac Arrest from VF/VT refractory VF:** Initial: 1–1.5 mg/kg IV, additional 0.5–0.75 mg/kg IV push, repeat in 5–10 min, max total 3 mg/kg. ET: 2–4 mg/kg. **Perfusing stable VT, wide complex tachycardia or ectopy:** (up to 1–1.5 mg/kg may be used) IV push; repeat 0.5–0.75 mg/kg q5–10min; max total 3 mg/kg. Maint: 1–4 mg/min (30–50 mcg/min).

(continued)